MILADY'S AESTHETICIAN SERIES

Microdermabrasion

2ND EDITION

MILADY'S AESTHETICIAN SERIES

Microdermabrasion

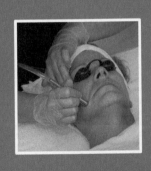
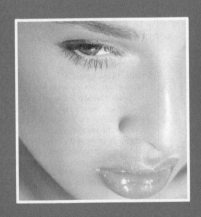
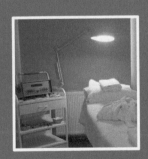

PAMELA HILL, R.N.

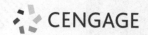

Milady's Aesthetician Series: Microdermabrasion

Edition: 2

Pamela Hill, R.N.

President, Milady: Dawn Gerrain

Publisher: Erin O'Connor

Acquisitions Editor: Martine Edwards

Product Manager: Philip Mandl

Editorial Assistant: Elizabeth Edwards

Director of Beauty Industry Relations: Sandra Bruce

Senior Marketing Manager: Gerard McAvey

Production Director: Wendy Troeger

Senior Content Project Manager: Nina Tucciarelli

Art Director: Joy Kocsis

For product information and technology assistance, contact us at
Professional & Career Group Customer Support, 1-800-648-7450
For permission to use material from this text or product,
submit all requests online at **cengage.com/permissions**.
Further permissions questions can be e-mailed to
permissionrequest@cengage.com.

Library of Congress Control Number: 2009923905

ISBN-13: 978-1-4354-3865-1

ISBN-10: 1-4354-3865-5

Cengage
200 Pier 4 Boulevard
Boston, MA 02210
USA

Cengage products are represented in Canada by Nelson Education, Ltd.

To learn more about Cengage platforms and services, register or access your online learning solution, or purchase materials for your course, visit **www.cengage.com**.

Notice to the Reader

Publisher does not warrant or guarantee any of the products described herein or perform any independent analysis in connection with any of the product information contained herein. Publisher does not assume, and expressly disclaims, any obligation to obtain and include information other than that provided to it by the manufacturer. The reader is expressly warned to consider and adopt all safety precautions that might be indicated by the activities described herein and to avoid all potential hazards. By following the instructions contained herein, the reader willingly assumes all risks in connection with such instructions. The publisher makes no representations or warranties of any kind, including but not limited to, the warranties of fitness for particular purpose or merchantability, nor are any such representations implied with respect to the material set forth herein, and the publisher takes no responsibility with respect to such material. The publisher shall not be liable for any special, consequential, or exemplary damages resulting, in whole or part, from the readers' use of, or reliance upon, this material.

Contents

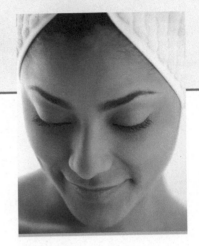

■ **Chapter 4**

■ **Chapter 5**

■ Chapter 9

■ Chapter 10

Preface

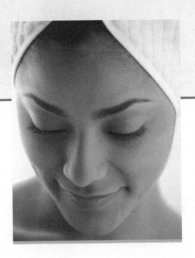

There just isn't enough information. Why isn't there more information? Why can't you tell us more? As the leader of a network of medical skin care clinics, I have heard these questions asked over and over. For the last seventeen years I have spent my days managing medical spas. Part of my job as the President and CEO was the development and oversight of the training programs for our facilities. Needless to say, I have met and trained many clinicians. What I notice is that my first-rate, curious clinicians (aesthetician or nurse) can never get enough information. They are always looking for more information, improved technology to provide advanced results, a new book and more and more! While these questions are obvious signs of a good clinician, they are wrought with peril since unbiased information isn't always available.

This book is intended for those who are studying to become first-rate clinicians, as well as the clinicians who thirst for more information, expanding on what they already know. That said, this text is written to expand on the basic knowledge of aesthetician training, and take it from a conceptual level to the practical level.

I have researched and written this book so that I could satisfy that hunger that makes a great aesthetician, particularly in the area of microdermabrasion. Microdermabrasion has developed into one of the most popular procedures in the skin care industry. However, only minimal research exists on the efficacy of microdermabrasion. The research that does exist has shown remarkable results in the improvement of both the epidermis and the dermis. Microdermabrasion can provide extraordinary results for qualified candidates. The treatment can also provide extraordinary results for those who are not necessarily qualified, but have realistic expectations. This book takes modern research, facts, and opinions, and shapes them into a start-to-finish model. This model has one fundamental intent: ideal results for the clinician and the patient alike.

This *clinical handbook* for microdermabrasion is my answer to the chants for more information. The chapters are organized, one on top of the other, with *essential, must-have information* on microdermabrasion. To this effect, general knowledge is expanded upon, and insightful hints and recommendations allow you to optimize your knowledge and achieve the optimal, replicable results which will insure your success. Each chapter has questions and "Top 10 Tips to Take to the Spa," which will help you well beyond your training, and give you the knowledge that is helpful well beyond the classroom. Also, you will see several case studies of our patients, how we selected them, what we accomplished, and how their result evolved. The book was developed to help you learn the basics of microdermabrasion while adding information that will allow you, the clinician, to develop, refine, and redefine your microdermabrasion skills.

Good luck!

About the Author

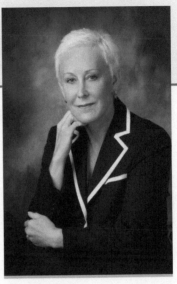

Pamela Hill

Pamela Hill, RN, CEO, received her diploma from Presbyterian/ St. Luke's Hospital and Colorado Women's College. She followed through to practice as a registered nurse for more than 20 years with her initial emphasis in cardiac surgery and then in cosmetic surgery and medical skin care. In 1992, Ms. Hill founded Facial Aesthetics®, a network of medical skin care clinics in association with John A. Grossman, M.D. Since then, Ms. Hill has been an industry pioneer in the growth and development of the medical spa industry. As the president and chief executive officer of Facial Aesthetics®, Ms. Hill has been a proactive member and pioneer in the evolution of the medical spa model and the integration and union of cosmeceuticals and nonsurgical skin care. In addition to her leadership in the medical spa industry, she has also been actively engaged in the research and development of the successful Pamela Hill Skin Care product line.

Ms. Hill has devoted her passion for nonmedical skin care to the instruction of a higher level of education and skill for those aspiring to be the aestheticians of tomorrow. To further this mission, Ms. Hill founded the Pamela Hill Institute® in 2004.

Reviewers

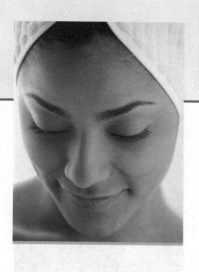

The author and publisher wish to thank the reviewers for their assistance and expertise in reviewing this text. We are indebted to them.

Darlene Purdy, Henderson, Nevada

Jean Harrity, Cary, Illinois

Ruth Ann Holloway, Providence, Utah

Tracy L. Johnson, Flowery Branch, Georgia

Sheryl Baba, Hyannis, Massachusetts

Acknowledgments

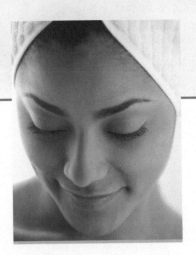

It is hard to know where to begin to thank those who have been instrumental in helping me achieve the goal of publishing *Milady's Aesthetician Series: Microdermabrasion, 2nd edition*. When I accepted the opportunity to create a *medical aesthetic series*, my husband wondered whether I had lost my mind. He worried that I would have time to do little else but sit in front of my computer; he was right. Therefore, my first thanks goes to my husband. Always at my side, he has been my best critic, my beacon of light, my teacher, and my best friend, without whom this book would not exist.

There are many other people to thank, including the staff at all of my clinics, who supported me, taught me, and rallied me on to the goal line. However, two individuals at my clinics stand out. First, thanks to Carmella, the aesthetician who took care of the patients represented in this text, saw the patients, worked on the programs, and ensured the photographs were taken. Without her help we would not have achieved our goals. In addition, Christian Sterling was in the "writing dugout." He has been with me each day, documenting references, conducting research, and helping me stay focused. Without these two very dedicated colleagues, this book would never have been completed.

Additional thanks go to those at Milady who believe in my message and supported me through this process.

Milady and the author would like to thank the following for contributing to this series:

Larry Hamill Photography, Denver, CO

The owner, Edit Viski-Hanka, and her entire staff at Edit Euro Spa in Denver, CO, for allowing us to use their beautiful location for our photo shoot.

Aesthetic Technologies for graciously allowing the use of the Parisian Peel® Prestige™

Models who participated in the photo shoot:

Jessica Anderson Barbour	Julie O'Toole
Marnie Brooks	Jeffrey Robison
Tina Marie Castillo	Melissa Ryan
Beverley J. Grant	Kathryn Staples
Velma Guss	Christian M. Sterling
Alysa K. Hill	Kavina Trujillo
Patricia Iannacito	Lawrence P. Trujillo, Jr.
Rosalyn Kurpiers	Nina Tucciarelli
Sandra D. Martinez	Karyn Turner
Connee McAllister	Phyllis Walsh
Patricia J. McIntyre	Pamela Whatcott
Polly McKibben	Lisa Williams
Barbara J. Miller	Donna R. Wilson
Susan Nathan	Sandra Vinnik
Janene T. Newell	Edit Viski-Hanka

Introduction to Microdermabrasion

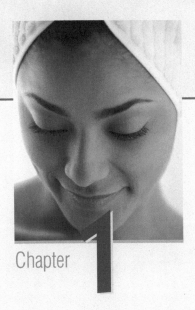

Chapter 1

After completing this chapter you should be able to:

1. Describe the history of microdermabrasion.
2. Discuss the value of clinical training for microdermabrasion.
3. Discuss variations in licensure regulations and insurance requirements.
4. Name the career options available with microdermabrasion training.
5. Understand the key points of professional ethics.

INTRODUCTION

nonsurgical aesthetic skin care
Any noninvasive procedure that is intended to improve overall skin health and appearance.

microdermabrasion
Nonsurgical aesthetic skin procedure that uses tiny crystals to strike and exfoliate the skin.

downtime
Industry jargon for recovery time.

Lines, wrinkles, and sagging skin were once considered irreversible consequences of the aging process. Earlier generations begrudgingly accepted them as a rite of passage into the golden years, wearing their lines proudly as testament to their survival of war, depression, and oppression. Today, such is no longer the case. Nowadays, the signs of aging are unwarranted and unwanted. As the Baby Boomers pass into their own golden years, they have been responsible for the creation of a multibillion-dollar industry called **nonsurgical aesthetic skin care**. Wanting to sustain a youthful appearance, Baby Boomers and the generations that follow them have forced our industry to develop products and services to meet their needs. Among those services is **microdermabrasion**. Microdermabrasion can be a simple procedure or a single step in a multifaceted treatment. It is a treatment with great range and the opportunity to improve the skin with little or no **downtime** to the client—just what the doctor ordered!

In the early 1990s, microdermabrasion was considered to be a new treatment with its fair share of naysayers and skeptics. Since then, microdermabrasion has been scientifically and histologically proven to improve the appearance of the stratum corneum and the integrity of the underlying layers of the skin. With proper programs and a monthly commitment from your client, a remarkable difference in the skin can be made.

Microdermabrasion has expansive appeal to young and old alike. With many positive attributes to recommend it—low complication rates, rapid and predictable results, no anesthesia requirement, low discomfort, safety, and little client downtime—clients and aestheticians alike prefer microdermabrasion as a monthly skin treatment.

Progress in medical science and **cosmeceutical** research has made great strides in our ability to treat the skin and generate nonsurgical results. Looking good means looking younger, and our society puts a high price on the commodity of youth.

Evolution of Skin Care

Skin care has held a place in every culture (including Egyptian, Greek, Roman, Indian, and African) through to the present day (Figure 1–1). From decorating and celebrating to masking and concealing, every culture throughout time has placed a value on faces and how they look. Today, a much more scientific and medical approach is used which not only enhances the appearance of our faces but also improves it down to the cellular level. Presently, the medical and aesthetic arts continue to converge. Although the two seem distant cousins, both are of ancient origin.

The Chinese were the first to understand medical fundamentals that are still practiced today. Traditional Chinese medicine dates back over 5,000 years to the writings of Fu Xi. His texts, called the *Trigrams*, relied on the theories of **yin and yang**. Yin and yang represent harmony between nature and its daily phenomena. The Yellow Emperor of the Han Dynasty later wrote of the need for a "positive physician-client relationship." The Chinese methods involving **Chi**, the balance of

cosmeceutical
A product that does more than decorate or camouflage but does less than prescription drugs; term originally coined by Dr. Albert Kligman.

yin and yang
Concept originally devised by Fu Xi that describes the harmony between nature and its daily phenomenon.

Chi
Concept originally theorized by the Yellow Emperor of China's Han Dynasty. According to Chi, nature has a delicate balance, and it describes illness as an imbalance.

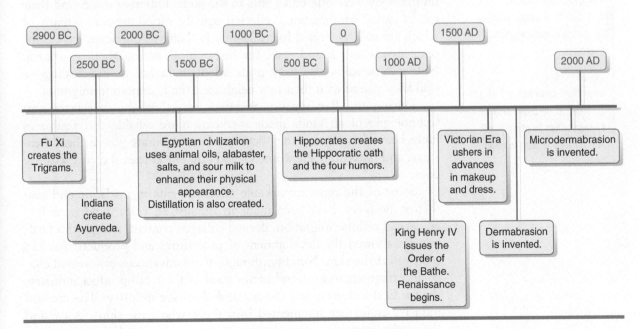

Figure 1–1 Evolution of skin care; line depicts the progress of skin care.

nature and imbalance of illness, are important foundations on which contemporary Western medicine was constructed.[1]

In ancient Egypt, materials were commonly used to enhance the skin's appearance. Ancient Egyptians routinely used animal oils, alabaster, and salts to this effect. Some Egyptian women even soaked in sour milk, unaware that the lactic acid was the source of their positive results. In addition, the Egyptians are credited for inventing the process of distillation, which they used to extract oils and other essences for use in both ceremonial and aesthetic contexts.[2]

Simultaneously, physicians in ancient Greece were making medical and aesthetic advancements of their own. **Hippocrates** had named the **four humors** (blood, phlegm, yellow bile, and black bile), the balance of which he hypothesized defined a person's character. Hippocrates also created the **Hippocratic oath**, which is still taken today by doctors and requires that those in attendance work cohesively (a point that has modern-day relevance for students reading this text). Concurrently, the Greeks also used accessories and adornments to enhance their physical appearance, including using pigments such as vermilion to enhance facial coloration.

From then on, many other cultures compounded previous knowledge and learned their own techniques in both medicine and aesthetics. The Indian concept of **Ayurveda**, or *science of living*, became part of the foundations of Western medicine. In Africa, colorful decorations on the body were offered as gifts to the gods. Different colors and their use in varied combinations reflected equally varied meanings, many of which are still celebrated today. Similarly, Native Americans wore elaborate beads and headdresses for hierarchical and aesthetic purposes. Native Americans also were quite adept in herbal wound healing—a skill they shared with their new neighbors, the European immigrants.

During the Renaissance, amazing breakthroughs in science and technologies of all kinds made medicine more reliable and aesthetics more beautiful. During the Victorian Era, elaborate gowns, headdressings, and makeup made women stand out—or at least the very wealthy ones.

Some of the most remarkable advancements in medicine and aesthetics, however, have been made in the last 25 years. Understanding epidermal cellular migration, dermal collagen content, and wound healing has allowed the development of procedures and products that can truly affect the skin. Notably, though, these advancements created chaos and fragmentation in industries such as the retail product industry, the medical industry, and the spa and skin-care industry. The medical industry is further fragmented into those who treat skin disease and those who treat skin aging, leaving consumers many choices. Combine

Hippocrates
Greek physician and "father of medicine," who created the Hippocratic oath and theorized the four humors.

four humors
Early medical concept originally postulated by Hippocrates, which stated that the character of a person is determined by the specific balance of the four fluids (black bile, yellow bile, blood, and phlegm) that he perceived as running through the body.

Hippocratic oath
Oath taken by all doctors relating to the practice of medicine; created by Hippocrates.

Ayurveda
Indian theory dating back to 2500 B.C. and known as *the science of living*. Ayurveda defines the essentials that were perceived as being necessary to health.

these choices with the abundance of products and services that claim to fight the effects of aging, and consumers may wonder: Where do I go and for what? For all of these reasons and much more, advanced skin care has "gone medical" and is creating a name for itself.

HISTORY AND ORIGINS OF MICRODERMABRASION

The idea of "sanding" the skin to improve its appearance is a longstanding technique used by plastic surgeons and cosmetic dermatologists. Whether the physician is using a small wire brush or pieces of actual sandpaper to abrade the skin in combination with chemical peeling, surgeons have had success with sanding the skin to improve its appearance.

Although microdermabrasion is not a surgical resurfacing tool, it has its origins in surgical resurfacing procedures such as dermabrasion. Microdermabrasion and dermabrasion have one broad similarity: Both procedures start from the premise that sanding the skin will improve its appearance. Obviously, it is the depth of the procedures and the number of treatments that significantly differ.

Like dermabrasion, microdermabrasion also resurfaces the skin, but the apparatus (crystals versus wire brush or sandpaper) is different and the depth is more superficial. Microdermabrasion also has much broader applications, addressing fine lines, dyschromias, texture issues, acne scarring, small scars, and solar keratosis.

Microdermabrasion was originally developed in the early 1980s. Early microdermabrasion machines were simple but had several problems. The machines were created as open systems, which meant that the user poured the crystals from a storage container into the machine and discarded the crystals by letting them flow into a trash receptacle. This open system was problematic for two reasons. First, the crystals could spill and the crystal dust could land on the floor, counter, and chair of the treatment room. Second, there was also concern that the aluminum oxide crystals, or corundum, might precipitate Alzheimer's disease in aestheticians or clients who inhaled particles. Although this concern was disproved, aestheticians are still encouraged to wear masks when doing microdermabrasion. Next-generation machines had several improvements, including a closed crystal system, use of disposable tips and filters, and the addition of equipment such as ultrasound to improve the absorption of topical products.

Today, each microdermabrasion machine seems to have special elements such as ergonomically correct handpieces, infusion systems,

Dermabrasion is a rarely-used skin resurfacing technique developed in the early 1900s. The procedure uses a small wire brush or diamond-coated wheel to resurface the skin. The wheel turns very quickly, producing injury to the skin at the papillary dermis and sometimes deeper.

dermabrasion
Predecessor to microdermabrasion that used a wire brush or a diamond-coated wheel to resurface the skin from the papillary dermal level.

open systems
In microdermabrasion, the first machines allowed for the escape of crystals and crystalline dust particles. Originally these particles were thought to be a risk factor for Alzheimer's disease, but this has since been disproved. Most modern machines are closed systems that do not allow particulate emission.

aluminum oxide crystals
Common type of abrasive crystals used for microdermabrasion.

corundum
Naturally occurring aluminum oxide.

ergonomically correct
Being consistent with body contouring so as not to inflict long-term damage (as with repeated use of poorly designed office equipment or devices).

stratum corneum
Superficial sublayer of the epidermis; varies in thickness over the body.

stratum granulosum
Thin, clear sublayer of the epidermis.

exfoliate
To remove dead skin cells and other debris from the skin's surface to give it a healthier sheen.

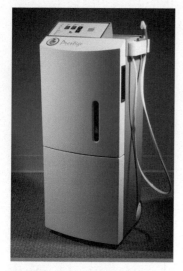

Figure 1–2 Medical microdermabrasion machine using crystals. (Photograph courtesy of Parisian Peel®.)

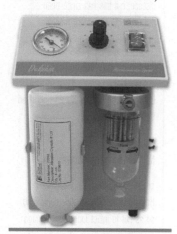

Figure 1–3 A compact medical microdermabrasion machine. (New Delphia on photograph identification)

completely enclosed crystal systems including filters, and compact units that can be carried without difficulty by the aesthetician. Whatever you desire in a microdermabrasion machine, no doubt you will be able to find the machine to fit your needs.

Microdermabrasion Defined

The truest definition of *microdermabrasion* is "polishing" of the skin, specifically the **stratum corneum** and **stratum granulosum**. The process involves vacuuming fine aluminum oxide crystals through a handpiece held at a 45-degree or 90-degree angle. As the crystals move through the system, striking the skin, they **exfoliate** and then are returned to the enclosed disposal canister.

In the microdermabrasion treatment, several varying components will have an effect on the end result: the type of crystals used, the machine and its functional use (speed, the handpiece, tips and infusion serums), and of course, the aesthetician (Figure 1–2). These components are discussed here but will be described in greater depth in subsequent chapters.

The type of crystals used for microdermabrasion varies (Figure 1–3). In addition to aluminum oxide crystals, salt crystals or sometimes diamond-encrusted tips can be used. Microdermabrasion with salt crystals is known as a *salt peel;* diamond-encrusted tips more closely resemble a traditional dermabrasion apparatus.

The machine and how it is operated will also have an effect on the result. Misusing the machine could injure the client and the aesthetician. The most common mistake made in the use of a microdermabrasion treatment machine is in the treatment depth, which is controlled by three variables: (1) the strength of the flow of the crystals, (2) the speed of the handpiece over the skin, and (3) the number of passes made. These details will be discussed in depth later in the text.

The third and most important determining factor for positive results is aesthetician training. Improper training or misuse of equipment will have negative consequences for the aesthetician, client, and spa. This is why regimented and thorough training is a necessary component to any microdermabrasion treatment plan.

Benefits of Microdermabrasion

The most common, expected, and visible result a client will see after microdermabrasion treatment is obvious—a deep exfoliation that leaves the skin healthier and more refreshed. It appears this way because older, drier, dead skin is removed at a pace that the natural sloughing process cannot match. The loosening and removal of this debris makes room for newer and more vital skin cells to reveal themselves.

Many aestheticians using microdermabrasion as a primary spa treatment will report auxiliary benefits. Among the additional benefits the client may see are tighter skin, reduction in T-zone oiliness, and possible *temporary* pore size reduction. From a scientific point of view, the skin might be tighter. More than one study has demonstrated that microdermabrasion acts not only on the epidermis but also the dermis.[3] Additionally, one might be convinced that regular microdermabrasion treatments reduce the oiliness found in the T-zone. Finally, many clients and aestheticians alike hope that pore size will decrease. Although aestheticians may initially see a reduction in the size of the pores, the reality is that pores will not shrink. One can think of pores like the lines of the hand. Once the imprint has been established, it is there to stay.

> The most important thing to know about microdermabrasion is that it works. Microdermabrasion has been proven to improve the quality of the dermis and epidermis.

Microdermabrasion versus Other Treatments

Microdermabrasion is often compared with other treatments such as **glycolic acid, Jessner's solution,** and **trichloroacetic acid (TCA)** peels, and surgical laser resurfacing treatments. These comparisons are really not appropriate—because of its unique benefits, microdermabrasion is in a class by itself (Table 1–1). However, many of these peels and advanced treatments such as LED and FotoFacial™ are being combined with microdermabrasion to create a treatment plan that is more advanced than microdermabrasion alone. Combining these techniques creates an improved outcome for the client.

Light and moderate-depth peels have many of the same indications as microdermabrasion treatments, including light acne scarring,

glycolic acid
Alpha hydroxy acid derived from sugar cane; it has a small molecular size that allows for easier penetration into the skin.

Jessner's solution
Peel solution for the skin that is 14 percent resorcinol, 14 percent salicylic acid, 14 percent lactic acid in ethanol.

trichloroacetic acid (TCA)
Chemical used in peel solutions that dissolve aging cells to make room for newer, healthier ones.

Table 1–1 Comparison of Treatments

Treatment	What It Does Do	What It Does Not Do
Trichloroacetic acid (TCA) peels	Flattens scarring Reduces rhytids Improves photo damage Improves hyperpigmentation	Reduce pore size Eradicate all rhytids Remove telangiectasia Remove deep scarring
Jessner's solution and glycolic acid peels	Reduces rhytids Improves photo damage Improves hyperpigmentation	Reduce pore size Eradicate all rhytids Remove telangiectasia Remove deep scarring
Dermabrasion	Flattens scarring Reduces rhytids Improves photo damage Improves hyperpigmentation	Reduce pore size Eradicate all rhytids Remove telangiectasia Remove deep scarring

Continued

Table 1–1	Comparison of Treatments – *cont'd*	
CO₂ laser	Removes some acne scarring	Reduce pore size
	Removes coarse static rhytids	Eradicate all rhytids
	Reduces coarse dynamic rhytids	Remove telangiectasia
	Improves photo damage	Remove deep scarring
	Improves hyperpigmentation	
Erbium laser	Removes some acne scarring	Reduce pore size
	Removes coarse static rhytids	Eradicate all rhytids
	Reduces coarse dynamic rhytids	Remove telangiectasia
	Improves photo damage	Remove deep scarring
	Improves hyperpigmentation	
Microdermabrasion	Flattens scars	Reduce pore size
	Reduces fine dynamic rhytids	Eradicate all rhytids
	Improves photo damage	Remove telangiectasia
	Improves hyperpigmentation	Remove deep scarring

dyschromia
Discoloration of the skin.

deep-epidermal wounding
Injury that reaches deep into the epidermis, as with peeling solutions.

papillary dermal wounding
Any injury to the skin that reaches deep enough to cause bleeding.

epidermal cells
Cells found in the outermost layer of skin.

keratolysis
Separation of the skin cells in the epidermal layer.

post-inflammatory hyperpigmentation (PIH)
Dyschromia associated with injury to the skin.

CO₂ laser
Aggressive type of laser used for skin resurfacing that vaporizes skin and causes thermal injury, allowing for improved collagen production.

erbium laser
Less aggressive type of laser that causes less thermal injury while still causing epidermal and papillary dermal injuries.

hypopigmentation
Lack of production of melanin from melanocytes.

dyschromia, rough texture, and fine lines. Peels, however, create **deep-epidermal wounding** and **papillary dermal wounding**, something that microdermabrasion is not intended to do. Peels use a solution to *melt* **epidermal cells** and exfoliate the skin rather than the *mechanical means* of the microdermabrasion treatment. Peels act differently on the skin by causing separation of the layers of the epidermis (**keratolysis**) and then sloughing off those necrotic layers. Additionally, peels require some downtime for the client to peel and heal. Due to penetration depth, peels can also pose a slightly higher risk of scarring, infection, and **post-inflammatory hyperpigmentation (PIH)**. However, both light to moderate peels and microdermabrasion create enough minor injury to stimulate collagen remodeling in the dermis and new collagen formation.

Resurfacing lasers cause epidermal and papillary dermal injury. Three major types of skin-resurfacing lasers exist: (1) the **CO₂ laser** (2) the **erbium laser** and (3) Fractionated. The CO₂ laser vaporizes the skin and in doing so causes a thermal injury, which in turn causes additional improvements in the dermis through collagen formation.

Unfortunately, because of the aggressive nature of CO₂ laser, the skin is at great risk for **hypopigmentation**. The erbium laser can also cause epidermal and papillary dermal injury, but this "lighter" laser does so with little thermal injury; therefore the result is somewhat less than the CO₂ laser-resurfacing procedure. The erbium laser also creates a slightly lower risk of hypopigmentation. Fractionated under the trade names Fraxel or DOT cause a pixel injury to the skin. In this fashion it leaves some areas of the skin untouched promoting faster healing.

None of these surgical resurfacing procedures are valid comparisons to microdermabrasion because of the length of downtime, pain, required anesthesia, potential for complications, and possible scarring.

▪ TRAINING

Because microdermabrasion treatments are technique-sensitive, aestheticians must understand the process of microdermabrasion, the importance of home products for the skin, and proper management of aftercare (all important factors for success) before they attempt the procedure (Table 1–2). The training process for microdermabrasion should not be left to the microdermabrasion machine vendor, although the vendor is a good resource of information about how a particular machine functions and for troubleshooting. Many states now have a required number of hours in microdermabrasion theory and practical application to achieve licensure. This is a step in the right direction but still does not provide the medical spa, physician, or employer with the level of confidence necessary. The medical spa should take training very seriously and have access to a trainer who will follow the spa's protocol for learning.

Microdermabrasion training should take place in a dedicated class that addresses theory and hands-on practice. The classroom work should include a review of the anatomy and physiology of the skin, the basics of wound healing, the indications and contraindications of treatment, and the fundamentals of at-home skin programs. The course

technique-sensitive
Exact protocols and processes must be observed to obtain an optimal outcome; however, because of individual variations in pressure or style, different aestheticians may get different results, even if protocol is observed.

anatomy
Study of the body and how its structures work in relation to each other.

physiology
Study of body function.

Table 1–2 Classroom and Clinical Training

Classroom Training	Clinical Training
Anatomy/physiology	Equipment
Indications	Consultation
Contraindications	Technique
Wound healing	Home care
Home care	Spa-specific information
Policy and procedure	Models

spa protocols
Any set of rules or guidelines established by a spa for safe practice; guidelines will vary by location but are expected to be observed by aestheticians working within the individual spa.

should require familiarity with spa protocols for microdermabrasion and the variety of available treatments and programs. Once the student completes the classroom work and has passed the recommended examination, he or she can move on to hands-on, clinical training.

The clinical-training program should focus on *technique*. Critical to the aesthetician's ability to replicate the treatments are his or her use of the handpiece, the pressure of the handpiece against the skin, and the number and direction of passes. The ability to reproduce a treatment comes with practice; therefore, extra time should be built into this arm of the training process. The aesthetician should not provide microdermabrasion treatments to clients until he or she has completed a thorough clinical-training program. Too frequently, this potentially harmful piece of equipment is put into the hands of untrained personnel. Although complications are generally minimal from microdermabrasion, we should not be misled into thinking that complications are nonexistent.

Classroom Training

As previously mentioned, classroom training is the starting point. This section of the training program should start with a review of basic information. The review process can be accomplished through a simple workbook, online courses, DVDs or traditional classroom sessions. It is important that it is done and that the aesthetician proves his or her work by passing a simple examination with a score of at least 80 percent.

Anatomy and physiology reviews should include information about the layers of the skin and their physiology. Because microdermabrasion affects both the epidermis and the dermis, both layers and all the sublayers of the skin should be reviewed. The anatomic structures identified as the appendages of the skin should be relearned in greater detail. A broad theoretic understanding of the indications and contraindications for microdermabrasion should be discussed. Aestheticians should also learn about the principles of wound healing so that they are aware of the potential injuries and how to manage the care. A thorough discussion of the spa's policy regarding the home care products and pre-treatment will help the aesthetician to be prepared when he or she greets his or her first client in the treatment room. Finally, some of the classroom time should be spent reviewing the spa's microdermabrasion policy and procedures, as well as the aesthetician's expectations.

appendages
Anatomic structures associated with a larger structure; for the skin, appendages include hair follicles and sweat glands.

indications
Any sign or circumstance that a particular treatment is appropriate or warranted.

contraindications
Any sign or symptom that a particular treatment that would otherwise be advisable would be inappropriate.

Clinical Spa Training

In the spa segment of the training, the aesthetician should be working one-on-one with the spa educator or instructor to master the use of the

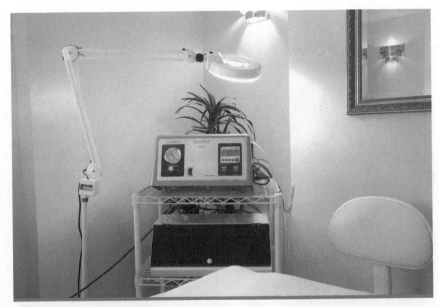

Figure 1–4 Salon microdermabrasion machine using crystals. (Photograph courtesy of Edit euroSpa.)

microdermabrasion equipment. The clinical spa training should be directed at three specific processes: (1) the consultative process, (2) the microdermabrasion technique, and (3) the pre- and post-treatment homecare programs (Figure 1–4). When learning about the consultative process, the aesthetician should take the specifics learned in the classroom, such as indications and contraindications, and apply them appropriately to specific skin types and clients' complaints. When focusing on the microdermabrasion technique, aestheticians should work on the specifics of the treatment, including pressure, stroke angles, number of passes, and tautness of the skin (see Chapter 9) while performing a treatment (Figure 1–5). Finally, home adjunct therapy for the client is a critical component of the long-term success of the spa program.

The spa must require at least 10 *model clients* with varying skin types and concerns to be treated before treatment of *clients*. A spa examination is also required to ensure the aesthetician understands his or her particular machine and the application of the microdermabrasion treatment.

Training Protocols

Training protocols are those documents that help you to understand the processes deemed acceptable for training. Protocols address subjects such as who can be trained, how the training takes place, and the necessary test scores to be approved as a skilled microdermabrasion

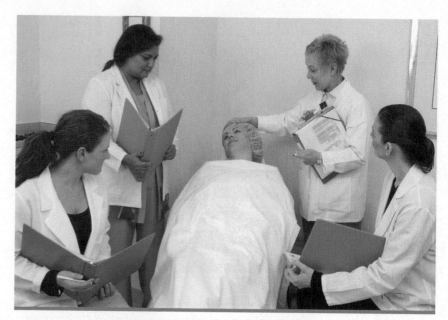

Figure 1–5 Clinical training is an important beginning step in providing microdermabrasion treatments.

aesthetician. Each spa should have a protocol to guide its behavior and options for training.

Training Requirements

The protocols should list the training requirements. These training requirements are the specific actions that must take place for the aesthetician to be placed into a training program and, after completing the training, to be released to treat clients. Three important points regarding training requirements bear repetition: (1) the aesthetician must have a current and valid license in the state in which he or she is practicing, (2) the physician or spa manager should recommend that the aesthetician be trained for the procedure, and (3) the aesthetician must score at least 80 percent on the theoretic testing and at least 90 percent on the spa testing.

Evaluating Aesthetician Skills

Although testing is a great tool to evaluate the student through the treatment-related educational process, it is not always an accurate indicator of the aesthetician's true spa abilities. A simple checklist for the aesthetician and the spa instructor might be useful. This *skill list* should include tasks such as draping the client, client communication skills, home program evaluation, and the ability to orient to the physical space.

Microdermabrasion Protocol Training

Standard policy and procedure

Pamela Hill Institute

Training and certification for microdermabrasion

Date of Origination: June 1996

Creator: Pamela Hill, RN

Date of Review: June 1997

Revisions by: S. Smith M.E.

Date of Revisions: June 1998, June 1999, June 2000, June 2001, June 2002, June 2003, June 2007, June 2009

Policy #: 01-001

Attachments: Policy and procedure document for microdermabrasion, certificates of completion, written test, spa test

Title of Policy: Training and certification for microdermabrasion

Policy: All spa staff will be licensed and insured in the state of employment. Certification through the company training program is required prior to client care.

Purpose: To ensure that all spa staff employed by the company are properly trained and certified in the techniques, policies, and procedures through the company training programs

Scope: All spa personnel

Definition: Spa aesthetic personnel

Procedure Indications: All aestheticians seeking certification will be recommended to the training program by their supervisors.

Testing if Necessary: Score of 80 percent or greater on the written examination is required before proceeding to spa training. A score of 90 percent or greater on the spa examination is required to treat clients.

Required Reading: Articles and technical information, provided by the instructor

Classroom Training: The training will consist of two classroom days. The curriculum for these days includes a review of anatomy and physiology of the skin, wound healing, principles and techniques of microdermabrasion, and home care regimens for microdermabrasion. A written test will be administered at the conclusion of the 2-day classroom course. A score of at least 80 percent is required to move to the spa training.

Spa Training: The aesthetician will be responsible for finding 10 models on whom to practice the microdermabrasion treatment. These models should have different skin types and different skin problems. It is preferable that the models have not had any previous skin care or treatments. A full consultation is done, followed by a treatment. The aesthetician will need to prove competency in consultation skills, the development of home programs, and the techniques of microdermabrasion described in the policy and procedure document. A passing score of 90 percent is required on the training to be released to treat clients.

Aesthetician Requirements: Licensed professional

Aesthetician Required Training: Certificate of completion in a microdermabrasion course with a state-recognized school or company training program

Table 1–3 Additional Aesthetician Skills		
Spa Skills	**Score 1–10**	**Recommended Improvements**
Communications Skills		
Clarity		
Education		
Sales abilities		
Safety Skills		
Wears protective gear		
Understands machine		
Charting		
Understands the record		
Makes appropriate notes		
Takes pictures		
Products		
Understands product lines		
Professionalism		
Appropriate to client		
Appropriate to peers		

These skill sets and those identified in Table 1–3 will help the aesthetician expand his or her knowledge.

Continuing Education

Educational updates can take place by three methods: (1) an annual recertification process through the spa, (2) **continuing education units (CEUs)** obtained at meetings, or (3) online study and education. Annual recertification processes within a spa usually have two phases. The first phase is through self-managed workbook reading and quizzes. These workbooks can be printed or put on your intranet (an efficient

continuing education units (CEUs)
Any certified training or event that is intended to build or add skills.

way of managing the process). The second phase is the spa recertification. This recertification is the process by which the spa educator or physician observes the aesthetician treating clients. The educator uses a score sheet to evaluate the aesthetician in all areas of the treatment room, including the actual treatment, cleanliness of the room, professionalism with the client, and so forth. The score on this evaluation must be at least 90 percent. If the aesthetician does not achieve a passing score, a problem-solving document called a **progressive improvement plan (PIP)** should be implemented to help the aesthetician improve his or her treatments.

    The next approach to ensuring educational updates is by requiring recognized CEUs. For example, for nurses in some states such as California, this is a requirement to renew the registered nurse (RN) license. This concept is now being translated to aestheticians as some states begin to require continuing education to renew licensure. CEUs can be obtained at annual meetings of professional organizations. Each year, one or two people can be selected from the spa to attend the annual meetings. Although expensive, these meetings are usually very illuminating and help the aesthetician to stay current on the newest products and services. If some aestheticians at the spa cannot attend the meeting, the returning aesthetician should give a report and provide copies of any relevant handouts.

    Finally, learning can take place through a variety of Web sites or DVDs that are dedicated to education on the Internet. These sites provide recognized CEUs or simple educational information.

progressive improvement plan (PIP)
Administrative document that is intended to record a problem and the actions that will be taken to improve the problem and prevent its reoccurrence.

> Ongoing education is the most important thing you will do for your career. It is your annuity for increasing wages, enhancing treatment results, and improving yourself.

▪ CAREER OPPORTUNITIES

Career opportunities abound for the educated and skilled medical aesthetician and cosmetic nurse (Table 1–4). Creating a **career plan** for success is the first step to realizing your dream. Many professionals in the area of self-improvement recommend identifying the goal and working backward to achieve that goal.

    Using this technique, identify where you want to be in five years and what you want to be doing. Then create a list of objectives to achieve the goal. For example, if you are currently an aesthetician without medical experience and you would like to be in a medical office as a microdermabrasion specialist, identify objectives that will allow you to meet the goal. Find out where to gain the training, expertise, and experience that will allow you to be a valued employee in a medical setting. Identify internships or learning situations that will help you to perfect your spa skills. Take communication courses that will help you to learn how to communicate with clients, peers, and superiors in a medical setting. Take sales

career plan
Action taken by an aesthetician to set goals and to ensure their realization.

> Ongoing training should be part of a yearly *self-improvement* plan. After you graduate from school, plan to take at least one course a year about a new subject that will add depth and power to your résumé.

Table 1–4 Career Opportunities	
Medical Office	Plastic surgery
	Dermatology
	Family practice
	Gynecology
	Otolaryngologist (ear, nose, and throat [ENT])
	Dentistry
Spas	Salon spas
	Fitness club spas
	Country club spas
	Holistic spas
	Day spas
Resorts	Destination spas
	Resort/hotel spas
	Cruise ship spas

courses that will help you to make a contribution to your employer and to yourself. Learn the basics of building a business. Create a professional résumé, and practice interviewing skills that will help you to get the job.

Marketing yourself to a business will become an important skill in acquiring the right job. Whether you want to land a job in a medical spa, a destination spa, or a holistic spa, the tactics you use to get there will be the same. Remember, just as you are looking for the perfect job, the employer is looking for the perfect employee. Not every opportunity will be a good match for you or the employer, and that is okay. Understanding the components of a good match will be the key to long-term success. By marketing yourself, you will have a sound understanding of what positions will be a good match for you personally.

Several components of marketing yourself should be addressed, including your value and values, your integrity, your skills, and your needs. Before looking for a job, it would be worthwhile to write out information for each category. This exercise will help you to ask potential employers the right questions, which will assist in your own determination. You can also use it to practice interviewing with a friend. Remember, you are interviewing the employer as much as the employer is interviewing you, so you should be well-prepared.

Values are defined as "the abstract concepts of what is right, worthwhile, or desirable; principles or standards."[4] Ask questions about the business's philosophies and goals (businesses should have both financial and nonfinancial goals). Specifically ask about client care philosophies; then discuss those values with which you can identify. Important values to you may include being on time, following company protocol, the quality of client care, or even volunteering at the local women's shelter. Think twice about taking a position where your values differ from those of the spa or employer.

Under the subject of your value, you will want to itemize specifics such as the location of your primary education. Some schools have more prestige than others; build on this if it is possible. Include a list of advanced education, including college (name, location, and degree), and any advanced aesthetic education classes (with whom and where). Finally, include experience in the field in which you are looking to be employed.

Integrity is different from *values*. Integrity is defined as "uncompromising adherence to moral and ethical principles; honesty."[5] In this category you will want to ask questions about client care, such as how complications are handled, how unhappy clients are dealt with, and how fee disputes are managed. In addition, ask direct questions about the ethical principles of the company. There should be a written philosophy. Usually it is in the **mission statement**. Then consider if these ethical principles are similar or the same as your own—they should be.

Your skills are important to an employer, but sometimes the position is not exactly what you are looking for. You may be underqualified or overqualified. You need to assess this with the employer. Ask questions about the specific skills needed, and respond with information about your skills. If you are underqualified but otherwise a match, what training will be available to help you become qualified? How quickly will that happen and who will do the training? Will there be a pay raise once the training is complete? These are important questions to ask before committing to a position. What you hear at the interview and what happens in a job is not always the same thing. It is in your best interest to put into writing some of what would otherwise be a "handshake" deal. This approach eliminates any future misunderstandings or hard feelings. If the employer is unwilling to do this, maybe it is not a match.

Your needs are especially important, but they are not exclusive of the employer's needs. The best situation is when you find a *need match*. List your needs, such as salary (pay rate, pay schedule, and commission), benefits, vacation time, sick day policies, hours to be worked, desired job description, and any other important needs you may have. Before the interview, decide which ones you can compromise on and which ones will be deal-breakers. Making this decision in advance prevents you from "giving in" on certain points during the interview, only to regret it later.

Once you have your credentials, your résumé, and your marketing plan, you are ready to go get the job for which you are uniquely qualified.

mission statement
Written statement of a business's individual philosophy.

Medical Offices

Busy aesthetic medical offices are always looking for proficient aestheticians and cosmetic nurses. Often, a physician will be looking for an employee who can multitask and take on additional job responsibilities. Depending on the scope of the practice, you may have an opportunity that will allow you to learn more and expand your skills. Some medical offices are willing to train untrained aestheticians or cosmetic nurses. However, the market is very competitive, and soon those who hold advanced education certificates will become the employees of choice. So what are the advantages and disadvantages of working in a medical office?

Working in a medical office has many rewards, among them prestige, advanced knowledge, complex treatments, and the chance to work with other medical professionals. Medical professionals are unlike other professionals because their training has spanned life and death, and their commitment to their clients is extremely strong. The ability to make a difference in the lives of clients is both meaningful and rewarding, as is the chance to learn and become more skilled at your chosen profession. Working in a medical office requires expert skills, willingness to learn, compassion, understanding, and expert professionalism; the payoffs are unlike those of any other profession.

The downside to working in a medical office includes dealing with office politics (although all offices seem to have politics), being "low man on the totem pole" (the aesthetician or cosmetic nurse sometimes feels out of the loop and unimportant), adhering to many new rules that have little or no apparent meaning, learning a new business sector, and building the nonsurgical aesthetic business in isolation. Physicians, nurses, and clients do not tolerate mistakes; therefore, a medical office can be an intense and intimidating place in which to work. In addition, physicians are often busy doing surgery or seeing clients and do not have time to dedicate to the growth and development of the aesthetic arm of a business, even though it is important to them. This means they will be looking to the aesthetician or cosmetic nurse to do this. Understanding all of the potential pitfalls of building a nonsurgical aesthetic business will be important in this situation. If you learn how to maneuver through the rough spots, you will find this a rewarding and financial profitable career.

Salons and Spas

Salons and spas offer a sense of well-being and luxury to the client. As treatments have become more sophisticated and our tools have become

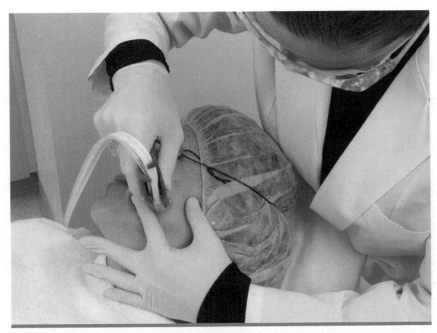

Figure 1–6 Microdermabrasion treatments are *technique sensitive*. Proper training should always take place before treating patients.

more advanced, we have the opportunity to provide our clients with treatments that may supplement medical treatments (**lymphatic drainage**) or help to reduce stress (**reflexology**). As the medical spa has become more popular and more aestheticians have the desire to work in the medical spa, other types of spas are looking for qualified and valuable employees (Figure 1–6). Many different types of spas exist; among them are salon spas, resort spas, cruise ship spas, day spas, club spas, destination spas, and holistic or mineral bath spas (Figures 1–7 and 1–8). Each spa has a different focus and requires the aesthetician to understand the advanced treatments he or she will be providing. Especially popular in resort spas and destination spas are body treatments and nutritional counseling. Cruise ship spas are looking for employees with excellent customer-service skills and great technical skills.

Spa directors expect their employees to be professional, educated, and willing to work hard to build their clientele. Having some experience or education in marketing will give you an opportunity to excel and build your clientele more quickly. Like the medical spa, it is important for the aesthetician to acquire advanced education and refine his or her techniques to be successful in the specific spa in which he or she happens to have interest.

lymphatic drainage
Drainage of lymphatic fluids.

reflexology
System of massage in which certain body parts are massaged in specific areas to favorably influence other body functions.

The aesthetician must be properly licensed by the state in which he or she plans to work.

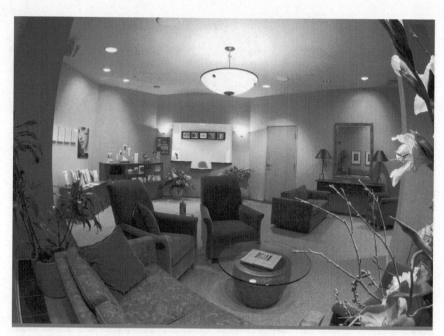

Figure 1–7 Medical spas are comfortable and also have facilities conducive to more technical procedures. They may resemble a physician's office. (Photograph courtesy of Facial Aesthetics.)

▪ LICENSE AND INSURANCE

Whether you are an aesthetician, nurse, physician's assistant, or medical assistant, you should be licensed in the state in which you work. Confirmation of licensure should be provided to the employer and kept in the employee record. Many aestheticians like to keep their licenses hanging in their treatment rooms for all to see. In some states, this is a requirement. Unlicensed aestheticians should not be working in a medical setting (or at all, for that matter), and the license should be obtained before employment.

Several types of insurance are necessary for a spa business. For the aesthetician, the most important insurance policy will be the malpractice policy. This is the insurance policy that covers your actions when treating clients. If something goes wrong, this is the policy that will protect you. When working in the medical office, sometimes the physician will have a broad policy under which you will be covered. This is also true in the luxury spa. For you, as the individual aesthetician, getting proper coverage is a fact-finding mission. First, speak with your employer and find out what the status of coverage will be for your position. Second, find a reputable company and have a consultation with one of the agents. Take his or her counsel and then consider a discussion with an attorney to ensure your best interests are evaluated.

Liability Issues

Liability issues for the aesthetician are an important factor in preparing for a career. In the U.S., people are more litigious than ever before. If something goes wrong, the client is always looking for someone to blame, and a lawyer is always available to take the case. Whether a case ever comes to settlement or trial, the stress of being blamed will be unbelievable; it is a situation in which no aesthetician should be caught.

Many potential liability risks exist for aestheticians. The most common occurrences that place the aesthetician at risk for lawsuits are scars, burns, product reactions and allergic reactions, infections, and failure to keep information confidential. When speaking specifically of microdermabrasion, the greatest risk of liability is corneal abrasion.

Scarring is an obvious concern, especially in the medical spa. No one is exempt from causing a scar; even improperly done extractions can cause scarring. Although medical aestheticians are more at risk, all aestheticians should be aware that any day they work they could cause a scar.

> Before you begin your employment, be sure to research state regulations as they pertain to your license and specific place of employment. Next, call an insurance agent to make sure you have the proper coverage for the procedures you will be doing.

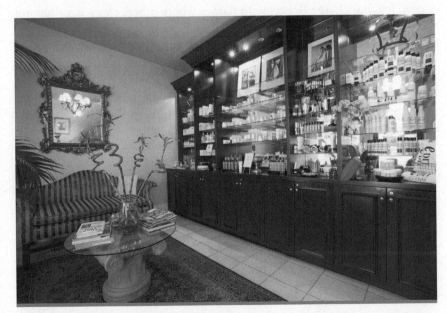

Figure 1–8 Traditional spas offer nonmedicinal treatments in a professional and aesthetically pleasing environment. They may also be more luxurious and have a retail focus. (Photograph courtesy of Edit EuroSpa, Denver, Colorado.)

With aggressive tools (such as peel solutions or microdermabrasion) the aesthetician needs to follow protocol carefully and ensure that he or she is skilled in the treatments being provided. Burns are usually caused by paraffin, peel solutions, and improperly used equipment. Product reactions and allergic responses are also a worry, especially if the response is extensive. Further, it can be considered negligence if the client told you in advance of allergies but the information was lost or disregarded. Product allergies can leave significant erythema and may require an emergency room visit if severe.

Infection may be a result of an aesthetician's failure to provide an adequate standard of care. Infections can happen in a variety of ways: failure to properly clean and sterilize implements, including extractors, microdermabrasion tips, brushes, electrodes, tweezers, bowls, reusable masks, or anything that touches the skin; failure to wear gloves during treatments (including spa treatments); or a lack of understanding about the sterilization and contamination process. The transmission of hepatitis C, **human immunodeficiency virus (HIV)**, which is the cause of **acquired immunodeficiency syndrome (AIDS)**, and **herpes simplex (HSV)** should all be of great concern to the aesthetician.

Failure to keep confidential client information is a subject for clients and the public. Talking about a client by name in front of another client, leaving charts or records on counters or desks where clients have access, leaving charge tickets with names where others can see, or having a signed guestbook at the front desk are all examples of a failure to keep information confidential. In the medical setting a federal regulation exists that all offices and medical professionals must follow; it is called the **Health Insurance Portability and Accountability Act of 1996 (HIPAA)**. No federal regulations exist for spas, but a standard of ethics and professionalism directs spa and salon employees to keep clients' information confidential.

Aside from the potential for scars mentioned previously, microdermabrasion has a risk for corneal abrasion. This can happen in two ways: (1) the goggles are not properly fitted to protect the eyes from crystals during treatment, or (2) crystals are swept into the eyes after the treatment. When a corneal abrasion occurs, an emergency room visit is usually necessary, followed by the care of an ophthalmologist. Of course, this visit puts the aesthetician at risk; therefore, great care must be taken by the aesthetician to protect the client's eyes.

▪ REGULATORY AGENCIES

The agencies that regulate the licenses of aestheticians are not federalized, and laws vary from state to state. Therefore, it will be important

hepatitis
Caused by multiple viruses defined as hepatitis A, B, or C; it is a contagious inflammation of the liver with possible chronic consequences, particularly with hepatitis C.

human immunodeficiency virus (HIV)
Virus that causes acquired immunodeficiency syndrome (AIDS); see *acquired immunodeficiency syndrome (AIDS)*.

acquired immunodeficiency syndrome (AIDS)
Opportunistic infections that occur as a result of the final stages of HIV and the associated compromise of the immune system.

herpes simplex (HSV)
Infectious disease caused by HSV-1, characterized by thin-walled vesicles that tend to occur repeatedly in the same place on the skin's surface.

Health Insurance Portability and Accountability Act of 1996 (HIPAA)
Federal regulation that dictates procedural protocols to protect client privacy.

for you to check with the licensing agency in your state to determine if, aside from general licensure, any specific requirements exist for your job. For example, you might need a certificate indicating that you have completed a course on microdermabrasion to perform the treatment.

■ PROFESSIONAL CODE OF ETHICS

The first question to ask is "Why have a code of ethics?"[6] Two types of ethical codes exist: (1) personal ethics and (2) **professional ethics**. Although they may overlap, each document is important. Individually, the code of ethics is a very personal document that discusses how you will live your life and what your priorities are in daily decision making.

Creating a code of ethics is not an easy task. In the absence of a national code of ethics for medical aestheticians, cosmetic nurses, and physicians' assistants, creating one in your workplace is imperative. For a code of ethics to be meaningful, the group that is going to use the document must develop it. It may feel like an overwhelming task because the subject matter can be broad and diverse, especially if the group writing the code is large. The focus of the code should be based on moral principles, and the group writing it should begin by asking certain questions: "Why a code of ethics?" "What is the purpose of our organization?" "For what will this code be used?"

For the code to be useful, it must reflect the qualities of the group (Table 1–5). This can be difficult, because each person within the group

professional ethics
Set of guidelines that should set a framework for professional behavior and responsibilities.

Belonging to a professional organization can be educational and a great place to network, but finding a good fit is important. Usually the physician you are working with belongs to a professional organization. If associations exist for ancillary staff, consider these organizations first.

"A Code of Ethics is a means of uniquely expressing a group's collective commitment to a specific set of standards of conduct while offering guidance in how to best follow those codes."[7]

Table 1–5 Writing a Professional Code of Ethics	
Component	**Considerations**
Preamble	What is the purpose of the organization?
Statement of intent	What is the purpose of the code itself?
Fundamental principles	What population is affected by your organization? What is your organization's area of expertise?
Fundamental rules	What unethical situations does your organization want to prevent? What are the likely problem situations in which unethical solutions might arise?
Guidelines for the fundamental principles and fundamental rules	How can these unethical situations be prevented? How can you prevent conflicting principles?

has different qualities and moral viewpoints. However, finding a place of compromise is always the best option. The code of ethics must be broad enough to take into consideration the number of people using it but specific enough to direct behavior. If the code fails to provide substantive guidance for the organization, it creates confusion. As for the skin care industry at large and your business specifically, a few tips can be offered (see Table 1–5).

Higher Standard of Professionalism

When you work in the medical office, more is expected of you by both the client and the physician. You are expected to adhere to a higher level of professionalism and customer service than is familiar to you in the spa setting. You must train yourself to refrain from laughing, joking, and loud behavior. Clients may think you are talking or laughing about them. In addition, that kind of "party" atmosphere does not reflect positively on your image or your profession. In fact, it could negatively reflect on you in the eyes of the client. Your ethical conduct should be present in your contact with clients, their charts or records, and your communication with others about the client. The information you pass along about the client to colleagues or others involved in their care should be complete but comply with the HIPAA regulations (see following). The client list of the medical spa belongs to the physician and, according to the laws of HIPAA, the information should never leave the medical office.

Professionalism in the Medical Setting

As a professional you must commit to the aesthetics industry, your career, and your clients by behaving in the most upright manner. Your behavior is evaluated each day by your clients, your colleagues, and your physicians. Adhere to the written code of ethics in your office, and take the time to create your own individual code. This will help you through the rough decisions you may have to make on your own or in coordination with your manager. Just as important, try to find a mentor inside your office, and create a relationship of trust and learning. A mentor is a "wise and trusted counselor or teacher."[8] This person will help you to learn, and you can model your behavior and professionalism after him or her.

Finally, a word on ethics and clients. Although it may feel like the client you meet and treat *belongs* to you, the reality is that this client belongs to the medical spa and physician. Without the physician's license you would be unable to extend your services. Therefore, if and when you leave the employ of the spa, it is inappropriate and unethical

Proper Handling of Medical Information

Access to Medical Records—Clients are entitled to have copies of their records and to look at their medical records.

Notice of Privacy Practices—Medical facilities are required to communicate with clients in writing about how their medical information will be used and what their rights are under the law.

Limits on the Use of Personal Medical Information—This section of the law deals with insurance plans and how the client's information is communicated between insurance companies and medical professionals.

Prohibition on Marketing—Restrictions exist concerning how client information can be used for marketing purposes.

Stronger State Laws—The national law does not affect stricter state laws. However, all states must abide by the national law.

Confidential Communications—Clients can dictate where and how they are contacted.

Complaints—All clients may file a complaint if they feel their privacy has been violated.

Here are a few basic tips that will help you to avoid trouble with HIPAA:

- Do not talk about clients within earshot of other clients (especially at the front desk and near or in the waiting area).
- Do not share information about the client with others, including the client's family.
- Do not fax medical records.
- Do not gossip about clients.
- Do not leave charge tickets where other clients can see names.
- Do not make a computer screen available for the client to see.
- Do not release information over the phone.
- Do not release copied information without a signed release by the client.
- Take only the record for the client you are treating into the treatment room.
- Chart immediately and file the chart; do not leave charts lying about.
- Be an ethical professional and consider how you would like to be treated.

to take a list of client names and phone numbers to contact for your next job. This is poor judgment, and if you are a medical professional (RN, physician's assistant), your professional license may be at risk. This behavior will not gain you points in the medical and professional community. If the physician you are going to work for asks you to do this, you should be concerned. All you have is your reputation. You may some day require the referral of your current manager or physician or need to work with them on some professional level, such as on a committee. Do not embarrass yourself by doing something inappropriate or, worse yet, illegal.

Health Insurance Portability and Accountability Act of 1996

When working in a medical office, it is important for the aesthetician to understand all of the laws and regulations that affect the practice. Among these rules and laws is HIPAA. Passed by Congress in 1996 and signed into law in January of 1997, the purpose of this law is to protect the privacy of clients' health information. Uniform standards regulate how health information changes hands. This information is protected by stringent rules that apply to information in the chart, on the computer or fax, and by spoken word. Seven categories of the law exist with which you should concern yourself: (1) access to medical records, (2) notice of privacy practices, (3) limits on use of personal medical information, (4) prohibition on marketing, (5) stronger state laws, (6) confidential communications, and (7) complaints.[9]

Professionalism in the Spa Setting

Because many laws exist that regulate the medical setting, focus should be more on the behavior required there than in the spa setting. However, the same level of professionalism is required at the spa, and codes of ethics and codes of conduct are vitally important there. To say simply that good customer service and the golden rule are adequate is a failure to appreciate the magnitude of these principles.

• CONCLUSION

Career opportunities abound for the trained and focused aesthetician. Options exist beyond working in the regular day spa, and it is up to the aesthetician to evaluate the opportunities and act on them. Recognizing the importance of HIPAA, ethics, and professionalism will ensure that you are well-respected within the spa. Continuing to manage your career after graduation by taking continuing education courses will allow you to maintain and expand your skills while increasing your success as an aesthetician.

▷ ▷ ▷ Top 10 Tips to Take to the Spa

1. Baby Boomers were the driving force behind aesthetic skin care; however, now your client population will be of all ages.

2. The origins of microdermabrasion are found in traditional dermabrasion; however, microdermabrasion is far more superficial and nonabrasive.

3. Three different kinds of microdermabrasion crystals are used: aluminum oxide, salt crystals, and diamond-encrusted tips. All work in basically the same fashion, by polishing the skin.

4. Microdermabrasion is in a class by itself. Although it is compared with light peels and laser treatments, no other medical spa treatment provides the same level of exfoliation and improvement in the skin's tone and texture.

5. Microdermabrasion is a technique-sensitive procedure; repetitive practice is necessary to achieve a predictable result. Practice as much as you can.

6. Continue your education through courses at conferences and programs that are available through manufacturers and colleges.

7. Be aware of the potential liability issues when treating a microdermabrasion client.

8. Be professional.

9. Be ethical.

10. Keep your client information confidential.

Chapter Review Questions

1. What is nonsurgical aesthetic skin care? List three reasons why it might be preferred over more invasive types of skin care?

2. What is microdermabrasion, and why does it qualify as a non-surgical aesthetic skin care treatment?

3. Why does microdermabrasion have such mass appeal?

4. Choose one step in the evolution of skin care. Explain why you think they might have significance to the field of aesthetics.

5. How are dermabrasion and microdermabrasion different from one another?

6. How might newer "closed system" machines be preferential to the older "open system" machines?

7. Explain the term *corundum*. Go into depth about the materials used as corundum and their pros and cons.

8. What three factors affect treatment depth in microdermabrasion?

9. True or false: Microdermabrasion can loosen and remove the debris of older and dead skin, allowing room for newer and more vital skin cells to reveal themselves.

10. True or false: Microdermabrasion improves only the epidermis, but does not affect the dermis.

11. True or false: It is not recommended to use microdermabrasion in conjunction with other treatments.

12. Define the term *technique-sensitive* in the context of microdermabrasion.

13. Which is more important, employer training or vendor training of microdermabrasion? What are the benefits of each? The negatives?

14. What components of classroom training would benefit an aesthetician? Why?

15. Explain the training protocols for microdermabrasion. What are they, and how would a student of microdermabrasion benefit from them?

16. How does ongoing or continued education benefit a student of microdermabrasion?

17. From where you are now, write about the aesthetic sector in which you imagine yourself. What are you doing to enable that to happen?

18. List some of your personal values as they might apply to your future as an aesthetician.

19. What are the liability issues associated with performing microdermabrasion? How can these issues be prevented?

20. What is the regulatory body in the state in which you intend to practice microdermabrasion?

21. Write your own code of ethics.

22. Would you consider working in a medical environment? What might the benefits of doing so?

23. Explain HIPAA. Why might that apply to aesthetics?

24. Why might you benefit from membership in a professional organization?

Chapter References

1. D'Angelo, J., Dean, P., Dietz, S., Hinds, C., Lees, M., Miller, E., & Zani, A. (2003). A journey through time: Esthetics then and now. In *Milady's standard: Comprehensive training for estheticians* (pp. 4–23). Clifton Park, NY: Thomson Delmar Learning.

2. Rubin, M. (1995). *Manual of chemical peels: Superficial and medium depth.* Philadelphia, PA: Lippincott, Williams & Wilkins.
3. Guttman, C. (2002, August). Histologic studies: Microdermabrasion not just superficial. *Cosmetic Surgery Times* [Online]. Available: http://www.cosmeticsurgerytimes.com
4. *Webster's College Dictionary.* (1992). New York: Random House.
5. *Webster's College Dictionary.* (1992). New York: Random House.
6. MacDonald, C. (2004, March 9). *Why have a code of ethics?* [Online]. Available: http://www.ethicsweb.ca
7. Olson, A. (2004, March 11). *Authoring a code: Observations on process and organization* [Online]. Available: http://www.iit.edu
8. *Webster's College Dictionary.* (1992). New York: Random House.
9. United States Department of Health and Human Services. (2004, March 9). *Fact sheet* [Online]. Available: http://www.hhs.gov

Anatomy and Physiology of the Skin

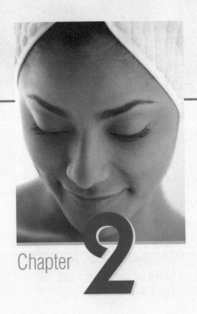

Chapter 2

Key Terms

absorbents
adipose cells
amino acids
anagen phase
apocrine sweat glands
astringents
avascular
basal cell carcinoma
catagen phase
ceramides
cleansing agents
collagen
cornified
dermal-epidermal
   junction
dermis
desmosomes
desquamation
eccrine sweat glands
elastin
emollients
epidermis
extrinsic aging
fibroblasts
filaggrin
glycosaminoglycans
   (GAGs)

ground substance
histamine
hyperpigmentation
hypodermis
integumentary
   system
intrinsic aging
keratin
keratinization
keratinocytes
keratolytics
lamellar granules
Langerhans' cells
lipids
mast cells
melanin
melanocytes
melanoma
melasma gravidarum
Merkel cells
natural moisturizing
   factor (NMF)
organelles
papillae
pathogens
pheromones
pilosebaceous unit

postmitotic cells
psoriasis
rete pegs
reticular dermis
reticulin
rhytids
sebaceous glands
skin turgor
slough
squamous cell
   carcinomas (SCCs)
stem cells
stratum basale
stratum lucidum
stratum spinosum
subcutaneous
suppurate
telogen phase
transepidermal water
   loss (TEWL)
urticaria pigmentosa
vesicles
vitiligo

Learning Objectives

After completing this chapter you should be able to:

1. Define the layers of the skin.
2. Discuss and define the importance of melanocytes, keratinocytes, and fibroblasts.
3. Understand the importance of glycosaminoglycans.
4. Describe the difference between intrinsic and extrinsic aging.
5. Describe transepidermal water loss.
6. Understand the constituents of natural moisturizing factor.

INTRODUCTION

The skin and its appendages—nails, hair, nerve endings, sweat and oil glands—collectively encompass the **integumentary system**, sometimes referred to as *integument*. Skin is vital to our survival, as it keeps our bodies and its various components intact and, just as important, provides our immediate contact with the environment. Our skin senses vital information about the world in which we live; therefore, it ensures our survival.

Although seemingly uniform and simple in its presentation and purpose, it is far more complex and varied than it appears. Skin varies in thickness and in sensitivity. During development in the womb, parts of it develop from brain tissues and become attached to the brain through nerves, which conduct pleasure and pain.[1] These signals are vital to our success as a species. Although not all of the sensations humans feel are pleasurable, they are all purposeful. If we could not sense cold air, we would all freeze to death. If we could not feel a cut, we could bleed to death or die from infection. These sensations are sensed by nerves, which in turn send the information to our brains for processing and translation. The skin overall possesses most of the nerve endings that transmit vital information about our environment to the brain. Relatively few are found on our posterior sides; however, in lips, fingers, and genitals they are abundant.

Because the skin is our outermost organ, it also serves as a unique identifier, which we see and use to associate and differentiate one person from another. Being the psychosocial creatures we are, we have put great emphasis on how others perceive the way we appear. The way we dress,

integumentary system
Skin and its appendages (nails, hair and sweat and oil glands).

"The beauty of a face is a frail ornament, a passing flower, a moment's brightness belonging only to the skin."[2] The skin is the largest human organ. It is our protection from outside elements, it identifies us, and it defines our beauty.

Table 2–1 Fun Facts About the Skin[3]

Humans shed millions of dead skin flakes every minute.
In adults, the skin usually covers about 2 m^2 (about the size of a shower curtain) and weighs about 7 lbs. It also has 300 million skin cells.
The skin is between 1.5 mm and 4 mm thick, about as thick as a few sheets of paper.
The thickest areas of the skin (plantar and palmar regions) contain no hair follicles or sweat glands.
Millions of coiled sweat glands discharge sweat and salts to the surface, where evaporation begins to cool the body in seconds.
Just below the surface, the dermis feeds miles of blood vessels with nutrients.
The brain and skin become connected very early in fetal development. Even in the womb, a baby's hand can feel its way to the mouth.
Touch is the first sense to develop.
The skin's array of nerves is sensitive enough to feel the weight of a mosquito as it lands.

decorate, and posture ourselves conveys gender, age, strength, and most noticeably, attractiveness.

The appearance of the skin has become a synonym for beauty in our society, and we strive to optimize it. New scientific developments promise creams to "turn back the clock" that are longer-acting, stronger, or faster. Some consumers are extraordinarily sophisticated in finding the newest treatments and the latest products to counteract the aging process. Others are overwhelmed by the options available to them. Either way, we can do things to maintain and even regain beautiful skin (Table 2–1). To do so we must ask ourselves questions: How do we determine what works best? Why does it work? How much change is possible? Even the savviest consumer needs help answering these questions. Most of them will turn to you for advice. It is here that our quest begins.

▪ SKIN PHYSIOLOGY

As discussed, the skin does much more than just hold in the other organs. Not much thicker than a sheet of paper, skin is quite complex. In general terms, it protects, senses, and aids temperature regulation, excretion, immunologic response, and metabolism (Figure 2–1).

As an aesthetician in the field of dermal techniques, it is important for you to be familiar with the skin, its layers, and the cells within them. A deeper understanding of skin structure and function will help you to be a better aesthetician. In turn, this will provide your client improved results and safer care.

An active organ, the skin provides protection, conveys sensation, sends signals, regulates temperature, produces vitamin D_3, and helps rid our bodies of unneeded or threatening components.[4] It is elastic–it stretches when we frown or smile or bend, and regains its normality when we relax.[5]

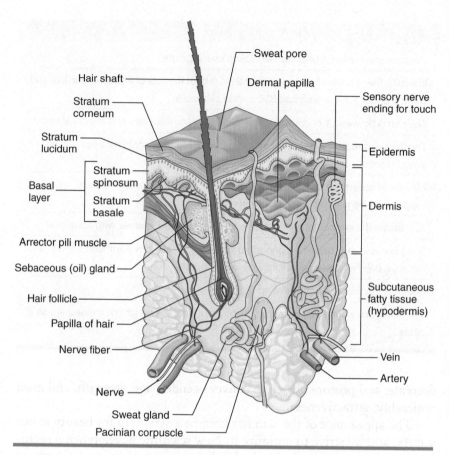

Hair shaft

Stratum
corneum

Stratum
lucidum

Basal
layer

Stratum
spinosum

Stratum
basale

Arrector pili muscle

Sebaceous (oil) gland

Hair follicle

Papilla of hair

Nerve fiber

Nerve

Sweat gland

Pacinian corpuscle

Sweat pore

Dermal papilla

Sensory nerve
ending for touch

Epidermis

Dermis

Subcutaneous
fatty tissue
(hypodermis)

Vein

Artery

Figure 2–1 Having a thorough understanding of the different layers of skin is a vital part of aesthetician training.

Protection

Protection is one of the skin's main functions. Skin acts as a barrier against intruders such as water, ultraviolet light, bacteria, and fungi. It protects vital organs against minor trauma. The skin is a mostly-waterproof sheath that guards against too much moisture entering or escaping from the body. It also secretes acids that could otherwise allow bacteria and viruses to penetrate our skin and cause disease or even death.[6] Likewise, the skin acts as armor against foreign matter. The final way the skin protects us is against the damaging effects of solar rays. The pigment melanin is produced as an active response to ultraviolet light, thus preventing cellular damage. This will be discussed in more detail later in this chapter.

Sensation and Communication

Skin is capable of receiving a diverse amount of tactile information from a variety of receptors. Neural receptors, some of them quite elaborate, mediate touch, position, pressure, temperature, and pain. The communication goes two ways and occurs instinctively. The skin releases signals such as blushing, **pheromones** (unique chemical signals), and body odor.

The four senses recognized by the skin are (1) touch (pressure being sustained by contact), (2) cold, (3) heat, and (4) pain.[7] Nerves that receive and send these sensory signals to the brain show a variety of sensory endings, including expanded tips (Merkel's disks and Ruffini's endings), encapsulated endings (Pacinian corpuscles, Meissner's corpuscles, and Krause's end-bulbs), and simple naked nerve endings. Many sensory nerves terminate around hair follicles. Expanded or encapsulated nerve endings can also occur in areas of the body removed from the skin—explaining *deep* pain we can feel, such as in response to a kidney punch.

pheromones
Chemical substances that, when released, may affect the behavior or physiology of a recipient.

Thermoregulation

Skin is critical for regulating body temperature.[8] The body's optimal internal (or *core*) temperature is maintained by actions of blood vessels in the lower layer of the skin. Blood vessels will insulate the body's core temperature from both internal and external temperature variations by constricting and relaxing blood flow. When we are exposed to cold, blood vessels in the lower layer of the skin constrict. This allows the blood to bypass that which would cool it as the skin cools to the outside temperature. When it is warm, those blood vessels dilate and heat is radiated outward. Perspiration evaporates off the surface of the skin and cools us. To this effect, body heat is conserved.

Although normal core body temperature is 37° C or 98.6° F, skin surface is normally cooler, around 33° C or 91° F.[9] The surface temperature of the skin depends on the temperature of the air that touches it and the amount of time spent in that air. Weather factors such as wind and humidity affect skin temperature, and temperature at different points of the skin surface can differ dramatically. After exertions on a windy and snowy day, one climber on Denali reported the temperature of his big toe to be 42° F at the same time that the surface of his chest measured 88° F.[10]

Metabolism

Blood vessels within the lower layer of the skin also provide nutrition for the skin. Blood flow carries vitamins, minerals, and oxygen that are critical to skin's health and appearance. Oxygen requirements for skin are *greater* than that of connective tissue, and if not enough oxygen is supplied, the health of the skin may suffer. This is why smoking cigarettes may cause problems with healing. Skin health not only affects how we look but also how quickly and smoothly injuries such as cat scratches and paper cuts heal.

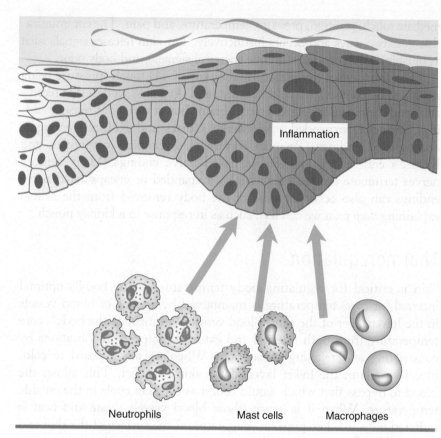

Inflammation

Neutrophils   Mast cells   Macrophages

Figure 2–2 Skin contains specialized cells, particularly mast cells and Langerhans' cells, which protect the body within by defending the skin against microorganisms.

Immunologic Response

Skin contains specialized cells to protect it and all of the elements it contains. **Mast cells** and **Langerhans' cells** defend the skin against microorganisms. Langerhans' cells detect antigens in the uppermost layer of the skin. Mast cells are poised to create an inflammatory response should the skin be injured (Figure 2–2).[11] This is evidenced by allergic reactions (Figure 2–3). Mast cells are responsible for **histamine** and related responses to mosquito bites and bee stings.

Excretion

The skin releases fluid and toxins through the sweat glands. These same glands are important regulators of body temperature, as mentioned previously.[12]

mast cells
Large tissue cell present in the skin that produces histamine and other acute symptoms of allergic reactions.

Langerhans' cells
Cells possessing processes (dendrites) that detect pathogens; involved in immune response. Type of macrophage common to the epidermis.

histamine
Amino acid histidine, found in the body and released from mast cells as part of an allergic reaction.

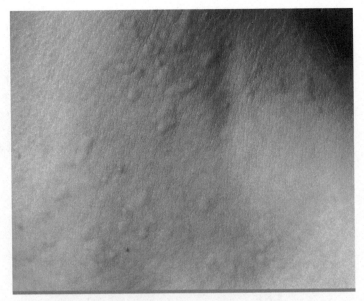

Figure 2–3 In allergic reactions manifested in the skin, such as hives, a large number of mast cells are seen.

▪ SKIN ANATOMY

If one of the skin's main functions is to act as a barrier against intruding substances, then how do lotions that we apply absorb into the skin? The main answer is the appendages. *Appendages* are smaller parts of a greater part. For the skin, they include the pilosebaceous unit (hair follicle and accompanying **sebaceous glands** and arrector pili muscle), sweat glands, and nails.[13] Appendages originate in the uppermost layer of the skin (the **epidermis**) but extend in pockets of epidermis into the lower layer, the **dermis**.

External substances such as skin creams, ointments, and salves can enter the skin through the appendages of the hair and sweat glands (Figure 2–4), through the intercellular spaces between the **cornified** cells, or smaller molecules can pass through cells at the surface of the skin.

Sweat Glands

You can think of sweat glands as simple tubes. They are vital for regulating body temperature. Because of the composition of what they carry to the surface, sweat glands also influence water balance and ionic penetration.

Ordinary **eccrine sweat glands** are located over most of the body, and large **apocrine sweat glands** are concentrated in axillary (underarm),

sebaceous glands
Small glands usually located next to the hair follicle in the dermis that release fatty liquids onto the hair follicle to soften hair and skin.

epidermis
Top layer of the skin.

dermis
Second layer of skin that is responsible for attaching the skin to the body.

cornified
Hardening or thickening of the skin.

eccrine sweat glands
Smaller of the sweat glands that reside all over the body.

apocrine sweat glands
Larger of the sweat glands that are housed in axillary (underarm), pubic, and perianal areas.

The skin's appendages are important in healing, especially superficial healing and protection of the skin. When the skin is superficially injured over a limited surface, it can grow back quickly because of epithelial cells remaining in deeper hair follicles and sweat glands.

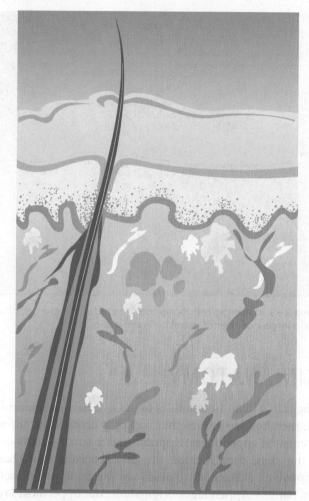

Figure 2–4 It is important for an aesthetician to understand how the skin accepts products topically.

pubic, and perianal areas.[14] The latter develop at puberty.[15] Although sweat from the apocrine glands is initially odorless, it can mix with bacteria on the skin and acquire an odor.

Normal, healthy adults secrete about one pint of sweat per day (more with physical activity).[16] Because of daily loss of water, everyone needs to actively replace water lost inside the body, regardless of their activity level. However, the more active you are, the more water that needs to be replaced. As much as four cups of water can be lost during hard exercise. To avoid dehydration, water should be consumed regularly throughout the day and more before, during, and after exercise.

When a person has become thirsty, they are already dehydrated, so it is important to consume fluids regardless of thirst. Symptoms of dehydration include dizziness, disorientation, and clumsiness.[17]

Hair Follicles

Hair is a type of modified skin. It grows everywhere on a person's body except the palmar and plantar regions of hands and feet. Hair follicles are densest on the head, neck, and shoulder regions, where there can be as many as 300 to 900/cm². Conversely, about 100/cm² are found on the torso and limbs.[18] Hair follicles are tubular. They protrude deep into the skin to develop and nourish the hair. The hair follicle contains epidermal cells, whereas the hair itself is **keratin**. Hair follicles have several distinct anatomic components, including *the bulb, the root,* and *the papilla.*

The hair follicle, gland, nerve, and muscle are called the **pilosebaceous unit** (Figure 2–5). Hair follicles are associated with sebaceous glands (small masses of cells and fat) that lubricate the hair; nerve endings that detect motion of the hair shaft and control piloerection ("goose bumps"); and smooth muscle, which actually creates the goose bumps.[19] The sebaceous glands, which are most active, reside on the face, chest, and back.

All hair goes through an **anagen phase** (growth), a **catagen phase** (transitional), and a **telogen phase** (resting)—the hair grows, resides for a while, and then falls out.[20] This growth cycle varies in different parts of the body. For instance, the entire cycle takes 4 months for eyelashes and 3 to 4 years for scalp hairs.

keratin
Protein cell found in the skin, hair, and nails. Insoluble in water, weak acids, or alkalis.

pilosebaceous unit
Hair follicle and accompanying sebaceous glands and arrector pili muscle.

anagen phase
Hair growth phase in which growth is actually occurring.

catagen phase
Intermediate stage in the hair growth phase.

telogen phase
Stage of hair growth during which the hair is at rest.

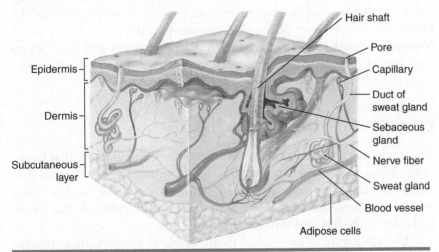

Figure 2–5 The skin's appendages include the pilosebaceous unit (hair follicle, accompanying sebaceous glands, and arrector pili muscle) and sweat glands.

As we will see, this process of division, growth, and maturation somewhat resembles that of the skin's top layer. In both cases, cells go through a process of hardening and then *sloughing*, or being shed (Figure 2–6). However, when cells at the bottom of the hair follicle **slough**, they create a column of keratinized (hardened, "horny") cells. This is the hair that grows up through the shaft and extends through the follicle. Hair growth is a complex process, but understanding this process is key to the success of hair removal with lasers or light. Lasers are known only to be effective on hairs in the growth (anagen) phase.

Nails

Like hair, nails are also a type of modified skin.[21] They are formed from hardened cells in the top layer of skin. Nails on the fingers and toes protect their sensitive tips. They provide support for the tips of our digits and assist in picking up objects. Although effective, they are not necessary for living (and neither are the details of their histology necessary for us to know).

> **slough**
> To cast off skin, feathers, hair, or horn.
>
> **subcutaneous**
> Beneath the skin.
>
> **avascular**
> Lacking in blood vessels; thus having a poor blood supply.

▪ LAYERS OF THE SKIN

The skin is comprised of two main layers: (1) the epidermis and (2) the dermis. The epidermis, or top layer, is tough and, because of its exposure, constantly being worn down and replaced.[22] It contains no blood vessels or nerves and is vital in preventing loss of moisture from the body. The deeper layer of the skin, the dermis, and the **subcutaneous** (meaning *beneath the skin*) fat beneath it lend strength and elasticity to the skin. Within both layers of skin are sublayers, with cells that perform specific functions.

Epidermis

The epidermis is the skin that we see. It contains tiny pockets that house sweat glands and pilosebaceous glands.[23] Compared to the dermis, it is often very thin, approximately 0.12 mm, but its thickness also varies dramatically over the body.[24] It is thickest on the palms of the hands and soles of the feet and thinnest on the eyelids.

The epidermis is **avascular**, (without blood vessels), impermeable to water, physically tough, and dry at the surface to impede the growth of microorganisms. It is continually replacing itself. When the epidermis is injured or diseased, its replacement speeds up in response; this is

> As the outermost layer of the skin, the epidermis shields us from the environment, potential injury, bacteria, pollution, and almost everything else that might penetrate it. The dermis is the support, providing the epidermis with strength and stability.

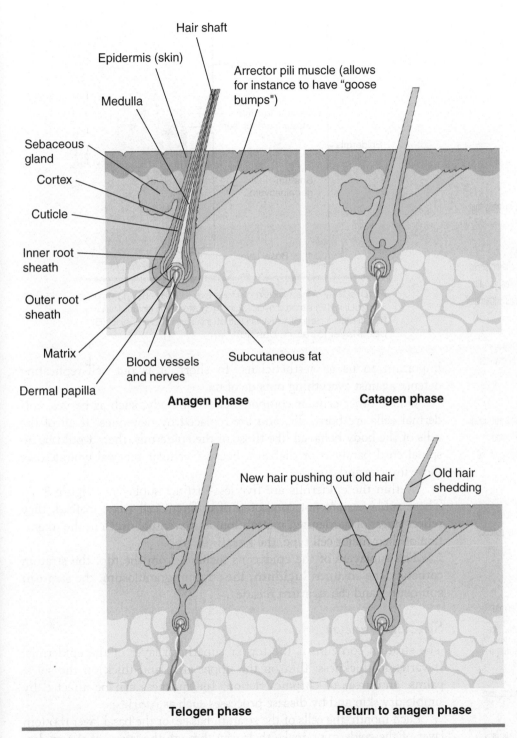

Hair shaft

Epidermis (skin)

Medulla

Arrector pili muscle (allows for instance to have "goose bumps")

Sebaceous gland

Cortex

Cuticle

Inner root sheath

Outer root sheath

Matrix

Dermal papilla

Blood vessels and nerves

Subcutaneous fat

Anagen phase

Catagen phase

New hair pushing out old hair

Old hair shedding

Telogen phase

Return to anagen phase

Figure 2–6 Hair goes through three distinct phases during its life cycle: (1) the anagen phase (growth), (2) catagen phase (transitional), and (3) telogen phase (resting).

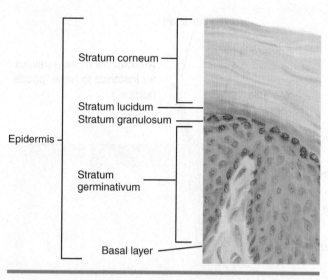

Stratum corneum

Stratum lucidum
Stratum granulosum

Epidermis

Stratum
germinativum

Basal layer

Figure 2–7 The epidermis has five sublayers: (1) stratum corneum, (2) stratum lucidum, (3) stratum granulosum, (4) stratum germinativum (stratum spinosum), and (5) basal layer (stratum basale).

keratinocytes
Any cells in the skin, hair, or nails that produce keratin.

stratum lucidum
Sublayer of the epidermis characterized by the appearance of granules and the disappearance of the nucleus within the skin cells.

stratum spinosum
Sublayer of the epidermis intertwined with desmosomes.

stratum basale
Lowest layer of the epidermis (or basal layer); houses germinal cells and regenerating cells for all layers of the epidermis.

psoriasis
Chronic skin disease characterized by inflammation and white scaly patches.

Psoriasis is a genetic malfunction of the epidermal cellular reproduction rate. The accelerated process creates a phenomenon known as *psoriasis plaques*. Psoriasis can also be environmentally precipitated, but people usually are genetically predisposed.

important to us as aestheticians. In short, it is our self-replicating defense against everything outside of us.

Unlike other cellular components of the body, such as nerves, epidermal cells are born, die, and are replaced by new ones. If all of the cells of the body behaved like those of the epidermis, there would be no spinal cord paralysis or diabetes, because cellular renewal would solve those injuries and diseases.

Within the epidermis are five less-distinct sublayers (Figure 2–7). These sublayers are not composed of different cell *types*; instead, they reflect *stages* of hardening, maturation, and eventual death in the migration of their major cell type, the **keratinocyte**.[25]

The sublayers of the epidermis include, from the top, the stratum corneum, the **stratum lucidum**, the stratum granulosum, the **stratum spinosum**, and the **stratum basale**.

Stratum Corneum

The stratum corneum is the top or superficial layer of the epidermis. It varies in thickness: thin on the upper arm, and thick on the soles, palms, and areas of chronic friction. Its thickness can be affected by simple dry skin and by disease processes such as **psoriasis**.

Each month, the cells of the stratum basale, or the basal layer (bottom layer of the epidermis), make their way through the layers of the epidermis into the stratum corneum. The cells begin as healthy plump cells with fully functioning nuclei. However, as they near the summit, they shrivel and flatten out.[26] The cells complete their gradual transition to death and are soon sloughed off, but this is what makes them protective. It is actually this layer that is "polished" by microdermabrasion.

Although it is drier than lower skin layers, the stratum corneum contains a compound, **natural moisturizing factor (NMF)**, that helps to keep the skin soft and moisturized even in dry climates.[28] NMF is composed of **amino acids** and **filaggrin**, water-soluble chemicals capable of absorbing large quantities of water. The presence of NMF in the stratum corneum is critical for soft and flexible skin. Although NMF is contained only in the uppermost layer of the skin, its existence is made possible by ingredients provided by deeper structures.[29]

NMF gives the cells of the stratum corneum their ability to bind with water. NMF is found only in the stratum corneum and is solely responsible for the regulation of water in the very superficial layers of the stratum corneum. Not surprisingly, its presence is diminished by age and excessive exposure to soap. This is key to understanding the phenomenon of dry skin.

It is worth noting that NMF and TEWL have nothing to do with water loss associated with sweating. It is a common misconception that drinking water will improve hydration levels of the skin. This is simply not true. Drinking water improves water level inside the body, but is used up there. The best way to rehydrate the skin is by applying a topical moisturizer.

Stratum Lucidum

This thin, clear band (*lucidum* means *clear or bright*) of closely packed cells is most prominent in areas of thick skin and may be absent in other areas.[30]

Stratum Granulosum

Like the other sublayers of the epidermis, this layer signals transition of the cells within it.[31] It is in this layer that the keratin loses nuclei and **organelles**, becoming flat before moving farther up into the stratum corneum. It is called the *stratum granulosum* because of the granules that now appear in the cells. In effect, these granules write the death warrant of the cell, because as the granules grow in size, the nucleus—the power-generator of the cell—disintegrates and dies.[32]

Stratum Spinosum

Stratum spinosum means *spiny layer*. Cells in this sublayer are intertwined with tiny structures called **desmosomes**. Under the microscope, desmosomes resemble hair combed with an eggbeater, which is why this part is often called the *prickly-cell* layer. The hair-like desmosomes

Unbeknownst to us, our bodies gently and constantly lose water via evaporation through a process called **transepidermal water loss (TEWL)**.[27] When too much water evaporates, not only our skin but also our bodies suffer ill effects. Preventing excessive water loss is important both to the skin and to the body as a whole.

In the stratum corneum, filaggrin assists keratinocytes in creating the NMF. Later, it combines with other cells found within the granular layer to create strength and stability for the epidermis.

natural moisturizing factor (NMF)
Compound found only in the top layer of skin that gives cells their ability to bind with water.

amino acids
Organic compound that contains an amino group and a carboxylic group.

filaggrin
Synthesizes lipids (fats) that are thought to serve as "intercellular cement"; important component of NMF.

transepidermal water loss (TEWL)
Process by which our bodies constantly lose water via evaporation.

organelles
Microorganisms responsible for functions within the cell.

desmosomes
Small hair-like structures in the spiny layer of the epidermis.

A vital function of the spiny layer (stratum spinosum) is to provide components of NMF (natural moisturizing factor).

The cells of the basal layer form the lowest portion of the epidermis, attaching to the dermis below and the spiny layer above. This is the layer that generates the epidermal cellular process.

lamellar granules
Control lipids that produce NMF.

lipids
Fat or fat-like substances, insoluble in water.

keratinization
Progressive maturation of the cell in the movement through the stratum corneum.

ceramides
Class of lipids that do not contain glycerol.

stem cells
A stalk-like cell that is unspecialized; gives rise to specialized cells.

postmitotic cells
Cells that have completed mitotic division.

melanocytes
Cells in the epidermis that produce pigment.

Merkel cells
Cells that are usually close to nerve endings and may be involved in sensory perception.

desquamation
Shedding of cells, such as at the stratum corneum.

permit materials to move around them in the intercellular space. Lamellar granules are also found here. These granules control lipids that migrate to the stratum corneum and become another component of NMF.

In this, the first leg of the journey, keratinocytes depart the basal layer and show the first signs of keratinization. Here also we find lamellar granules, organelles that deliver fats to the stratum corneum. These granules contain the lipids and other components such as cholesterol, fatty acids, ceramides, and enzymes necessary to produce NMF. Once these granules reach the stratum corneum, they release their contents and cause the NMF to form.

Stratum Basale

The "basement" of the epidermis is appropriately called the *basal layer*. It anchors the epidermis to the dermis. This layer contains germinal cells, cells of regeneration, for all sublayers of the epidermis. It is here that few different basal cell types are housed, including stem cells, amplifying cells, and postmitotic cells. Basal cells remain in the basal layer, creating a solid skin foundation, and keratinocytes begin their upward migration to the stratum corneum.

Specialized Epidermal Cells

Four specialized cells exist within the epidermis: (1) keratinocytes, (2) melanocytes, (3) Langerhans' cells, and (4) Merkel cells (Table 2–2).

Keratinocytes

The majority of cells in the epidermis are keratinocytes. These cells are generated in the basal sublayer but are destined, half the time, to depart. Fifty percent of the keratinocytes produced remain in the basal sublayer of the epidermis (and are then, as you saw previously, identified as basal cells). The others, retaining their keratinocyte identity and a certain apparent ambition, begin moving up, passing through the remaining sublayers to the surface, becoming hard and cornified and finally being sloughed off.[33]

During differentiation, keratinocytes go through critical changes. The shape flattens, then organelles are "lost" and fibrous proteins are shaped, and, finally, as the cell becomes dehydrated, the cell membrane thickens.

The process of moving from the basal layer to the stratum corneum and then sloughing off is called desquamation. It takes approximately 28 to 35 days in younger people and up to 45 days as we age. When it

Table 2–2 Specialized Epidermal Cells

Cell Type	Location	Function
Keratinocytes	Generated in the strata basale; half begin to migrate upward, eventually to be sloughed off	Basic skin cells that collectively make up skin; undergo desquamation
Melanocytes	Between epidermis and dermis	Secrete pigments that give skin, hair, and eyes their color
Langerhans' cells	Strata spinosum and strata basale	Patrol epidermis for foreign invaders; ingest them for removal by the lymphatic system
Merkel cells	By nerve endings throughout epidermis	Exact function unclear; likely involved in sensation

takes longer, it shows. Delays in the migration process and extrinsic factors such as smoking, solar damage, and pollution cause our skin to turn sallow and gray. It causes the complaint so often heard from our clients: "My skin just looks dull and dirty."

Melanocytes

Located in or near the basal layer, melanocytes occupy the junction between the epidermis and the dermis (Figure 2–8). They secrete the pigment **melanin** that lends color to skin, eyes, and hair. Melanin protects the skin from ultraviolet light and is produced in response to it. Melanin is also produced in response to genetic and hormonal cues, such as a pregnancy. Skin color is not determined by melanocyte concentration or quantity but rather by the degree of melanocyte activity. Men and women of all races have roughly equal amounts of melanocytes (Figure 2–9).

After melanocytes have produced melanin, they transfer it to keratinocytes via small appendages that act like eyedroppers. Regardless of whether they carry cargo, keratinocytes continue their migration toward the surface.[34] In this cellular relationship, *melanocytes* are the melanin-*making* cells and keratinocytes are the melanin-*receiving* cells; although melanocytes produce melanin, in the end keratinocytes contain it. The proportion of melanocytes to keratinocytes varies from 1:4 to 1:10, depending on age, with melanocyte proportion decreasing with age. Therefore, our ability to protect our skin with melanin decreases as we get older.

The more rapidly the keratinocyte moves to the stratum corneum, the more youthful skin appears. Through the use of microdermabrasion, our objective is to increase the migration rate of keratinocytes to the stratum corneum without injuring the skin.

Home-care products such as alpha hydroxy acids, Retin A®, and retinol serums penetrate the skin and cause a slight amount of irritation. This irritation causes the skin to react as if it were injured, stimulating the production and migration of keratinocytes toward the stratum corneum.

melanin
Pigment that protects skin from ultraviolet damage.

Although melanocytes partially protect the skin from ultraviolet radiation, do not be fooled into thinking that those who tan easily or have darker skin types are protected from skin cancers.

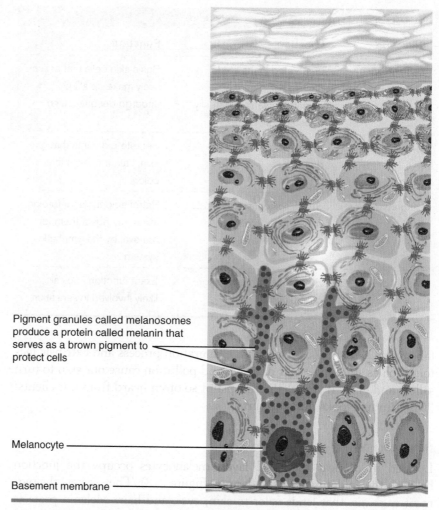

Pigment granules called melanosomes produce a protein called melanin that serves as a brown pigment to protect cells

Melanocyte

Basement membrane

Figure 2–8 The melanocyte is responsible for the skin's pigment.

hyperpigmentation
Overproduction and overdeposits of melanin.

Both injury and inflammation can cause increases in melanin production. Such an injury is known as post-inflammatory **hyperpigmentation** (PIH) and is a recognized complication of both microdermabrasion and peeling. Pigmentation in both its over- and underproduction will be discussed later in the chapter (see *Pigmentary Disorders*).

Langerhans' cells

Found in the lower layers of the epidermis, Langerhans' cells engage in surveillance against would-be intruders.[35] Although smaller in breadth than keratinocytes, they stretch fingerlike processes between keratinocytes to the surface, where they scan like periscopes. Upon encountering "bad bacteria," they *acquire* them and transport the offenders to T lymphocytes in the regional lymph nodes for disposal.

Light skin   **Dark skin**

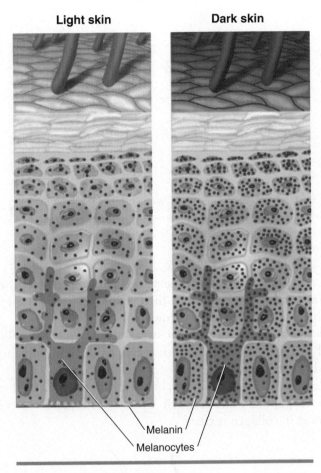

Melanin

Melanocytes

Figure 2–9 Melanocytes are packed more densely in African-American skin.

Merkel cells

Merkel cells are associated with the nerve endings found in the epidermis. Their specific function remains unclear, but because they are numerous about the lip, hard palate, palms, finger and footpads, and proximal nail folds, they are likely involved in sensation.[36,37]

Dermis

In our continued exploration of the skin, we encounter the second, deeper layer—the dermis (Figure 2–10). The dermis provides the vital function of attaching skin to body.

The dermis is criss-crossed with three types of fibers that lend strength and elasticity. These fibers—reticulin, collagen, and elastin—form a network that creates stability for the skin. Type I collagen runs throughout the dermis and is responsible for its tensile strength and

reticulin
Water-soluble protein in the connective tissue framework of reticular tissue.

collagen
Water-soluble protein found in connective tissues. Particularly, type I collagen forms a network in the epidermis and is credited with providing skin with its tensile strength and firmness.

elastin
Protein responsible for giving tissue its elastic qualities.

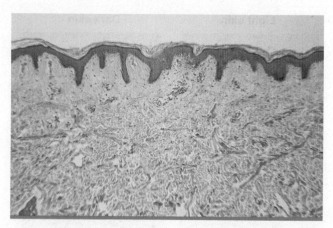

Figure 2–10 Specialized cells in the dermis include mast cells and fibroblasts.

providing skin its youthful appearance of tightness, firmness, and fullness.[38] The combined strength of these tissues anchors the epidermis above to the subcutaneous tissue below.

Epidermal appendages such as sweat glands and hair follicles are embedded in the dermis, which also serves as the end point for blood vessels and nerves (Figure 2–11).[39]

The dermis, which varies but is about 2 mm thick, is further subdivided into the papillary and reticular layers.[40] This subdivision is based on differences in collagen texture.[41]

> On its superficial side the dermis holds the epidermis at the **dermal-epidermal junction**. On its distal side it attaches to subcutaneous tissue.

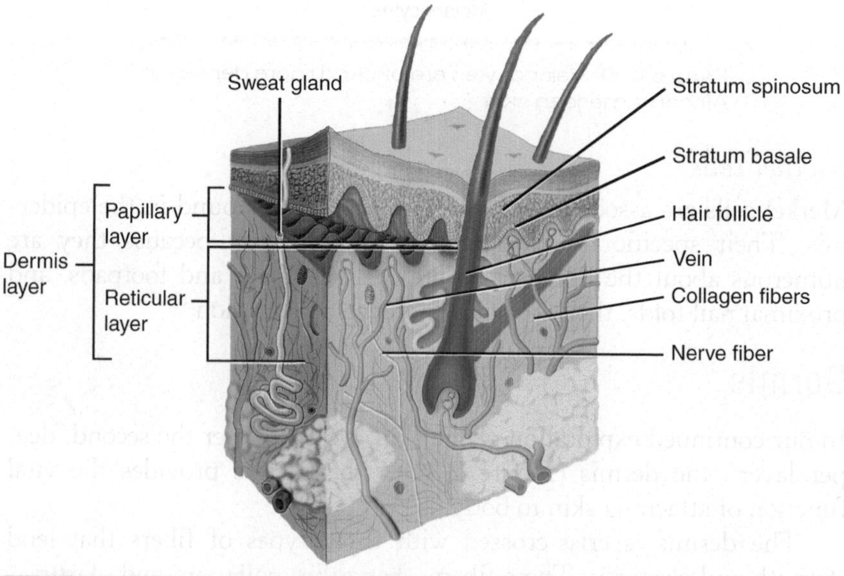

dermal-epidermal junction
Superficial side of the dermis, connected to the epidermis by subcutaneous tissue.

Sweat gland
Papillary layer
Dermis layer
Reticular layer
Stratum spinosum
Stratum basale
Hair follicle
Vein
Collagen fibers
Nerve fiber

Figure 2–11 The dermis has two layers: (1) the papillary dermis and (2) the reticular dermis.

Papillary Dermis

Papillary dermis, the most superficial layer of the dermis, is the first skin layer to contain capillary blood vessels, small nerves, and lymphatic vessels.

Because the papillary dermis contains blood vessels and blood vessels provide temperature changes when they constrict or dilate, it is the papillary dermis that is specifically responsible for thermoregulation of the body. When you are performing microdermabrasion and encounter *pinpoint* bleeding—fine individual points of bleeding—you have arrived at the papillary dermis. Does that not increase your respect for the thickness of the epidermis?

In addition to its *holding* properties, the papillary dermis has another very important function in regulating the appearance of skin surface—it houses **glycosaminoglycans (GAGs)**. GAGs are a variety of chains made of polysaccharide, a type of complex carbohydrate. Attracted almost fanatically to water, GAGs are thought capable of binding up to 1,000 times their weight in water.[45] Think for a moment about the padding this provides. This moisture-attracting property makes them one of the most important components in our study of the skin. Unfortunately, many histology studies of the skin show a decrease in the number of GAGs with age.[46]

Reticular Dermis

Reticular dermis is located beneath papillary dermis and rests on the thick pad of fat known as subcutaneous tissue. Here lies the real anchor of the skin.

Within the **reticular dermis** are structures called **rete pegs**. These "pegs" extend up into the epidermis (and similar structures extend from above down into the dermis) to hold the dermis to the epidermis. These structures are responsible for holding the epidermis and dermis together to create the skin. Capillary networks run through rete pegs like tiny elevators, bringing nutrients to the epidermis. It is widened vessels in the rete pegs that cause broken capillaries. People with transparent or very light skin may flush or blush, causing a dilation of the capillaries in the rete pegs.

Specialized Dermal Cells

Many specialized dermal cells exist. Their functions range from directing the production of collagen and ground substance to providing nutrients and removing waste from the skin (Table 2–3).

Collagen in the papillary dermis is finely textured.[42] It contains projections, called **papillae**, which fit the dermis to the epidermis.[43] We are accustomed to using these uniquely individual ridged patterns in foot- and fingerprinting.[44]

glycosaminoglycans (GAGs)
Polysaccharide chains, most prominent in the dermis, that bind with water, smoothing and softening the surface from below; most abundant GAG is hyaluronic acid.

reticular dermis
Sublayer of the dermis that connects the dermis to the epidermis and is home to the skin's appendages (nails, hair, glands).

rete pegs
Anatomic feature that holds the dermis and epidermis together.

papillae
Projections from the dermis into the epidermis that hold them together.

Collagen in this layer (*reticular* means *like a network*) is larger and more coarsely textured.[47] In the example of a cow's skin after tanning, it is the cow's dermis that makes the leather.[48]

The reticular dermis houses the appendages of the skin, nerves, and blood vessels. It is loaded with collagen, blood vessels, and nerve endings.

Table 2-3 Specialized Dermal Cells

Cell Type	Location	Function
Fibroblasts	Reticular dermis, papillary dermis	Direct the production of collagen, reticulin, and ground substance
Mast cells	Papillary dermis	Protect skin against invasion and infection
Ground substance	Reticular dermis, papillary dermis	Provide nutrients and remove waste

fibroblasts
Cells that produce connective tissue.

ground substance
Consists mainly of GAGs (hyaluronic acid, chondroitin sulfate, and dermatan sulfate); involved in maintenance and repair of dermis.

urticaria pigmentosa
Allergic reactions such as hives with a large number of mast cells.

hypodermis
Layer of subcutaneous fat and connective tissue lying beneath the epidermis.

adipose cells
Cells that contain stored fat in connective tissue.

Fibroblast cells

Fibroblasts are the command cells for the dermis. They direct the production of collagen, elastin, and reticulin and the **ground substance** for the dermis. In response to injury, fibroblasts proliferate to manufacture new collagen, from which scarring occurs.[49]

Mast cells

Along with lymphocytes and macrophages, the mast cells reside in connective tissue of the dermis, usually in the neighborhood of blood vessels. These cells protect against injury and invasion. Release of histamine by mast cells produces the inflammation that ousts intruders and begins wound healing.[50] In allergic reactions manifested in the skin, such as hives, large numbers of mast cells exist. We would see this in a condition such as **urticaria pigmentosa**.

Ground substance

Through diffusion, ground substance provides nutrients to and removes wastes from other tissue components.[51] It is integral to the healing process. As a wound heals, the available ground substance creates a moister wound that will heal more quickly. It is constantly undergoing synthesis and degradation. The ground substance of the dermis consists largely of GAGs. Age probably brings a decrease in the ground substance.

■ HYPODERMIS OR SUBCUTANEOUS TISSUE

Under the reticular dermis lies the **hypodermis**, or subcutaneous fat (Figure 2–12). It is made up of clumps of fat-filled cells called **adipose cells**. It is the "cushion layer" of the skin and helps protect internal organs from blows; it also acts as an insulator, conserving body heat.[52]

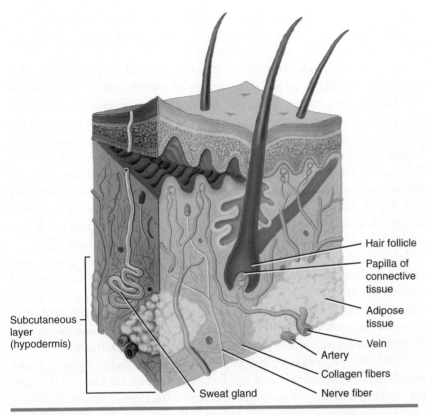

Figure 2–12 The hypodermis, or subcutaneous fat, is found beneath the reticular dermis.

The attachment of subcutaneous tissue to reticular dermis is not tight or rigid. Rather, it is loose, allowing the skin a degree of shifting movement over muscle and skeletal structures. The subcutaneous tissue is criss-crossed with connective tissue to fibers and layers interspersed with fat to hold it together. When pockets of fat accumulate between the connective tissue bands beyond the ability of the connective tissue to hold it smooth, the appearance is called *cellulite* or *orange-peel skin*. Because women generally have thinner skin and less rigid connective tissue bands than men, *cellulite* is generally more apparent in women. It is also more likely to appear in certain areas of the body as well, such as the hips, thighs, and buttocks.

SKIN HEALTH OVER TIME

As children, we take our soft, pliable, quickly healing skin for granted. We play outside, cavort in any available water, and roam hills, valleys,

Women generally have thinner skin and less rigid connective tissue bands than men. It is for this reason that cellulite generally is more apparent in women.

and flats. During this time, our skin is absorbing the effects of this mild trauma. The effects are not all bad, but they are certainly cumulative. Every bit of exposure has its consequences.

In reality, we cannot completely avoid the sun. Many people are idolaters of the sun. In an earlier time, people of wealth and leisure valued a pale, tanless complexion. It was in the late twentieth century that sun-bronzed skin took on its sexy aura of vigor and well-being. It connoted the ability to spend leisure time on beaches, golf courses, and tennis courts. Within boundaries, sun exposure is not all bad; in fact, we need the sun. Although we can get some vitamin D from plant and animal sources, sunlight on our skins is responsible for up to 90 percent of the vitamin D upon which our bodies depend.[53] In tight conjunction with calcium, neither one of which works well without the other, vitamin D gives our bones tensile strength[54] (thus the process of enriching milk with vitamin D).

Without question, however, many people get more sun exposure than is necessary for bone health. People who work outside are hard-pressed to avoid the effects of UV exposure, even with generous applications of sunscreen. Even if the sun never touches us, we are bombarded with tiny molecular renegades (radiation) that do their damage. As long as we live, we cannot completely avoid damage to the skin, and it will age.

The aging process is both complex and simple. Simply put, it is the degradation of the dermis and epidermis over time that leaves the skin thin, lacking elasticity, lined, and speckled with pigmentation. A reduction in **skin turgor** occurs.[55] Loss of adhesion between the layers of the epidermis and between the epidermis and dermis create a greater tendency for injury and more visible effects of gravity (wrinkles and folds). Decreases in filaggrin and NMF mean dry and flaky skin. Wound healing slows from a slowing in Langerhans' cells production.[56]

To further understand the changes in our skin over time, we use the terms **intrinsic aging** and **extrinsic aging**. Intrinsic aging occurs by virtue of genetics and gravity—it is unavoidable. Extrinsic aging is the portion for which we are responsible. It is aging attributable to external factors such as the sun, pollution, and smoking.

Intrinsic Aging

Because genetics play a noteworthy role in the aging process, some of those effects are out of our hands. The longer one lives, the more likely it is that one will face one's mother or father in the mirror one day. Intrinsic aging happens over time and regardless of resistance (Figure 2–13). Clients seen for problems such as deep smile lines or, more typically, vertical upper lip lines will report that either their mother or father had the same aging symptoms.

skin turgor
Flexibility of the skin.

intrinsic aging
Changes that would occur over time without the effects of any environmental factors.

extrinsic aging
Changes that are brought on by the effects of the environment and our choices relating to them, specifically sun exposure.

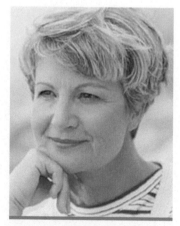

Figure 2–13 Those who have had limited or restricted access to sunlight will primarily exhibit intrinsic aging. This woman is in her 70s.

Although most of intrinsic aging is beyond our control, it does not mean that we should throw up our hands and consider it a lost cause. Advanced skin care techniques, among them microdermabrasion in the clinical setting and sophisticated home-care regimens, can blunt the onset of the inevitable.

Extrinsic Aging

Exposure to such environmental hazards as wind, severe temperature changes, sun, smoking, and pollution accelerate the aging process and increase the potential for skin cancers (Figure 2–14). To the aesthetician, extrinsic aging may be considered the type of aging over which we have complete control. We can protect our skin from extrinsic aging by using sun block or staying out of the sun altogether. Simply being outside, unprotected, will age the skin more rapidly. Wind and extremes in temperature will age the skin more rapidly than skin that is not exposed to temperature or wind extremes. An age-controlled comparison of an Iowa farmer's skin to that of a non-gardening suburban mother who shuns the outdoors would reveal a dramatic difference in extrinsic aging.

Although microdermabrasion is very effective in treating solar damage specifically and extrinsic aging in general, the most important task for the aesthetician is education of the client. All clients should be reminded of potential injuries to the skin that occur with extreme or prolonged exposure to the sun, wind, temperature extremes, and pollution. The most significant factor in extrinsic aging is the sun.

Extrinsic aging magnifies **rhytids** (wrinkles), a dull, dry, and sallow appearance of the skin, actinic keratosis (overgrowth of skin layers), and irregular pigmentation. Over time, skin that is consistently exposed or has extreme exposure to the environment may develop skin cancers. Although **basal cell carcinomas** (BCCs) are the most common, more serious squamous cell and **melanoma** cancers are on the rise. Recent statistics tell the story of decades of sun worship. The American Cancer Society tells us that as of this writing over one million cases of skin cancer have been diagnosed yearly. Most of these cases are considered sun-related. Of the million diagnosed cases each year, over 55,000 of those will be melanoma, and of those diagnosed with melanoma, nearly 10,000 will die!

Pigmentary Disorders

Melanin production can increase or decrease beyond normal, creating a mottled appearance in the skin. These problems can be congenital or

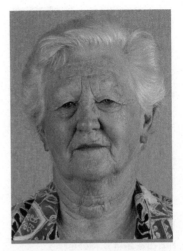

Figure 2–14 Yesterday's tan will eventually appear as tomorrow's extrinsic aging. This woman is also in her 70s.

rhytids
Wrinkles.

basal cell carcinoma
Slow-growing tumor that generally does not metastasize; the most common form of skin cancer that usually occurs in regions of repeated sunburn.

melanoma
Malignant, darkly pigmented mole or tumor of the skin.

A simple yet effective way to manage extrinsic aging is to avoid smoking. It is also thought that secondhand smoke contributes to extrinsic aging.

Over time, skin that is consistently exposed or has extreme exposure to the environment may develop skin cancers.

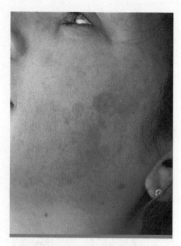

Figure 2–15 Melasma appears as a dark spot or dark areas on the face and neck.

melasma gravidarum
"Mask of pregnancy" from an overproduction of melanin.

vitiligo
Skin disorder characterized by white patches surrounded by otherwise normally pigmented skin; most common on dark-skinned individuals from tropical regions.

squamous cell carcinomas (SCCs)
Malignant cancer of the epithelial cells.

acquired. It is the responsibility of aestheticians to avoid the latter pitfall in their treatment of clients.

Hyperpigmentation

Hyperpigmentation results from increased deposition of melanin. It is one of the most common problems seen in the medical spa. This irregular pigmentation has origins in solar exposure, pregnancy, medications, and birth control. It can be frustrating, yet is a simple problem to solve.

Hyperpigmentation occurs when melanocytes are overstimulated in a haphazard fashion. Such is the case in melasma gravidarum, commonly known as the *pregnancy mask* (Figure 2–15). This results not only from pregnancy but also with the use of birth control pills.

Unfortunately, hyperpigmentation can also result from aggressive or mismanaged peeling, microdermabrasion, and intense pulsed light (IPL) therapy (e.g., FotoFacial)—essentially, from any procedure in which the skin is overstimulated or injured. Hyperpigmentation is especially common in certain skin types. These skin types should be treated with care both in the spa and at home to avoid hyperpigmentation.

Hypopigmentation

Hypopigmentation occurs when melanocytes no longer produce melanin, leaving areas of the skin without pigment. Diseases such as vitiligo and leukoderma (in association with inflammatory diseases such as atopic dermatitis) are two relatively common disorders that create hypopigmentation.

Just as with hyperpigmentation, hypopigmentation can also occur when skin has been damaged through aggressive treatment. Any treatment that affects melanocytes may result in hypopigmentation. White spots are indicative that melanocytes have been damaged and will no longer produce pigment. This can be seen after a deep dermabrasion, chemical peels, and laser resurfacing. Microdermabrasion is a less common cause.

Skin Cancers

If you discover a suspicious mole or lesion, you ought to recommend that a physician examine it. This protocol should be part of the policy and procedures at your spa. Take photographs of these particular moles or lesions. Make notes regarding the length of time the lesion or mole has been present, if it is changing, and any other pertinent information. Moles or lesions for which you should be on the lookout include melanomas, BCCs, and squamous cell carcinomas (SCCs). When the

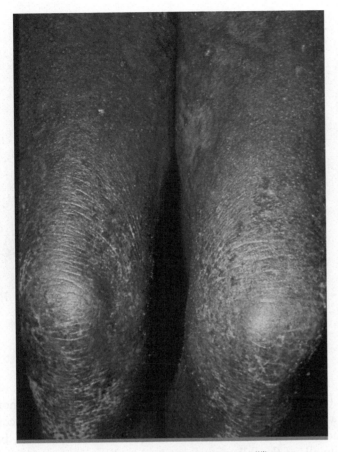

Figure 2–16 Melanocyte inactivity causes vitiligo.

Vitiligo affects approximately 4 percent of the world's population (Figure 2–16).[57] Affecting the melanocytes of the skin, vitiligo causes hypopigmentation that is irreversible. Those afflicted with vitiligo are often physiologically affected and self-conscious of their appearance.

physician sees a client, a copy of the physician's report should come back to you and be placed in your skin care record. If a biopsy or lesion removal is done, file a copy of that pathology report in the skin care chart. Remember, you cannot, as an aesthetician, diagnose a client. You may inform the client that he or she has a cause for concern, and that he or she ought to see a physician for an accurate diagnosis. If you are employed at a medi-spa with an on-site physician, summon the physician to have a look.

Basal Cell Carcinoma

BCC is the most common skin cancer, often found in areas of repeated sunburns and sun exposure (Figure 2–17). A BCC is a slow-growing tumor and generally does not metastasize. It can, however, cause a good deal of disfigurement if left untreated or treated ineffectually. In the U.S., the incidence of BCC annually is nearly 900,000 (550,000 men

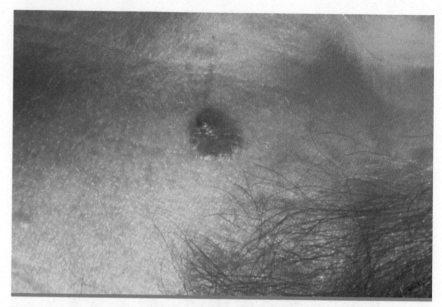

Figure 2–17 Basal cell carcinomas (BCCs) result from chronic sun exposure.

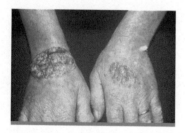

Figure 2–18 Squamous cell carcinomas (SCCs) from chronic sun exposure and irritation.

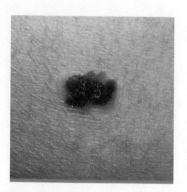

Figure 2–19 Melanoma carcinomas from chronic and intense sun exposure.

and 350,000 women).[58] Six subtypes of BCC exist: (1) nodular, (2) pigmented, (3) superficial, (4) micronodular, (5) cystic, and (6) morpheaform. Each subset has its own distinct features. The most common appearance of BCC is as a pearly nodule. It can exhibit some, but not necessarily all, of the following features: bleeding, crusting, and a small center depression.

Squamous Cell Carcinoma

SCC is the second-most common skin cancer, with over 200,000 cases diagnosed annually (Figure 2–18).[59] Unlike BCC, SCC can sometimes metastasize if left untreated. As with BCC, chronic sun exposure seems to be the main precursor to SCC, although it has been found in areas without sun exposure, such as the mucous membranes of the mouth. Usually areas such as the inside of the mouth have been exposed to frequent and persistent sores, such as leukoplakia. On a rare occasion, SCC will spring up in an area of healthy skin. The hypothesis is that SCC may be passed genetically.

Melanoma

Melanoma is the most dangerous of all skin cancers because it will metastasize and cause death (Figure 2–19). It is important that you are always alert to the potential for melanoma. Melanoma is an irregularly shaped and irregularly colored mole, most commonly occurring on the back of the legs and trunk. Those who have had one to two significant sunburns are at risk for melanoma. Because these moles are not primarily located on the face, it is important for the aesthetician to be an *investigator,* asking the client about moles that are new or have changed. You can never be too careful when you suspect a melanoma and should refer the client to a physician. Remember the ABCDs of Skin Cancer, and you could save a life!

ABCD of Cancer

Asymmetry—Growth that, when divided in half, has two mismatched halves.

Border irregularity—Ragged or uneven edges that are blurred and poorly defined.

Color—Uneven black, brown, and tan coloring; other colors, like red, white, and blue, can also be interspersed in the growth; any change in the color of the preexisting mole or lesion.

Diameter—Any growth larger than the top of a pencil eraser, which is approximately 6 mm in diameter; any unusual or sudden increase in size should also be checked.

▪ PRINCIPLES OF TOPICAL THERAPY

The first principle for slowing the aging process is topical treatment, including **absorbents**, **astringents** (drying agents that shrink and contract the skin), **cleansing agents**, **emollients** (skin softeners), and **keratolytics** (agents that assist exfoliation of the keratinocytes).[60] Locally applied agents cleanse, debride (remove foreign material), protect the skin, and relieve the discomfort of dryness.

You will recall that, in the aging process, a slowing in the migration of keratinocytes from the basal layer to the surface causes skin to lose its fresh appearance and vitality. It follows that skin appearance can be much improved by accelerating the migration of those cells. Keratinocytes can be encouraged to move more quickly in several ways, including the use of stimulating home-care products such as alpha hydroxy acids, Retin A, and retinol serums. As discussed, when these products

absorbents
Products that pass through the skin.

astringents
Drying agents that shrink and contract the skin.

cleansing agents
Products that remove foreign matter and excretions from the skin's surface. Common ingredients in cleansers include detergents, surfactants, and antimicrobials.

emollients
Products that have a softening or soothing effect on the skin.

keratolytics
Products or agents that loosen horny skin layers.

penetrate the skin, they produce a tiny degree of irritation. This irritation causes the skin to react as if it were mildly injured, stimulating production of keratinocytes that then migrate toward the stratum corneum in a shorter period of time than usual. This may be demonstrated in some flakiness of the skin.

Home-care products are an essential component of a successful skin-care program. Clinical treatments do not work as well without a proper home-care regimen. When combined with a safe and regular clinical treatment such as microdermabrasion, skin will begin to reflect a more youthful appearance. Histology has shown microdermabrasion to be effective on both epidermis and dermis. According to Dr. Mark Rubin, "Although microabrasion is a very superficial treatment, findings from histologic studies show reproducibly that it yields tissue changes in both the epidermis and dermis that are consistent with skin rejuvenation."[61]

Recognizing When Something Is Wrong

Despite its significance in our health, appearance, and well-being, skin may be the most disregarded organ of the body. Damage can range from annoying to life-threatening (going beyond simple aging to include disease). Infections can be bacterial, fungal, parasitic, and viral. Various forms of dermatitis produce fluid-filled **vesicles** on the skin surface. Any slow-healing or encrusted lesions of the skin, as well as lesions that **suppurate** (discharge), should alert us to the strong possibility of **pathogens**. As aestheticians providing microdermabrasion, it is important for us to recognize potential skin problems, know the limitations of our treatments, and know when to seek help for our clients.

vesicles
Fluid-filled containers on the skin's surface.

suppurate
To form or discharge pus.

pathogens
Agents that cause disease, namely bacteria and viruses.

▪ CONCLUSION

On the surface the skin looks like an uncomplicated structure, simply meant to protect our inner organs from injury. However, as you can see, the skin is extraordinarily complex. Many cells work to keep the skin healthy and free from infection or disease. Without a doubt, you will return to this chapter and continue to expand your knowledge of the skin as you build your medical aesthetics career.

> > > **Top 10 Tips to Take to the Spa**

1. Skin appendages include hair follicles, sweat glands, and nails, and assist in epidermal healing.

2. The skin is a dynamic organ, changing daily.

3. The skin ages in two ways: intrinsically and extrinsically.

4. The epidermis is avascular.

5. The dermis houses all of the collagen, blood vessels, and nerves.

6. The keratinocyte is arguably the most important cell in the epidermis.

7. The stratum corneum (the outermost layer of the epidermis) is the layer of the skin that is "polished" by microdermabrasion.

8. The dermis and epidermis are both stimulated by microdermabrasion.

9. The stratum corneum houses NMF.

10. Because it is able to absorb water, NMF is responsible for the water content in the stratum corneum.

Chapter Review Questions

1. What are the three layers of the skin?

2. What are the melanocytes and where are they located?

3. What are the keratinocytes and where are they located?

4. What are the appendages of the skin?

5. Why are the appendages of the skin important?

6. What are the functions of the skin?

7. Name the five layers of the epidermis.

8. Is the stratum lucidum always a part of the epidermis?

9. Name the three special cells of the epidermis.

10. What are the layers of the dermis?

11. What are the specialized cells of the dermis?

12. What is intrinsic aging?

13. What is extrinsic aging?

14. What is hyperpigmentation?

15. What is hypopigmentation?

16. Name the three most common skin cancers?

17. What is NMF?

18. Why is NMF important?

19. What is TEWL?
20. Why is TEWL important?

Chapter References

1. Gray, J. (1997). *The world of skin care* [Online]. Available: http://www.pg.com
2. Moore, E. (Ed.). (1999). *Quotation finder*. Glasgow, Scotland: Harper Collins.
3. American Society of Plastic Surgeons. (2003, December). *2002 Quick facts on cosmetic and reconstructive surgery trends* [Online]. Available: http://www.plasticsurgery.org
4. Spense, A. P. (2004, February 22). *Basic human anatomy* (3rd ed.) [Online]. Available: http://www.sawyerproducts.com
5. Nemours Foundation. (2004). *Skin, hair, and nails* [Online]. Available: http://www.kidshealth.org
6. Merck & Co. (2001). *Resource library* [Online]. Available: http://www.mercksource.com
7. Ganong, W. F. (1989). Initiation of impulses in sense organs. In *Review of medical physiology* (14th ed.). Norwalk, CT: Appleton & Lange.
8. Merck & Co. (2001). *Resource library* [Online]. Available: http://www.mercksource.com
9. Students of Elert, G. (2001). *Temperature of a healthy human (skin temperature)* [Online]. Available: http://hypertextbook.com
10. Nova. (2000, November). *Surviving Denali* [Online]. Available: http://www.pbs.org
11. Gray, J. (1997). *The world of skin care* [Online]. Available: http://www.pg.com
12. Gray, J. (1997). *The world of skin care* [Online]. Available: http://www.pg.com
13. Gray, J. (1997). *The world of skin care* [Online]. Available: http://www.pg.com
14. Gray, J. (1997). *The world of skin care* [Online]. Available: http://www.pg.com
15. Nemours Foundation. (2004). *Skin, hair, and nails* [Online]. Available: http://www.kidshealth.org
16. Nemours Foundation. (2004). *Skin, hair, and nails* [Online]. Available: http://www.kidshealth.org
17. University of Iowa Healthcare. (2004, March 15). *Fluid replacement* [Online]. Available: http://www.uihealthcare.com
18. Elsner, P., & Maibach, H. L. (2000). *Cosmeceuticals: Drugs vs. cosmetics*. New York: Marcel Dekker, Inc.

19. Gray, J. (1997). *The world of skin care* [Online]. Available: http://www.pg.com

20. eMedicine.com, Inc. (2004). *Hair growth* [Online]. Available: http://www.emedicine.com

21. Nemours Foundation. (2004). *Skin, hair, and nails* [Online]. Available: http://www.kidshealth.org

22. Gray, J. (1997). *The world of skin care* [Online]. Available: http://www.pg.com

23. King, D. (2003, November 14). *Introduction to skin histology* [Online]. Available: http://www.Siumed.edu

24. Spense, A. P. (2004, February 22). *Basic human anatomy* (3rd ed.) [Online]. Available: http://www.sawyerproducts.com

25. King, D. (2003, November 14). *Introduction to skin histology* [Online]. Available: http://www.Siumed.edu

26. Lowe, N., & Sellar, P. (1999). *Skin secrets: The medical facts versus the beauty fiction.* New York: Collins & Brown.

27. Baumann, L. (2002). *Cosmetic dermatology practices and principles.* New York: McGraw-Hill.

28. Baumann, L. (2002). *Cosmetic dermatology practices and principles.* New York: McGraw-Hill.

29. King, D. (2003, November 14). *Introduction to skin histology* [Online]. Available: http://www.Siumed.edu

30. King, D. (2003, November 14). *Introduction to skin histology* [Online]. Available: http://www.Siumed.edu

31. King, D. (2003, November 14). *Introduction to skin histology* [Online]. Available: http://www.Siumed.edu

32. Spense, A. P. (2004, February 22). *Basic human anatomy* (3rd ed.) [Online]. Available: http://www.sawyerproducts.com

33. Moschella, S., Pillsbury, D., & Hurley, H. (1975). *Dermatology* (Vol. 1). Philadelphia: W. B. Saunders Company.

34. King, D. (2003, November 14). *Introduction to skin histology* [Online]. Available: http://www.Siumed.edu

35. King, D. (2003, November 14). *Introduction to skin histology* [Online]. Available: http://www.Siumed.edu

36. King, D. (2003, November 14). *Introduction to skin histology* [Online]. Available: http://www.Siumed.edu

37. Shea, C., & Prieto, V. G. (2003, October 13). *Merkel cell carcinoma* [Online]. Available: http://www.emedicine.com

38. Baumann, L. (2002). *Cosmetic dermatology practices and principles.* New York: McGraw-Hill.

39. King, D. (2003, November 14). *Introduction to skin histology* [Online]. Available: http://www.Siumed.edu

40. Spense, A. P. (2004, February 22). *Basic human anatomy* (3rd ed.) [Online]. Available: http://www.sawyerproducts.com

41. King, D. (2003, November 14). *Introduction to skin histology* [Online]. Available: http://www.Siumed.edu

42. King, D. (2003, November 14). *Introduction to skin histology* [Online]. Available: http://www.Siumed.edu

43. Nemours Foundation. (2004). *Skin, hair, and nails* [Online]. Available: http://www.kidshealth.org

44. Spense, A. P. (2004, February 22). *Basic human anatomy* (3rd ed.) [Online]. Available: http://www.sawyerproducts.com

45. Obagi, Z. (2002). *Skin health restoration and rejuvenation.* New York: Springer-Verlag, New York, Inc.

46. Baumann, L. (2002). *Cosmetic dermatology practices and principles.* New York: McGraw-Hill.

47. King, D. (2003, November 14). *Introduction to skin histology* [Online]. Available: http://www.Siumed.edu

48. Spense, A. P. (2004, February 22). *Basic human anatomy* (3rd ed.) [Online]. Available: http://www.sawyerproducts.com

49. King, D. (2003, November 14). *Introduction to skin histology* [Online]. Available: http://www.Siumed.edu

50. King, D. (2003, November 14). *Introduction to skin histology* [Online]. Available: http://www.Siumed.edu

51. King, D. (2003, November 14). *Introduction to skin histology* [Online]. Available: http://www.Siumed.edu

52. Nemours Foundation. (2004). *Skin, hair, and nails* [Online]. Available: http://www.kidshealth.org

53. Falkenbach, A. (2000). Muscle strength and vitamin D (letter). *Archives of Physical Medicine and Medical Rehabilitation,* 81 (241).

54. Rao, D. S. (1999). Perspective on assessment of vitamin D nutrition. *Journal of Clinical Densitometry,* 2(4).

55. Obagi, Z. (2002). *Skin health restoration and rejuvenation.* New York: Springer-Verlag, New York, Inc.

56. Bisaccia, E. & Scarborough, D. (2002). *The Columbia manual of dermatologic cosmetic surgery.* New York: McGraw-Hill.

57. Parsad, D., Sunil, D., & Kanwar, A. J. (2003, October 23). Quality of life in patients with vitiligo. *Journal of Health and Quality of Life Outcomes,* 1(1):58.

58. Revis, Jr., D. R. (2001, July). *Skin grafts, split thickness* [Online]. Available: http://www.emedicine.com

59. The Skin Cancer Foundation. (2004). *About squamous cell* [Online]. Available: http://www.skincancer.org

60. Berkow, R. (1992). *The Merck manual* (16th ed.). Rahway, NJ: Merck Research Laboratories.
61. Guttman, C. (August, 2002). Histologic studies: Microdermabrasion not just superficial. *Cosmetic Surgery Times* [Online]. Available: www.cosmeticsurgerytimes.com

Wound Healing

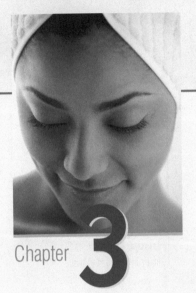

Chapter **3**

Key Terms

acute
atrophic scars
carbohydrates
chronic
epithelialization
epithelium
full-thickness wound
granulocytes
hypertrophic scars
inflammatory phase

insult
intense pulsed light
  (IPL)
ischemia
keloid scars
leukocytes
lymphocytes
macrophage
malnutrition
necrosis

neutrophils
partial-thickness
  wound
proliferative phase
protein
reepithelialization
remodeling phase
scars
wound
wound healing

Learning Objectives

After completing this chapter you should be able to:

1. Define the different types of wounds.
2. Discuss nutrition and wound healing.
3. Discuss the aged and wound healing.
4. Define a scar.
5. Name different events that lead to scar formation.

INTRODUCTION

The way skin heals itself is a multifactorial, multistage, and multilevel marvel that is easy to take for granted. Although we seldom give it a thought, wound healing is a complex subject with details that only a scientist or pathologist can fully understand or enjoy. However, as an aesthetician it is critical that you possess a basic understanding of the different types of wounds and the processes that they undergo to repair themselves.

Fundamentally, a wound is "... a disruption of normal anatomical structure which results from pathological processes beginning internally or externally to the involved organ."[1] Wound healing is "... the restoration of tissue continuity after injury."[2] Therefore, when an insult affects tissue it becomes inconsistent with the uninjured tissue nearby. For example, suppose you burn your hand. The contact with heat is the insulting event, and the specific area that has sustained the burn is the wound. The wound becomes red and painful. The wounded area is damaged and hence inconsistent with the normal tissue that did not come in contact with the offending heat source. In this chapter, we will examine the phases that most wounds will undergo to rebuild themselves in an attempt to become consistent once again. Remember, an injury, regardless of its origin, will heal according to the following steps. This is true for microdermabrasion as well as a burn.

BASIC PHASES OF WOUND HEALING

Wound healing basically traces three physiologic stages or phases: (1) inflammatory, (2) proliferative, and (3) remodeling or maturation. Although each stage has distinctive cellular events, they often work concurrently, overlapping at times. A good analogy would be to consider

wound
Disruption of normal tissue that results from pathologic processes beginning internally or externally to the involved organ.

wound healing
Restoration of tissue continuity after injury or trauma.

insult
Injury or a trauma to tissue.

Phases of Wound Healing[3]	
Inflammatory phase	Blood and tissue cells secrete substances to create inflammation, which helps overcome pathogens.
Proliferative phase	Scab and scar tissue build to protect and induce healing; remaining skin cells divide and produce new cells.
Remodeling phase	Scar tissue formed during healing is broken down; new skin begins to blend in with the old skin.

Table 3–1 Types of Wounds

Type of Wound	Description	Example
Contused (or subcutaneous) wound	Injury to tissue below the skin; skin is unbroken	Bruise, broken bones
Puncture wound	Injury caused by a sharp or pointed object, usually collapsed inward; deep tissue wounding (possibly penetrating additional organ tissues)	Stab wound, gun shot wound
Laceration	Unclean wound with jagged edges; can be of varying depths	Skinned knee
Incision	Clean cut caused by a sharp instrument	Surgical wound
Burn	Tissue injury as the result of excessive heat or acids; damage varies depending on insulting agent	Thermal, chemical

wound healing a symphony composed of several movements. Although each movement has its own theme, overlaps occur. Just as we can describe a symphony as separate movements,[4] we can describe the phases of wound healing as separate functions, working toward one goal: tissue continuity.

Insult

In the previous example we used the illustration of a burn. This is just one of many types of injuries, or insults, which can cause trauma to tissue. Several types of wounds exist, and the type of damage that has been sustained as a result of the insult characterizes each one (Table 3–1). In addition, these different injuries vary in the degrees of severity and in the specific phases that the tissue will undergo to repair itself. Likewise, multiple injuries sustained during one event will have consequences for each other.

Inflammatory Phase

Within hours of any skin injury, the first phase of wound healing, the **inflammatory phase**, has already begun, regardless of the type of wound. Early inflammatory wounds are red, warm, and swollen; the client feels pain. Blood flow and fluid increase at the site, and cells contained in both blood and skin are rapidly recruited in this first

inflammatory phase
Early wound healing phase during which blood and fluid collect and substances begin to fight infection and promote healing.

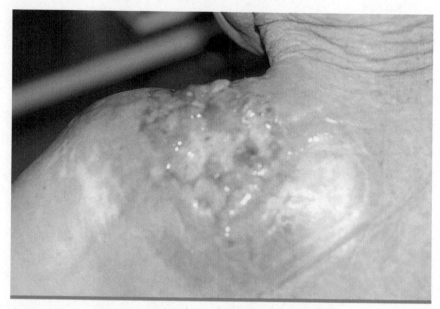

Figure 3-1 The inflammatory stage of healing.

leukocytes
White blood cells without granules involved in immune response; include lymphocytes and monocytes.

granulocytes
White blood cells involved in immune response; include neutrophils, eosinophils, and basophils.

neutrophils
Most common type of white blood cells that kill bacteria and discourage infection.

lymphocytes
White blood cells involved in the body's immune system; their numbers increase in the presence of infection.

macrophage
Part of the immune system in the skin; scavengers that clear debris in tissue injury.

defense. The motive behind the inflammation is to seek and destroy opportunistic pathogens that may find a vulnerable security lapse in the body's armor. The area is swarmed by an array of substances that inactivate bacteria, activate growth factors, and otherwise participate in the healing process (Figure 3–1).

If the injury penetrates the epidermis, damage to blood vessels also activates substances to control bleeding.[5] Blood coagulates and platelets aggregate to form a clot upon which inflammatory cells and fibroblasts accumulate.[6]

White blood cells, called **leukocytes** or **granulocytes**, are directly involved in immunity. Each has a specific and vital function in healing. **Neutrophils** are among the first healing cells on the scene, scavenging the wound for bacteria and devitalized cells and releasing oxygen-free radicals that kill bacteria.[7] Neutrophils usually reach the site of injury within 6 hours and are at full throttle by 24 hours, protecting against infection. Neutrophils that die in the wound release enzymes, dissolving unwanted cells. This produces a familiar substance called *pus*.[8] **Lymphocytes** arrive at about 72 hours and produce antibodies used to combat invaders (Table 3–2).

The blood acts mainly as a delivery device but does not act singularly in the process. Tissues are themselves supplied with their own inner "first-aid kits." A **macrophage**[9] is a cell stationed in connective tissue that actually has a limited, amoeba-like ability to move itself around

Table 3-2 Some Blood and Tissue Cells Involved in Healing

Blood cells:

White blood cells are infection fighters.[10] Two types exist: (1) those with granules (granulocytes) and (2) those without granules (leukocytes—*leuko* meaning *lacking color*).

Granulocytes—Neutrophils, eosinophils, and basophils.

Leukocytes—Lymphocytes and monocytes.

Tissue cells:

Macrophages—Cells in connective tissue that digest by-products of both defense and normal degeneration. They are found in high concentrations in different parts of the body.

Langerhans' cells—Macrophage cells in epidermis that perform surveillance for the immune system.

inflamed areas as it seeks suspicious substances to engulf.[11] When internal macrophages are activated, they secrete various growth factors. Their deficiency has been shown to result in defective healing. In addition, they play an important role in the transition from the inflammatory to the proliferative phase. Similarly, Langerhans' cells, macrophages specific to the epidermis, busily ingest old cells, abnormal cells, and unneeded cellular debris.

Proliferative Phase

About five days after the insulting event, the second phase of wound healing, the **proliferative phase**, begins.[12] By definition, the name means *the phase that builds upon, or compounds.* Granulation tissue, so called because of its granular appearance, is composed of fibrin, cellular components, and blood vessels. Their sheer bulk enables **reepithelialization**—or replacement of protective epithelial tissue—over the old wound site (Figure 3–2).

Collagen, which is prevalent in the dermis, is also a major component of the connective tissue that embodies itself around the wound. For the next 6 weeks, it will continue to embody the wound and act as a surrogate until the wound healing is complete. As collagen increases in the wound, so does its tensile strength,[13] making it less prone to reopening.

Healing of a wound begins not only from its edges but also from within any appendages lying within it that were not destroyed by the wound causing insult. As mentioned in Chapter 2, the appendages are rooted in the dermis, yet are enveloped by pockets of epithelial tissue extending back up to the epidermis. Wounds not deep enough to

proliferative phase
Phase of wound healing during which replacement of protective epithelial tissue occurs over the old wound site.

reepithelialization
Replacement of protective epithelial tissue.

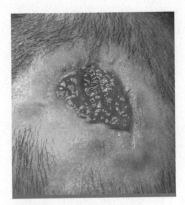

Figure 3–2 Proliferative stage of healing.

protein
Class of complex compounds that are synthesized by all living creatures; proteins are broken down into amino acids for use, including the rebuilding of tissue.

remodeling phase
Phase of wound healing during which collagen is assembled to replace skin.

The Truth about Collagen

Although the word *collagen* is no stranger to this text, the time has come to get a better picture of it. A major constituent of connective tissue, collagen is the most abundant **protein** in the body. Connective tissue includes skin, bone, ligaments, and cartilage. Collagen could, in fact, be considered the glue that holds the body's connective tissue together.[14] Because it contributes to a range of structures from brain to cornea, its components vary; at least 30 distinct types of collagen inhabit the human body. The most abundant in connective tissue form fibers that assemble themselves into networks capable of supporting more extensive structures; these are labeled type I through type V.[15] Those fiber-forming collagens are the ones with which we will be primarily concerned.

remove the pockets associated with them enable reepithelialization to proceed from remaining pockets. Therefore, appendages are very important to healing. Skin that has a greater density of appendages, such as the face, will tend to heal much more rapidly than areas with fewer such structures, such as the palmar and plantar regions.

Remodeling Phase

From 1 to 6 weeks after injury and in conjunction with the proliferative phase, collagen formation goes on at a furious pace. During that time, collagen is laid down in a microscopically haphazard pattern, like a box of matches spilled to the floor. In the remodeling phase that follows, collagen becomes more organized (Figure 3–3).

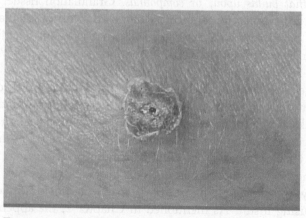

Figure 3–3 The remodeling stage of healing.

As type I collagen is gradually replaced by type III collagen, tensile strength increases. In particular wounds, this process may take as long as 1 to 2 years. This is why plastic surgeons may tell their patients that the scars from tummy tucks or face lifts take at least 6 months to 1 year to resolve, soften, flatten, and decolorize. During this same period, scars may widen and thicken.

Understanding the broad principles of wound healing—particularly as they apply to skin—and gaining the ability to apply this knowledge skillfully will ensure that your clients have the best possible outcome.

▪ TYPES OF WOUNDS

Obviously, microdermabrasion is intended to be a superficial process involving only the epidermis. Treatments including microdermabrasion and peels ideally involve superficial, controlled wounds. Nevertheless, we need to address the concept of wounds to include the unintended possibility that a deeper wound might occur. We define the depth of a wound as either partial-thickness or full-thickness.

Another definition and category that you need to know when considering wounds is time-related or *temporal*—how long they have been around. The descriptors are acute and chronic. Acute wounds are those of recent (or even emergent) occurrence. Chronic wounds are those that occurred days, weeks, or months ago. Chronic wounds might be such things as bedsores and leg ulcers, or virtually any injury that has not healed in an extended period of time. These wounds will not be discussed in this text.

Partial-Thickness Wounds

Depth of wound appears to have a *threshold level* above which, without other complications, the wound heals quickly and without scarring.[16] Shallow epidermal and dermal injuries that tend to heal without scarring are known as partial-thickness wounds (Figure 3–4).

Wounds created in the medical spa are not lacerations or incisions penetrating the skin, and they are intended to be only partial-thickness wounds. They do, however, often involve broad surface areas of the face or body. They result from treatments such as microdermabrasion; peels (glycolic, TCA, phenol); CO_2 and erbium lasers; intense pulsed light (IPL), also called *FotoFacial* or *PhotoFacial*®; laser hair removal; hyfr ecations; and shave excisions. These wounds heal quickly, usually within a week (Figure 3–5). They are superficial enough that only the process of reepithelialization is required.

scars
Marks left in the skin or on an internal organ as a result of deep tissue trauma; scars result from injury, disease, or medical procedures.

acute
Having a rapid onset with a short but severe course.

chronic
Disease or occurrence showing little or no change over a long period of time.

partial-thickness wound
Wound that penetrates only the epidermis or the upper layer of the papillary dermis; tend to heal quickly and without scarring.

intense pulsed light (IPL)
Machine that uses a variety of filters to diminish areas of color, both red and brown, on skin.

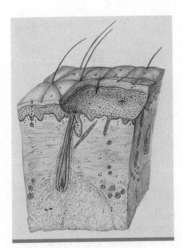

Figure 3–4 Partial-thickness wound.

TYPES OF WOUNDS

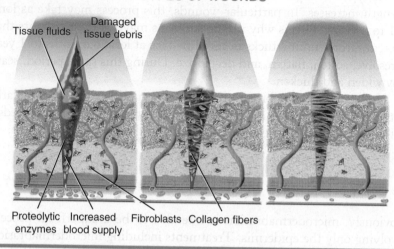

Tissue fluids — Damaged tissue debris

Proteolytic enzymes Increased blood supply Fibroblasts Collagen fibers

Figure 3–5 Wound healing is a multilevel marvel that is amazing and necessary to our survival.

Acute Partial-Thickness Wounds

Microdermabrasion wounds are usually simple injuries resulting (intentionally or unintentionally) from an aggressive hand. *Acute partial-thickness* describes a wound that is deeper than a simplified abrasion (as produced by successful microdermabrasion).

Abrasions should be familiar to you. It is the wound you sustained when you skinned your knee as a child or a rug burn you got from wrestling on carpeted floor. These wounds are usually epidermal with minimal papillary dermis involvement. Remember, the blood supply to the skin begins in the papillary dermis. Therefore, these wounds usually bleed or the capillaries appear ready to bleed.

Extraction wounds occur when the aesthetician is working hard to evacuate comedones or pustules. Aggressive or incorrect extraction techniques can cause a partial-thickness wound. If the wound is mishandled, a full-thickness wound followed by a scar is possible.

Full-Thickness Wounds

When wounds penetrate the dermis beneath a certain *threshold level,* wounds tend to heal more slowly and with scarring.[17] These are called **full-thickness wounds** (Figure 3–6). The resulting scar tissue is a variety of the original tissue, skin. It is neither as strong nor as aesthetically pleasing as the original.

full-thickness wound
Wound that penetrates to such a depth in the upper reticular dermis or subcutaneous tissue and is associated with slower healing; scarring will develop.

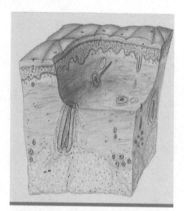

Figure 3–6 Full-thickness wounds are so called because they extend into the lower papillary and reticular dermis layers.

Full-thickness wounds are deeper, and it makes sense that their healing is far more involved and time-consuming. In this process, dead or dying cells are delineated and destroyed, precursors to collagen form and eventually collagen is created, the wound itself shrinks by contraction, and reepithelialization eventually occurs across the wound. We will discuss more about the process of wound healing in this environment later.

Full-thickness wounds in the medical spa could result from six possible scenarios: (1) microdermabrasion, chemical peel, or laser or IPL treatment that becomes infected; (2) overly aggressive instances of peels or laser therapy; (3) ischemic necrosis (deficient blood supply) from dermal fillers; (4) sclerotherapy; (5) deep hyfrecation; or (6) shave excision.

Acute Full-Thickness Wounds

Acute full-thickness wounds are those wounds that penetrate the epidermis and into the midpapillary dermis and beyond. These wounds are differentiated in their appearance and treatment protocols because they are localized; hence, the name. These wounds tend to bleed and ooze more than partial-thickness wounds. Likewise, they also take longer to heal than ordinary full-thickness wounds, and they will almost certainly result in a scar. These wounds need special attention and attentive care. Depending on protocol, clients with acute full-thickness wounds may be treated with oral antibiotics.

Aging and Wound Healing

It should not be much of a surprise that the process of skin healing slows down in the elderly. Diminished collagen production thins skin and slows inflammatory response to injury. Less collagen will not noticeably affect the healing of an acute partial-thickness wound; however, it is more profound in healing chronic full-thickness wounds. When a client has more than one health problem, for example, breast cancer and diabetes, healing of even acute partial-thickness wounds is likely to be noticeably compromised.

Therefore, it is important for an aesthetician to bear in mind two issues. First, take a complete health history to evaluate whether the client is a candidate for treatment. Then, having cleared the client for treatment, consider which treatments have the highest probability of success.

Nutrition and Wound Healing

Our society has a tendency to consider good nutrition to be a preventive measure against disease. Yet it is equally significant in regard to our capacity for rapid and effective wound-healing capacities. What we eat

malnutrition
Any condition that causes a lack of
nutritional substances for the body to
use and distribute.

supplies the building blocks for tissue repair. If the basic elements are not supplied through what we choose to eat, the healing process is impaired and the degree of impairment can be serious. This is simple, yet easily dismissed.

Malnutrition occurs in every corner of the world, not just in third-world countries. Economics is not always a factor. In the medical spa you may witness malnutrition in those who are anorexic and bulimic, as well as those who are elderly and in people with cancer or chronic illness.

As the body attempts to heal from an injury, proper nutrition plays a pivotal role. Under most circumstances, and certainly in the case of an epidermal wound, it should be easy for the healthy body to be effective in wound healing. Conversely, in the presence of malnutrition or diseases such as diabetes that impair circulation, wound healing can be seriously impaired.

To decipher what constitutes good nutrition, let us examine some familiar components of a healthy diet so that we can understand the role they play in wound healing.

Proteins

Proteins are made up of amino acids. Although it may seem redundant, our bodies break down proteins into amino acids before rebuilding these amino acids into proteins. This process is crucial for tissue repair. Tissue repair is an ongoing process in our bodies, even in the absence of wounds. Simply shedding our hair and skin cells requires the repair properties of protein.[18]

Amino acids are categorized as *essential* or *nonessential*. Essential amino acids must be obtained from what we eat—we cannot make them

Essential Amino Acids	Conditionally Essential Amino Acids
phenylalanine	arginine
valine	cysteine
threonine	glycine
tryptophan	glutamine
isoleucine	tyrosine
methionine	
histidine	
leucine	
lysine	

on our own.[19] If we do not ingest essential amino acids, of which nine are essential and five are conditionally essential, our bodies cannot build protein. Protein is easily obtained, primarily through meats, cheese, and eggs. Nonessential amino acids are found in our food and also occur naturally within our bodies.

Carbohydrates

Carbohydrates provide sugars that are easily broken down for use as an energy source. This fuel is either stored away for later consumption or used immediately, which helps spare protein for its ongoing role in building tissue.[20] Carbohydrates common in plant cell walls bring with them a bounty of other nutrients to feed and heal our bodies.[21] Whole grains, such as wheat, barley, and nuts, take longer to digest and keep us feeling satisfied longer.

Vitamins

Vitamins are found in everything we eat in varying degrees and also can be made within our bodies. Vitamins are defined as organic dietary components required for life, health, and growth. Unlike protein, fats, and minerals, they do not supply energy.[22]

One vitamin that is synonymous with good health, due to its antioxidant properties, is vitamin C. Our bodies do not manufacture vitamin C.[23] Therefore, we must consume it in our diets.

During its brief time inside our bodies, vitamin C is quite active and industrious. Just one of its critical tasks is to assist in making collagen. Collagen is required for blood vessels to function optimally—that is, to transport blood. Scurvy, the disease caused by vitamin C deficiency, slows wound healing because of poor collagen production; half of scurvy fatalities result from burst blood vessels.[24,25] Vitamin C, like many other antioxidants, can be ingested internally through food and supplements, and may also be applied topically. This will be discussed more thoroughly in Chapter 5.

Vitamin B is comprised of a spectrum of water-soluble vitamins essential to many aspects of health, including the fabrication of new tissue.[26] When scattered filaments of collagen "assemble themselves" into organized networks, they are assisted in that assembly by vitamin B. Vitamin B_6, pyridoxine, is involved in immune function, and vitamin B_{12} is vital for blood formation.[27]

Vitamin A, a fat-soluble vitamin, helps cells to reproduce normally (cell reproduction is heightened after injury).[29] Animal studies have shown vitamin E to diminish adhesions from surgical wounds but, provided in massive amounts, vitamin E can actually impair healing.[30]

carbohydrates
One of a group of chemical substances (including sugars) that contain only carbon, hydrogen, and oxygen. Common in fruits, grains, and nuts; carbohydrates are thought to be the most common chemical compounds on Earth.

Key nutritional components to the healing process include proteins, vitamins, major and trace minerals, proteins, and carbohydrates—all substances easily obtained through a healthy diet. One more essential component of good nutrition (and wound healing) is water, the "forgotten nutrient."

Water-soluble vitamins such as vitamins C and B complex are easily absorbed. They remain briefly in our bodies and are in high demand. To sustain optimal levels, they need to be taken in regularly.

Fat-soluble vitamins, such as vitamins A, D, E, and K, are poorly absorbed in the absence of bile and require intake of some dietary fat for their absorption.[28] They can also be toxic if taken in very large doses, so attending to recommended daily requirements is essential.

Vitamin K, another fat-soluble vitamin, assists the blood in clotting, a useful attribute in the presence of any bleeding wound.

Minerals

Minerals participate in nearly every process necessary for living and in several integral to healing.[31] The major minerals, such as calcium, are those present in your body in the greatest quantities. Trace minerals such as zinc are required in much smaller amounts.

Major Minerals:

Calcium, phosphorus, magnesium, sodium, potassium, and chloride

Minor Minerals:

Iron, zinc, iodine, copper, manganese, selenium, chromium, and molybdenum

Of these minerals, several stand out in connection with wound healing. Calcium plays a role in blood clotting; zinc is involved with enzymes that participate in wound healing; and copper helps to synthesize protein, which of course is necessary to repair tissue.[32]

Dietary Supplements

The issue of whether to supplement with vitamins and minerals is complex, highly individualized, and largely beyond the scope of this text. However, a few pointers can be provided. Vitamins C and B complex are necessary for healing, and supplementing with them for the purpose of healing is scientifically documented and generally accepted. However, the value of supplementing with fat-soluble vitamins to assist with healing of minor injuries in people not deficient in these vitamins remains unclear.[33] Certainly, occasions occur when supplementing with vitamin A may be recommended (for example, as a topical ointment for skin injuries in those taking oral corticosteroids). However, fat-soluble vitamins taken orally in excess can be toxic; therefore, under no circumstances would it be a good idea to take them in higher-than-recommended quantities.

When taking any supplement, be it vitamin or mineral, balance must be maintained, because these nutrients can work for or against each other in the body. Taking too much of one—or taking one at the wrong time with another one—could interfere with your body's ability to absorb that or other nutrients.[34] Furthermore, your body requires specific amount of vitamins. Taking too much is wasteful after a certain point and, as mentioned, toxic beyond that. Your body will excrete excess vitamins and mineral beyond what it needs.

SCARRING

Scars occur when both epidermis and dermis are injured and heal. You can be assured that a scar will occur if the wound has passed into the lower papillary dermis or the reticular dermis. The appearance of scarring, however, is variable and to some extent under our control.

Another aspect of scars, however, is not always obvious, especially to observers. That is the psychological effect of scarring upon the individual with the scar. Emotional responses to scarring fall along a continuum from almost complete apathy to almost complete hysteria, with many variations in between. People vary widely in their reaction to scars upon their own bodies, and that is something that the aesthetician would be wise to take into consideration and be sensitive to before performing any procedure with any possibility of scarring.

Normal Scarring

It may sound strange, but such a thing as *normal scarring* exists. Scarring as we now know it is the end point of the full-thickness wound-healing process, and normal scarring is the result of uncomplicated healing of such a wound. Normal scar tissue is decolorized and flat, nearly unrecognizable from the rest of the skin. When a wound is well taken care of, most scars will fade into unobtrusive components of skin surface (Figure 3–7).

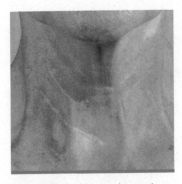

Figure 3–7 Normal scarring is the skin's best attempt to replicate the continuous tissue that is being replaced.

Events that Lead to Normal Scarring

Recall the three-step process of wound healing. If this process occurs without complication in a dermal injury, a normal scar results. In the simplest of terms, when dealing with injuries of the skin and absent of complicating factors such as infection, the type, size, cause, location, and especially *depth* of injury will determine whether a scar results. In general, injuries that penetrate only the epidermis will heal without a resulting scar. The epidermis is one of those infrequent body organs (also including gastrointestinal-tract epithelium, tracheobronchial epithelium, liver parenchyma, bone, and smooth muscle) that can regenerate themselves. Therefore, after a superficial injury (what we termed a *partial-thickness wound*) the epidermis simply reforms in the defect. This is called epithelialization. Within 24 hours, basal layer cells in injured healthy skin begin to multiply

epithelium
Membranous tissue covering internal organs and lining skin appendages.

epithelialization
Growth of new skin over a wound.

or proliferate and stream across the denuded surface to recreate an intact epidermal layer.

The dermis layer of the skin, beneath the epidermis, presents another story, because it cannot regenerate itself. Nevertheless, wounds that penetrate the epidermis and *only the upper part* of the dermis will also often heal without scar formation.

That may sound like a contradiction, but the singular anatomy of the epidermis and dermis enables it. Within the dermis are hair follicles, oil glands, and sweat glands. These appendages, you recall, originate in the epidermis. From that origin they penetrate down into the dermis while remaining enveloped in epidermal cells.

When a wound involves just the upper part of the dermis without scraping out these appendages, epithelial cells pocketing these appendages will proliferate and stream out of these structures to form a new, intact epidermis. With this kind of wound, still considered a partial-thickness wound, no true scar formation occurs, although additional collagen is stimulated to form in the dermis. This additional collagen will tend to tighten the skin and is, in part, the reason that we perform procedures that stimulate collagen (microdermabrasion, deeper dermabrasion, chemical peels, laser resurfacing).

However, generally speaking, dermal injuries will produce scars. When the dermis is completely penetrated or disrupted, even by hairline cuts from a surgical scalpel or laser beam, the dermis cannot regenerate and instead heals by the formation *of nonspecific connective tissue* (otherwise known as scarring) in what we termed a *full-thickness wound*. Scars need not be obvious. All things being equal, if the gap between the edges of the wound is very narrow, an excellent scar—a very unobtrusive one—should be all that remains.

Proper attention given to a wound reasonably free of complications should in most cases lead to normal scarring. Following are some examples.

Surgical Wounds

Although nobody likes scars, to some extent those scars resulting from surgeries, particularly major surgeries, are an expected result of those surgeries and tend not to produce as much agitation in clients as scars that are considered avoidable. At the same time, surgeons are constantly improving their techniques, decreasing the scope of their invasions, and developing better methods of covering their tracks.

Scars respond to products and interventions now known to improve their color, size, and feel.[35] Most of these postsurgical interventions are contingent on the client to perform but, as always, information that aestheticians can provide to clients will do clients a great service.

As to skin treatments performed in the medical spa, clients must be prepared before any procedure to understand the possibility that, despite our best intentions, some scarring is a possibility. Preparation will also help clients to understand what can be done to minimize scarring if it appears to be probable.

Injury

Injury covers a range of bodily damage with the potential to scar. Although the injuries or damages are not usually chosen by people, the extent of their disfigurement can be vastly minimized by the care that is given to them during healing. In most cases, clients with injuries will be under the care of primary-care doctors; however, should they happen to be simultaneously under your care in the medical spa, they may benefit from your sharing information about minimizing scar tissue. In fact, as an aesthetician in a medical spa specializing in skin care, you may be somewhat better informed regarding optimal healing techniques. However, while being generous in sharing requested information, be certain never to stray into medical advising.

Reducing the Probability of Normal Scarring[36]

Massaging creams

Sheets of silicone gel or mineral oil placed over scars

Taping of scars

Laser or dermabrasion treatment of scars

Steroid injection of scars

Abnormal Scarring

Wound healing requires the human body to undergo, in a timely and organized fashion, a multitude of events. When the healing process does not follow the normal pattern, failures in healing occur.

Sometimes, the fault for these failures lies with the client. Many people do not have the patience for scar resolution. They often want something done to remove a freshly created or still-healing scar, which of course is not possible. Clients also like to treat scars themselves. Clients use a variety of tactics on scars to try to resolve them, including nail files, glycolic acid, and vitamin E oil. None of these approaches provide favorable outcomes. Vitamin E is the most popular choice of home therapy. Unfortunately, evidence indicates that vitamin E oil has little or no benefit; of those who do use the product, approximately 33 percent develop dermatitis.[37]

The risk of abnormal scarring is much increased when healing of a deep skin wound is overextended—usually *over 3 weeks or longer.*[38] Various conditions can prolong healing. Skin that has been burned may be slow to heal. Similarly, a chronically inflamed earring piercing invites formation of an abnormal scar.

Failures in the process of normal wound healing are called **keloid scars**, **hypertrophic scars**, and **atrophic scars**.

Keloid Scarring

Keloid scars are defined by their growth outside the area of injury. They are seen most commonly on earlobes, shoulders, chest, and back—areas that may be subjected to a lot of skin tension—and usually accompany the healing of a deep skin wound.[39] They can form as long as one year after the original insult.

keloid scars
Scar formation in which tissue response is excessive in relation to normal tissue repair.

hypertrophic scars
Overly developed scar tissue that rises above the skin level, often overfed by an abundance of capillaries; will usually regress over time.

atrophic scars
Flat, small, round, and generally inverted scars; usually seen in acne or chicken-pox scarring.

Things that Make Healing Times Longer

Local infection

Inadequate wound closure

Presence of a foreign body

Certain medications

Smoking

Malnutrition or chronic disease

Advanced age

The word *keloid* means *crab claw,* and it describes the way lesions extend, sometimes like a starburst, from the scar into normal tissue.[40] The excessive development of both hypertrophic and keloid scars occurs in between 5 and 15 percent of human wounds. Why keloid scars develop is not fully understood. However, some hypothesize that for some reason, during the proliferation phase, fibroblasts, which form connective tissue, orchestrate an overabundance of collagen fibers.

Keloids are more commonly found in people with darker pigmentation; Hispanics, Asians, and those of African ancestry are more susceptible.[41] Fifteen percent of Hispanics and people of African ancestry report having keloids.

Keloid scars are difficult to treat. Most attempts at treatment are frustrating; however, because the scar can be so unsightly, many

Keloids and to a lesser extent hypertrophic scars seem to run in families. Although men and women are equally affected, women are more likely to seek treatment.

clients are willing to try just about anything to improve the appearance (Figure 3–8). Treatment options range from shriveling the scar with steroids to compressing it manually to removing it surgically.[42] Some physicians prefer to use silicone gel sheeting in combination with other treatments. Multipronged approaches may improve the chances of success.

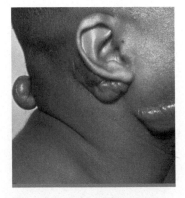

Figure 3–8 Keloid scarring is abnormal healing that extends beyond the boundaries of an insult.

Hypertrophic Scarring

A hypertrophic scar is excessive scar tissue that rises above the skin level yet, unlike keloids, stays within the confines of the original lesion or injury (Figure 3–9).[43] Hypertrophic scars are often overfed by an abundance of capillaries. In addition, in contrast to keloids, hypertrophic scars usually regress or resolve over a period of time.[44]

When hypertrophic scars are surgically removed, they may improve. Hypertrophic scarring will also respond to steroid injections and silicone gel sheeting applications.

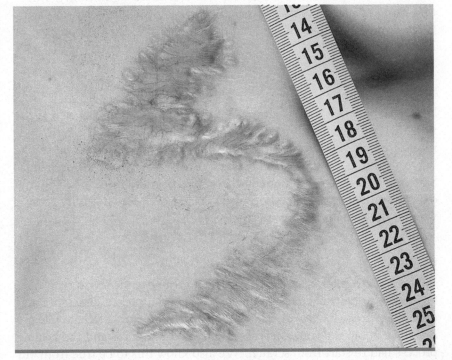

Figure 3–9 Red in color and raised hypertrophic scars are often confused with keloid scars.

Hypertrophic scarring crosses ethnic barriers and has been reported to be as high as 68 percent after surgical procedures or injury.[45]

Atrophic Scars

Atrophic scars are round and flat. We know these scars best as chicken-pox scars or acne scars. Because these scars can be shaped irregularly, each scar must be examined individually to evaluate the appropriateness of treatment. Atrophic scars are commonly treated in the medical spa with microdermabrasion and dermal fillers. Without complications, many of these scars will improve by themselves over time.

Events that Lead to Abnormal Scarring

If complications occur during healing, then the scar from a dermal wound could look worse.

Infection

Bacteria will always find a wound. *Staphylococcus* and *Streptococcus* live on the skin's surface; when an opening in the skin occurs, these bacteria rarely decline the invitation. Generally, the body handles these invaders; however, infection is always possible. Infections cause wounds to heal more slowly and, if left unattended, will scar more significantly. Infection can go so far as to cause tissue necrosis, the actual death of tissue. Clients must be urged never to underestimate the damage potential of infection.

Tissue Ischemia

Tissue ischemia is a local shortage of blood supply. This deficiency can be caused by several factors, including infection, poor client health, and, most often, smoking. It is critical for the client to understand that smoking can and does slow the healing process through tissue ischemia. Smoking causes constriction of the capillaries and a decrease in the oxygen content of the blood occurs. When blood does not fully serve a wound, the healing process is crippled.

Picking

When a client picks at a wound, it has a greater tendency to scar. You know this to be true from childhood. When you picked at scrapes and cuts, they took longer to heal and left deeper scars. When picking caused it to bleed again, the scab would need to reform and the healing process had to start from scratch. We also know this to be true from our experiences with acne. Picking disrupts the healing process and causes the cellular repair to begin repeatedly.

necrosis
Death of cells when tissue is deprived of blood supply.

ischemia
Localized restriction of blood flow usually caused by an obstruction of normal circulation.

■ CONCLUSION

Scar is the terrifying *S* word. Every aesthetician working in the aesthetic medical spa is frightened of creating a scar, and with good reason. Clients hate scars and, in reality, scars should not be a part of the aesthetician's eventual outcome. Interviews of people who had never undergone any type of medical skin care revealed the number-one reason they had avoided skin care at medical spas was the fear of scars.

Whenever the aesthetician feels the treatment he or she has done may have potential to scar, a physician should be notified immediately. We now know that avoiding scars can be possible. With a strong knowledge of anatomy and physiology and the principles of wound healing, the treatments we give our clients will leave them safe and beautiful.

In the end, however, client compliance to post-treatment home instructions may be as important as the spa care.

▶ ▷ ▷ Top 10 Tips to Take to the Spa

1. Try to observe many wounds so that you can tell the difference between full-thickness and partial-thickness wounds.

2. Observe and take note of different healing times and identify the reasons for each.

3. Know your wound-healing phases.

4. Understand the phenomenon of abnormal scarring.

5. Get comfortable about talking to clients about the possibility of scars.

6. Know what treatments might cause scars.

7. Understand how to treat wounds that occur in the medical spa.

8. Know when to ask for help.

9. Educate clients on wound healing.

10. Know why some wounds take longer to heal.

Chapter Review Questions

1. Why might understanding the process of wound healing be important to you as an aesthetician? Particular to microdermabrasion?

2. What is a wound? An insult?

3. What are the three stages of wound healing? Include significant physiological events and timelines in your description.

4. What are the most common types of wounds and wound depths to occur in association with microdermabrasion?

5. The inflammatory phase and infection share a few common characteristics. How would you decipher the difference between useful inflammation and infection?

6. How do white blood cells assist in wound healing? How might immunocompromisation, like that associated with chemotherapy or HIV/AIDS, be affected by their function?

7. How do tissue cells contribute to the healing process?

8. True or False: collagen, prevalent in the dermis, works for up to 2 weeks to wrap the wound.

9. True or False: collagen, an extremely rare protein, is found in connective tissue, and is an important component to both wound healing and youthful skin.

10. Match each of the following cells or cellular structures with its contribution to wound healing:

    a. Collagen

    b. Langerhans'

    c. Macrophages

    d. Lymphocytes

    e. Neutrophils

    f. Granulocytes

    g. Leukocytes

    ___ White blood cells involved in immune response; include neutrophils, eosinophils, and basophils.

    ___ Macrophage cells in epidermis that perform surveillance for the immune system.

    ___ White blood cells without granules involved in immune response; include lymphocytes and monocytes.

    ___ Part of the immune system in the skin; scavengers that clear debris in tissue injury.

    ___ White blood cells involved in the body's immune system; their numbers increase in the presence of infection.

    ___ Most common type of white blood cells that kill bacteria and discourage infection.

    ___ Prevalent in the dermis, it is also a major component of the connective tissue that embodies itself around the wounds.

11. True or False: The terms *acute* and *chronic* refer to wound depth.

12. True or False: microdermabrasion results in a partial-thickness wound, which heals quickly.

13. What is the difference between partial- and full-thickness wounds?

14. Explain how aging affects the wound healing process.

15. What nutrition-related factors will affect wound healing? As an aesthetician, what can you do to assist clients to heal better with regard to nutrition?

16. What is the difference between essential and nonessential amino acids?

17. Describe the difference between water-soluble and fat-soluble vitamins?

18. What trace minerals are necessary to successful wound healing? What do they contribute?

19. What is scarring? How does it occur?

20. What would constitute a normal scar? An abnormal scar? Why?

Chapter References

1. Lazarus, G. S., Cooper, D. M., Knighton, D. R. et al. (1994). Definitions and guidelines for assessment of wounds and evaluation of healing. *Archives of Dermatology, 130*, 489–493.

2. Goepel, J. R. (1996). Responses to cellular injury. In J. E. C. Underwood (Ed.), *General and systemic pathology* (2nd ed.) (pp. 121–122). London: Churchill Livingstone.

3. eMedicine.com, Inc. (2004). Wound healing, skin [Online]. Available: http://www.emedicine.com

4. Norman, R., & Bock, M. (March, 2003). Understanding wound management [Online]. Available: http://www.skinandaging.com/sa

5. eMedicine.com, Inc. (2004). Wound healing, growth factors [Online]. Available: http://www.emedicine.com

6. Huang, N. F., Zac-Varghese, S., & Luke, S. (2003). Apoptosis in skin wound healing [Online]. Available: http://www.medscape.com

7. eMedicine.com, Inc. (2004). Wound healing, growth factors [Online]. Available: http://www.emedicine.com

8. Thomas, C. L. (Ed.). (1997). *Taber's cyclopedic medical dictionary*. Philadelphia: F. A. Davis Company.

9. Thomas, C. L. (Ed.). (1997). *Taber's cyclopedic medical dictionary*. Philadelphia: F. A. Davis Company.

10. Kimball, J. W. (2003). *Blood* [Online]. Available: http://biology-pages.info

11. Thomas, C. L. (Ed.). (1997). *Taber's cyclopedic medical dictionary*. Philadelphia: F. A. Davis Company.

12. Clark, R. A. F. (1993). Basics of cutaneous wound repair. *Journal of Dermatologic Surgery and Oncology, 19*, 693–706.

13. Sholar, A., & Stadelmann, W. (2003). Wound healing, chronic wounds [Online]. Available: http://www.emedicine.com

14. Thomas, C. L. (Ed.). (1997). *Taber's cyclopedic medical dictionary*. Philadelphia: F. A. Davis Company.

15. Daresbury Imaging Group. (2005, May). Collagen [Online]. Available: http://detserv1.dl.ac.uk

16. Rutledge, B. J. (2004, January–February). Modeling dermal scars below and above the threshold [Online]. *Cosmetic Surgery Times*. Available: http://www.findarticles.com

17. Rutledge, B. J. (2004, January–February). Modeling dermal scars below and above the threshold [Online]. *Cosmetic Surgery Times*. Available: http://www.findarticles.com

18. Ganong, W. F. (1989). Energy balance, metabolism, & nutrition. In *Review of medical physiology* (14th ed.). Norwalk, CT: Appleton & Lange.

19. Ganong, W. F. (1989). Energy balance, metabolism, & nutrition. In *Review of medical physiology* (14th ed.). Norwalk, CT: Appleton & Lange.

20. Quinn, B. (2003). Nutrition and wound healing: What's the connection? [Online]. *Nutrition*. Available: http://www.wadsworth.com

21. Ganong, W. F. (1989). Energy balance, metabolism, & nutrition. In *Review of medical physiology* (14th ed.). Norwalk, CT: Appleton & Lange.

22. Ganong, W. F. (1989). Energy balance, metabolism, & nutrition. *In Review of medical physiology* (14th ed.). Norwalk, CT: Appleton & Lange.

23. Wooldridge, M. (1993). Linus Pauling lectures on vitamin C and heart disease [Online]. Available: http://www.lbl.gov

24. Bender, D. A. (2003). *Vitamins and minerals. Introduction to nutrition and metabolism* (3rd ed.). London: Taylor & Francis.

25. Wooldridge, M. (1993). Linus Pauling lectures on vitamin C and heart disease [Online]. Available: http://www.lbl.gov

26. Quinn, B. (2003). Nutrition and wound healing: What's the connection? [Online]. *Nutrition*. Available: http://www.wadsworth.com

27. Mead Johnson & Company. (2003). Vitamins, minerals, and water [Online]. Available: http://www.meadjohnson.com

28. Ganong, W. F. (1989). Energy balance, metabolism, & nutrition. In *Review of medical physiology* (14th ed.). Norwalk, CT: Appleton & Lange.

29. Quinn, B. (2003). Nutrition and wound healing: What's the connection? [Online]. *Nutrition.* Available: http://www.wadsworth.com

30. Healthnotes, Inc. (2002). Wound healing [Online]. Available: http://www.mycustompak.com

31. Mead Johnson & Company. (2003). Vitamins, minerals, and water [Online]. Available: http://www.meadjohnson.com

32. Mead Johnson & Company. (2003). Vitamins, minerals, and water [Online]. Available: http://www.meadjohnson.com

33. Healthnotes, Inc. (2002). Wound healing [Online]. Available: http://www.mycustompak.com

34. Mead Johnson & Company. (2003). Vitamins, minerals, and water [Online]. Available: http://www.meadjohnson.com

35. Romano, J. J. (2003). Scar treatment, therapy, and removal [Online]. Available: http://www.jromano.com

36. Bisaccia, E., & Scarborough, D. (2002). *The Columbia manual of dermatologic cosmetic surgery.* New York: McGraw-Hill.

37. Romano, J. J. (2003). Scar treatment, therapy, and removal [Online]. Available: http://www.jromano.com

38. eMedicine.com, Inc. (2004). Wound healing, keloids [Online]. Available: http://www.emedicine.com

39. eMedicine.com, Inc. (2004). Wound healing, keloids [Online]. Available: http://www.emedicine.com

40. eMedicine.com, Inc. (2004). Wound healing, keloids [Online]. Available: http://www.emedicine.com

41. eMedicine.com, Inc. (2004). Wound healing, keloids [Online]. Available: http://www.emedicine.com

42. eMedicine.com, Inc. (2004). Wound healing, keloids [Online]. Available: http://www.emedicine.com

43. Spas in Plastic Surgery. (2000, October). *Response to Tissue Injury, 27*(4). Philadelphia: W. B. Saunders Company.

44. eMedicine.com, Inc. (2004). Wound healing, keloids [Online]. Available: http://www.emedicine.com

45. Spas in Plastic Surgery. (2000, October). *Response to Tissue Injury, 27*(4). Philadelphia: W. B. Saunders Company.

Skin Typing

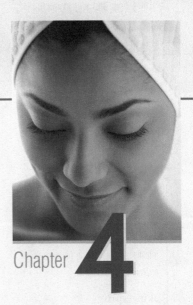

Key Terms

actinic keratoses

aging analysis

Fitzpatrick Skin
  Typing

Glogau classification
  of aging analysis

keratoses

lentigines

Rubin classification
  of aging
  analysis

skin condition

skin typing

telangiectasias

Chapter 4

Learning Objectives

After completing this chapter you should be able to:

1. Define and discuss the concepts of skin typing and aging analysis.
2. Define and discuss the Fitzpatrick method of skin typing.
3. Define and discuss the Glogau classification of aging analysis.
4. Define and discuss the Rubin classification of aging analysis.

INTRODUCTION

skin condition
Fundamental skin classification in which an individual's skin is grouped according to the degree of moisture retention, its reaction to products or environment, or both.

skin typing
More detailed skin classification that gives indications as to how a certain skin type will react to various treatment conditions.

aging analysis
Examines how aging physically presents itself in the skin, particularly, to what sorts of damaging conditions the skin has been exposed in the past and the results of that damage; considers both intrinsic and extrinsic aging modalities.

Fitzpatrick Skin Typing
Method of skin typing that considers skin's complexion, hair color, eye color, ethnicity, and the individual's reaction to unprotected sun exposure.

As you look around you, it is clear that everyone has different skin. The texture, color, thickness, and consistency will vary even on people who are closely related to one another. Therefore, the response to microdermabrasion, or any skin therapy, is different from client to client. The concept of biologic and environmental variables is one that is widely accepted in all health care, including medical skin care. For example, recommended drug doses are calculated according to the individual patient weight. To determine the *who, when, how,* and *why* of microdermabrasion, you also need to have specialized criteria. This allows you to try to predict the suitability of a client and the likely outcome. A variety of methods of classification have been developed to assist in this. The simplest of these, which we assume has already been completed at this point, is the classification of **skin condition** (normal, oily, dry, sensitive, or combination). The next level of skin analysis requires using two other categories of analytic system: (1) **skin typing** and (2) **aging analysis**.

SKIN TYPING AND AGING ANALYSIS

Evaluating the skin's condition, although an important first step, really does not provide enough information when doing advanced treatments such as microdermabrasion, peels, laser resurfacing, or true dermabrasion. As discussed, one person will not respond to a treatment exactly the same as the next person. Therefore, as an aesthetician you need to understand how individual skin types respond to different treatments— which skin types will allow aggressive treatments, and which require greater caution. This is among the benefits of the skin-typing classifications. Many years of clinical research and study have shown that factors exist that regularly and consistently affect the skin's response to injury. They include genetics, eye color, hair color, ethnic background, and true skin color. These factors were meshed into a classification system, developed by Dr. Thomas Fitzpatrick in 1975, commonly known as **Fitzpatrick Skin Typing**. It is perhaps the most widely used skin-typing classification applied today to predict the skin's response to a variety of therapies, from microdermabrasion to carbon dioxide (CO_2) laser resurfacing. Other skin classification systems include the Lancer Ethnicity Scale, which takes into account the person's ethnic heritage to determine potential healing capacities. Another classification system is the World Classification of Skin Type. This method is based on photosensitivity and the potential for post-inflammatory hyperpigmentation. Both of these systems have subcategories that assist the aesthetician in determining the potential treatment response. But, of all these systems, the Fitzpatrick System is by far the most widely used and the most familiar to aestheticians. A skin typing system helps the aesthetician to determine which clients have a greater risk of complications, including scarring and pigmentary problems from various treatments. The specifics of the Fitzpatrick classification and the means to determine a client's type are discussed at length.

The Fitzpatrick Skin Typing method, while not the only one used, is certainly the most common method to determine a client's suitability for a microdermabrasion treatment.

Although skin typing is an indicator of how an individual client's skin will respond to a particular treatment, aging analysis examines past environmental history, namely environmental damage (such as sun damage and free radical damage) that has been done to date and the visible results of that damage. The aesthetician uses this information to determine which treatment modality or modalities can be used to treat the damage and achieve a positive result. It evaluates the client's skin-aging pattern, both intrinsic and extrinsic. Remember that *intrinsic aging* refers to the changes that would occur to the skin over time without the effects of any environmental factors, while *extrinsic aging* refers to the changes that are brought on by the effects of the environment, especially, but not limited to, sun exposure. Aging analysis primarily evaluates *photoaging* or solar damage. However, the lines of expression are also considered.

Two aging analysis systems are commonly used: (1) the Glogau classification and (2) the Rubin classification. The **Glogau classification of aging analysis** is a system that measures the degree of photodamage and assigns a numeric designation based on that damage. According to the Glogau classification system, skin changes are classified as being *minimal, moderate, advanced,* or *severe.* The determination for each client is based on the following categories: client's chronologic age, pigment changes, **keratoses,** wrinkles, the use of makeup, and the extent of the acne scarring. It divides clients into four categories of increasing levels of photodamage.

Criticism of the Glogau system includes the fact that too many variables exist in each category, as well as determining factors that may be social or cultural in nature and have nothing to do with photodamage. Not all clients fit fairly into these categories in a meaningful way.

The **Rubin classification of aging analysis** is simpler; however, it examines only the aging associated with photodamage. Dr. Rubin classifies based on " . . . the level of photodamage based on the histologic

Glogau classification of aging analysis
System of aging analysis that calculates the degree of aging-related damage and assigns numeric typing; considers both intrinsic and extrinsic aging.

keratoses
Any condition of the skin characterized by excessive horny growth.

Rubin classification of aging analysis
System of aging analysis that calculates the degree of photodamage and assigns a numeric level; considers only extrinsic aging.

Dr. Thomas Fitzpatrick

Dr. Thomas Fitzpatrick is the former chairman of the Department of Dermatology at the renowned Massachusetts General Hospital in Boston, Massachusetts. He has been called the "father of modern academic dermatology" and "the most influential dermatologist of the last 100 years." The author of *Fitzpatrick's Dermatology in General Medicine*, he is best known for developing the Fitzpatrick phototype procedure for quantifying skin types and determining an individual's ultraviolet (UV) radiation (sun) susceptibility. During his career, he was interested in treating many diseases, including psoriasis and vitiligo. His treatment protocol used UVA (ultraviolet A) light. To quantify the amount of UVA exposure, it was important that a system be devised to set treatment parameters that would predict the client's response to UV light based on the type of skin he or she had.

depth of visible clinical changes."[1] The categories that Rubin uses are pigment changes, texture changes, and wrinkling. The aging analysis helps you to understand how "tough" the skin has become based on environmental damage.

This aging system, when meshed with the Fitzpatrick Skin Typing, will precisely evaluate the client, select an appropriate treatment modality, reduce risks, and increase your ability to predict the likely results of that plan.

Fitzpatrick Skin Typing

As discussed previously, in the Fitzpatrick System, each client is asked a series of questions related to skin color, unaltered eye and hair color, ethnic origins, and response to UV light (without any sun protection). Based on a series of questions we end up with six Fitzpatrick skin types (Fitzpatrick I through VI) that extend from very fair skin to very dark skin (Tables 4–1 through 4–6).

To determine classification, a number of questions are asked of each client, together with your own examination.

Add up the total scores for each of the three sections for your skin type score. This will give you a better evaluation of your skin type.

Now that you have your personal score, it is time to delve deeper into the categories and explore the meaning and necessity within the typing matrix.

Table 4-1 Fitzpatrick Skin-Typing Scale

Skin Type	Skin Color	Hair and Eye Color	Reaction to Sun	Common Ethnic Considerations
Type I	White	Blond hair & green eyes	Always burns, freckles	English, Scottish
Type II	White	Blond hair & green/blue eyes	Always burns, freckles, difficult to tan	Northern European
Type III	White	Blond/brown hair & blue/brown eyes	Tans after several burns, may freckle	German
Type IV	Brown	Brown hair & brown eyes	Tans more than average, rarely burns, rarely freckles	Mediterranean, Southern European, Hispanic
Type V	Dark brown	Brown/black hair & brown eyes	Tans with ease, rarely burns, no freckles	Asian, Indian, some Africans
Type VI	Black	Black hair & brown/black eyes	Tans, rarely burns, deeply pigmented never freckles	Africans

Table 4-2 Genetic Disposition[2]

	0	1	2	3	4	Score
What color are your eyes?	Light blue, gray, green	Blue, gray, or green	Blue	Dark brown	Brownish-black	
What is the natural color of your hair?	Sandy red	Blond	Chestnut/dark blond	Dark brown	Black	
What color is your skin (nonexposed areas)?	Reddish	Very pale	Pale with beige tint	Light brown	Dark brown	
Do you have freckles on exposed areas?	Many	Several	Few	Incidental	None	
					Genetic Disposition Total	

Skin Color

Skin color is essentially an inherited racial and ethnic characteristic; but even within the same race and ethnicity, some variability exists (Figure 4–1). This is the crux of the Lancer Ethnicity Scale. As mentioned, the Lancer

Table 4–3 Reaction to Sun Exposure[3]

	0	1	2	3	4	Score
What happens when you stay too long in the sun?	Painful redness, blistering, peeling	Blistering followed by peeling	Burns sometimes followed by peeling	Rare burns	Never had burns	
To what degree do you turn brown?	Hardly or not at all	Light color tan	Reasonable tan	Tan very easily	Turn dark brown quickly	
Do you turn brown with several hours of sun exposure?	Never	Seldom	Sometimes	Often	Always	
How does your face react to the sun?	Very sensitive	Sensitive	Normal	Very resistant	Never had a problem	

Reaction to Sun Exposure Total

Table 4–4 Tanning Habits[4]

	1	2	3	4	5	Score
When did you last expose your body to sun (or artificial sunlamp/tanning cream)?	More than 3 months ago	2–3 months ago	1–2 months ago	Less than 1 month ago	Less than 2 weeks ago	
Did you expose the area to be treated to the sun?	Never	Hardly ever	Sometimes	Often	Always	

Tanning Habits Total

system is specifically directed at the individual ethnicity and how that skin type will respond to the treatment. How, then, might you use the Lancer Scale? For example, the client might complete the Fitzpatrick Classification document to find that he or she is a Fitzpatrick III, but after asking the ethnicity of the client's parents the aesthetician finds that one of the parents is of African descent. This will change the Fitzpatrick Classification to a IV given the potential for post-inflammatory hyper-pigmentation or sensitivity due to higher pigment levels not uncovered

Table 4–5 Scores[5]	
Summary	**Score**
Total for genetic disposition (Table 4–2)	_____
Total for reaction to sun exposure (Table 4–3)	_____
Total for tanning habits (Table 4–4)	_____
Skin Type Score	_____

Table 4–6 Your Fitzpatrick Skin Type[6]	
Skin Type Score	**Fitzpatrick Skin Type**
0–7	I
8–16	II
17–25	III
25–30	IV
Over 30	V–VI

in the Fitzpatrick questionnaire. Using both scales together can assist the aesthetician in carefully selecting the treatment for the client.

Caucasian

When we think of Caucasian, we think *white*. However, white can come in a variety of shades, and this will affect whether the client is a Fitzpatrick I, II, or even III. In the Fitzpatrick I classification, the ethnic considerations are English, Scottish, Irish, Norwegian, Swedish, and Icelandic. These individuals have very fair skin, freckling, green or light blue eyes, and light hair colors.

Non-Hispanic Caucasian

This category of skin type has darker hair, mainly dark blonds, and brown. This *non-Hispanic Caucasian* category can also present several variations on the shades of darker whites and brown skin. They will probably fall into the Fitzpatrick III and IV categories. The eye color is blue, dark blue, and brown. This ethnic background is usually Mediterranean and Southern European. This would include Greeks, Middle Easterners, and Italians.

Hispanic

The Hispanic skin category has darker skin, darker hair, and darker eyes. Their hair is dark brown or black, and their eyes are brown. They

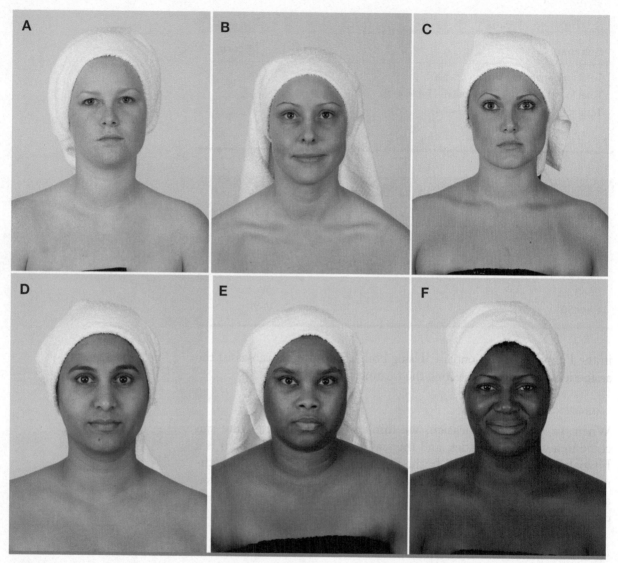

Figure 4–1 Assessing a patient's Fitzpatrick skin color is complicated and challenging. **A**, Fitzpatrick I; **B**, Fitzpatrick II; **C**, Fitzpatrick III; **D**, Fitzpatrick IV; **E**, Fitzpatrick V; **F**, Fitzpatrick VI.

will generally fall into the Fitzpatrick IV and perhaps V categories. Their ethnic background is Spain, Mexico, South America, and Central America.

African or African-American

The skin types of the African or African-American is darker. However, the skin will vary from light brown (like Hispanics) to very dark brown to a blue-black color. Their hair is always naturally black, but the eyes can be brown to black. In the darkest color, this skin is the Fitzpatrick VI; but they also can be Fitzpatrick V. Their ethnic background is African.

Asian and Pacific Islander

These skin types are light brown to brown in color; often the hair can be light brown or sometimes a dark red to dark brown. The eyes are brown and sometimes dark brown. These skin types have ethnic backgrounds in Japan, China, and the islands of the South Pacific, to mention a few.

American Indian or Alaskan Native

These skin types are light brown to brown. The hair color is brown to black. The eye color is brown to dark brown. These people are found in differing parts of the United States.

Choosing Skin Color

Aestheticians need to learn to choose skin color at a glance. As you begin the analysis of the skin in the spa, use these three easy steps: First, choose three areas of the body to evaluate. The face, under the breast or abdomen, and an arm are good choices. The face needs to be void of makeup. Next, look for freckles, telangiectasia, and skin tone. Finally, decide on a skin color based on what you see and what the client reports in terms of ethnic background.

Eye Color

Eye color is determined genetically, just like skin color. Three basic eye colors exist: (1) blue, (2) brown, and (3) green. These colors are further expanded: light blue, blue, blue-green, hazel, light brown, brown, and dark brown or black. Obviously the degree of color is determined genetically, but it also relates to the skin tone (Figure 4–2). If you are struggling to assess the correct Fitzpatrick skin type, looking at the eye color can help you to make the decision. Eye color is most helpful in analyzing Fitzpatrick I and Fitzpatrick II. These two skin types have varying colors of blue and green eyes that can be confusing to a beginner.

Hair Color

Hair color is probably the most difficult to appraise (Figure 4–3). Most women and some men color their hair to some degree, whether it is

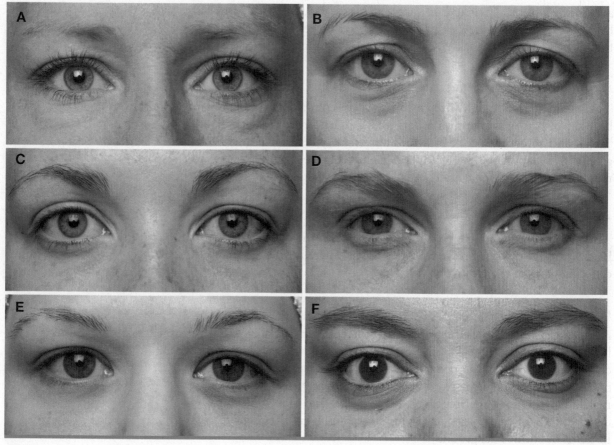

Figure 4–2 The primary eye colors (blue, green, and brown) include several variations. **A**, blue; **B**, blue/green; **C**, green; **D**, hazel; **E**, brown; **F**, dark brown/black.

highlights, full color, or a combination of both. Hair color can be determined at the roots, supposing they are present, or by eyebrows. If your client's hair color is altered, have the client try to describe the natural color. Hair color is going to be an indicator that you may or may not factor in, depending on the potential for error.

Response to Ultraviolet Light without Sun Protection Factor

Aside from identifying the skin type based on your skin analysis and the color of the eyes and hair, evaluating the skin's response to UV light is

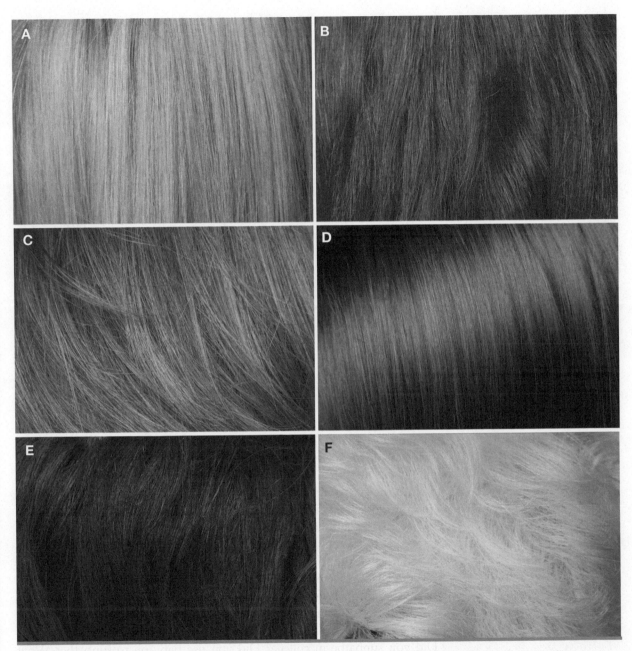

Figure 4–3 Many clients color their hair; therefore, you may not want to consider hair color as part of your assessment. *A*, light blond; *B*, red; *C*, dark blond; *D*, brown; *E*, dark brown/black; *F*, gray.

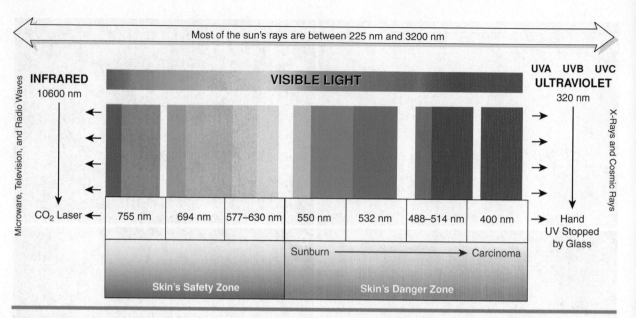

Figure 4–4 Ultraviolet A, B, and C light (UVA, UVB, and UVC) lengths are most toxic to the skin.

the single most important indicator of skin type (Figure 4–4). How you ask about the client's response to UV light is critical to the accuracy of the answer. It is also a question that requires client honesty, which can sometimes be lacking. You want to know how the skin responds to the sun *without* sunscreen. The problem is that no one wants to admit they go in the sun without sunscreen. Usually the client will tell you, "I never go into the sun," or "I never go in the sun without sunscreen." The best question to ask is, "Did you have a sunburn as a child?" or if he or she has ever had a sunburn that resulted in peeling of the skin. If the answer is yes, get the details. For example, you want to know if the sunburn produced blisters and, if so, where on the body. If it did not produce blisters, can the client remember how long it was sore or red? If he or she cannot remember, probe a little bit further. "As a child, did you vacation at the beach? How did your skin respond at the beach? As a child, did you swim during the summer? How did your skin respond at the swimming pool? Did you sunbathe in college? Did you use baby oil to sunbathe? What happened to your skin?" The next question to ask is if he or she has ever had a glycolic or trichloroacetic acid (TCA) peel. If the answer is yes, ask for the details. What was the strength, how long was the peel left on, and what were the results? Did he or she have any complications from the peel? Remember, Fitzpatrick analysis tells you how the skin responds to advanced skin care products and treatments.

Using the System

Now that you have collected all of the information, an analysis of Fitzpatrick Skin Type selection should be made using the following specific definitions. Your determination is based on what you see, the ethnic heritage (geographic origin of forbearers), eye color, and response to UV light. You should also factor in hair color if it is the natural color. There is a natural tendency to evaluate skin color when you are typing skin. Teach yourself to look at all of the characteristics associated with the Fitzpatrick Typing chart. The more difficult skins to type will be differentiated by the details of eye color and the skin's response to sun (especially as a child).

- *Fitzpatrick I* is the *very fair-skinned* individual. This person usually has very blond or red hair, light blue or green eyes, and burns within 10 to 15 minutes of being in the sun when exposed without sunscreen. This person tans by freckling. A good example of Fitzpatrick Skin Type I are the Irish, English, or Scottish.
- *Fitzpatrick II* is the *fair-skinned* individual. This individual has blond hair, sometimes *dark blond hair,* with blue or green eyes. They may tolerate a slightly longer period of time in the sun before burning, perhaps 30 to 40 minutes. This individual still freckles a lot and has a difficultly tanning. Good examples of Fitzpatrick Skin Type II are people of Northern European, Swedish, Finish, or Norwegian ancestry.
- *Fitzpatrick III* is still *white* but tans more easily than Fitzpatrick I and II. They will have fewer freckles than the Fitzpatrick I and II. Their hair can be blond, but is more likely to be a light brown to moderate brown color. The eye color is usually dark blue to brown. These individuals can be in the sun 60 to 70 minutes without sunscreen before they begin to burn. Examples of a Fitzpatrick Skin Type III are those of German, Northern Italian, and French ancestry.
- *Fitzpatrick IV* is *brown* and tans easily, usually without freckling. This individual can be in the sun without sunscreen and will rarely burn. The hair color is usually brown to dark brown, and the eyes are brown. Examples of Fitzpatrick Skin Type IV are Greeks, Southern Italians, some Asians, and some Hispanics.
- *Fitzpatrick V* is *dark brown*, tans easily, and generally does not have freckles. This person can be in the sun without sunscreen and will not burn. The hair is usually brown or black with brown eyes. Examples of Fitzpatrick Skin Type V include some Asians, some Hispanics, some Africans, and Middle Eastern Indians.

The Fitzpatrick Skin Typing system has six categories. Your determination is based on what you see and the questions you ask.

- *Fitzpatrick VI* is *black,* tans with ease, does not freckle, and is deeply pigmented. Their hair is black, and their eyes are brown or even black. Examples of Fitzpatrick VI are Africans.

Aestheticians should understand that identifying skin types is "as much an art as a science." Usually one component of the skin's characteristic will be more dominant than others, and this will be the determining factor in the skin type. Many times, a client simply will not fit into one category; he or she may seem to have attributes of several categories.

Mixed Skin Colors

As the world becomes more globalized, it has become a smaller place. A hundred years ago it was easier to assume that lighter skin came from one geographic region and darker skin came from another geographic region. Today, that is not the case. Increasingly, skin colors are melding together, along with ethnicities, societies, and economies. While this is a good thing for mankind, it makes skin typing more challenging for the aesthetician.

Mixed color is an important factor as you evaluate for skin typing. Therefore, it is incumbent on the aesthetician to use the Lancer Scale and to ask questions about the client's background. What is his or her ethnic history? Most clients are proud of their heritage and understand that genetics affect their appearance. However, before you begin asking the client questions about his or her background, explain why. You can do this by asking if the client looks more like his or her mother or father, explain how genetics affect skin color, then ask about the client's heritage. Even though the client may look more like one parent than the other, be sure to ask about the heritage of both parents.

What if your client is adopted? Unless the client happens to know the heritage of his or her birth parents, this piece of information is lost. In this case, it would be important to ask enough questions about previous sun exposure to give you an understanding of the skin type. What if he or she only knows one parent? Ask extensively about the known parent; this will help you to evaluate if the client resembles this parent. Then, as with adopted clients, you will need to use your clinical skills to come to an accurate conclusion. What you see and your analysis of what you see will need to guide you in these situations.

▪ AGING ANALYSIS

lentigines
Flat brown spots appearing on aged or sun-exposed skin; commonly called liver spots, they are not related to any liver disease.

Aging analysis is a method of categorizing clients based on their intrinsic and extrinsic aging factors. The analysis takes into consideration the kinds of lines, solar damage, such as keratosis and lentigines, and the condition of the stratum corneum. Of the *skin-aging systems,* both the Glogau and Rubin systems are widely used and well-respected.

The aging analysis is just as important as skin typing. The aging analysis helps you to understand the client's skin history. Through a group of well-organized questions, you will be able to ascertain the client's intrinsic aging history and the extrinsic aging history, that is, what role genetics are playing and how much sun exposure the client has had.

When the analyses are completed, the aesthetician will understand how the client's skin is going to behave under most circumstances. This will help the aesthetician to predict potential obstacles in the program, the possible outcome, and client compliance.

Advanced medical aestheticians use several methods of skin typing and aging analysis.

> Although plastic surgery, a facelift for example, may play a role in the aging analysis and the appearance of chronologic age, a facelift will not impact the quality of the skin.

Glogau Classification

The Glogau classification, as you know, is an aging classification used to determine the "past history" of the skin. This classification deals with the appearance of the skin involving both intrinsic and extrinsic aging history. Using all of the variables, we end up with four levels of aging. This can be a little more confusing than Fitzpatrick Skin Typing. Aestheticians should be familiar with the specific categories (Table 4–7).

> Aging analysis takes into consideration both intrinsic and extrinsic aging.

Dr. Richard G. Glogau

Dr. Richard G. Glogau is a clinical professor of dermatology at the University of California, where he is widely regarded as an expert in his field. He has garnered national and international recognition for his innovative work in dermatology, specifically in the areas of cosmetic surgery and skin cancer. Dr. Glogau lectures extensively on a wide range of topics in cosmetic dermatology, including soft tissue augmentation, photoaging, and resurfacing.

Pigment Changes

Pigment changes are most commonly changes related to sun exposure and aging skin. As you know, when the skin is exposed to the sun, long-term pigment changes are likely to present as freckles, lentigines, and telangiectasia (Figure 4–5, *A*). Some pigment changes, however, are secondarily related to the sun and caused by external factors such as

Table 4–7 Glogau Classification		
Damage	**Description**	**Characteristics**
Type I (mild)	No wrinkles	Early photoaging: Mild pigmentary changes No keratoses Minimal wrinkles Client age: 20s–30s Minimal or no makeup Minimal acne scarring
Type II (moderate)	Wrinkles in motion	Early to moderate photoaging: Early senile lentigines are visible Keratoses palpable but not visible Parallel smile lines beginning to appear Client age: 30s–40s Some foundation usually worn Mild acne scarring
Type III (advanced)	Wrinkles at rest	Advanced photoaging: Obvious dyschromia, **telangiectasias** Visible keratoses Wrinkles present even when not moving Client age: 50s or older Heavier foundation always worn Acne scarring present that makeup does not always cover
Type IV (severe)	Only wrinkles	Severe photoaging: Yellow/gray skin color Prior skin malignancies Wrinkles throughout—no normal skin Client age: 60s–70s Makeup cannot be worn (it cakes and cracks) Severe acne scarring

telangiectasias
Small visible capillaries; sometimes referred to as *broken capillaries.*

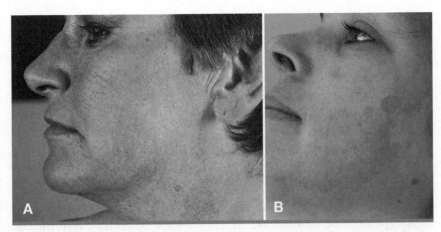

Figure 4–5 Melasma is a pigment change often thought of as "pregnancy mask."

medication or pregnancy (Figure 4–5, *B*). The origin of the pigment change is not specifically noted in the classification. If you are using this classification, you will want to note the origin of the dyschromia. This is best accomplished with a thorough health history. Most certainly, it is important to know what medications the client is taking, how those medications can affect the skin, and if the client is pregnant or breast feeding prior to microdermabrasion or any treatment.

Keratoses

Keratoses are different from pigment changes (Figure 4–6). Keratoses relate to the skin's response to the sun by the formation of rough, red, scaling patches. As you know, keratoses can become **actinic keratoses**. Actinic keratoses are sometimes called *precancerous* skin lesions and have the potential to develop into skin cancers, specifically basal cell carcinomas and squamous cell carcinomas. The number and location of keratoses are important in the aging analysis of the skin. In addition, you will be interested in the number of previous skin cancers or the suspicion of current skin cancers and their location.

Wrinkles

In this category you will be looking for how many wrinkles are present and where on the face they are present. The Glogau classification specifically speaks to the following categories: Type I, no wrinkles; Type II, wrinkles in motion; Type III, wrinkles at rest; and Type IV, only wrinkles. You will also want to advance your analysis and evaluate if the wrinkles are fine (small and only closely visible) or coarse (deep and noticeable) (Figure 4–7).

actinic keratoses
Potentially precancerous lesions of the skin, generally from sun exposure.

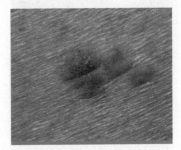

Figure 4–6 Keratoses are forerunners to basal carcinoma (BCC) and squamous cell carcinoma (SCC).

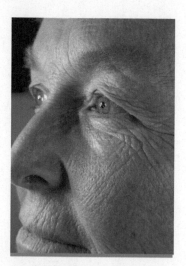

Figure 4–7 Wrinkles are most often associated with photodamage. This example of wrinkles includes static and dynamic wrinkles from aging and solar damage.

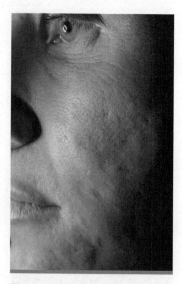

Figure 4–8 Acne scarring in this case will worsen with time as the skin becomes more lax.

Client's Chronologic Age

This category is fairly straightforward. How old is the client? However, since many clients will be age-conscious, do not ask them directly, or assume. Use the documentation provided, and avoid outwardly mentioning his or her specific age. Instead, refer to the age groupings specified by this classification.

This classification uses the age brackets of 20s to 30s for Type I, 30s to 40s for Type II, 50s to 60s for Type III, and 60s to 70s for Type IV.

Makeup

This is a tough category within the classification because it is not related to aging (intrinsic or extrinsic in the author's opinion). Nevertheless, in the Glogau aging classification it is a category that is used. The analysis assumes more makeup is used as the client grows chronologically older. As you know, makeup use is a personal choice, whether you are 20 or 70. Regardless, your client should remove all makeup prior to undergoing a skin analysis, for obvious reasons.

Acne Scarring

The category of acne scars can also be misleading. It assumes everyone has had acne, and that the scars get worse as we age. (Figure 4–8).

Using the Glogau Classification

Using the Glogau classification could be challenging for beginner and advanced aestheticians alike. The first question that should be asked when using this classification is, "What is my objective?" Multiple objectives exist within the classification system; among them is the evaluation of acne scarring, wrinkling, and solar damage (each a very different problem). The *type* is defined with two descriptors: (1) *mild, moderate, advanced,* and *severe* and (2) *no wrinkling, wrinkles in motion, wrinkles at rest,* and *only wrinkles.* If you are evaluating the client for a microdermabrasion program, the treatment approach might be somewhat different based on the classification you choose. Therefore, if you choose to use this classification, you will need to select the outstanding problem and classify it accordingly. For example, if the client's complaint is aging skin, select only those categories that apply, such as pigment changes, keratoses, wrinkling, and chronologic aging. Then classify your client accordingly. The following will make it simple:

- Type I (mild, no wrinkles)—This classification is for the mildest of problems. There are not any wrinkles present. Early signs of photoaging exist, including mild pigment changes. Signs of freckling should be looked for; no keratoses are seen. Mild to minimal acne scarring exists, and little if any makeup is worn. This client will be in his or her 20s or 30s.

- Type II (moderate, wrinkles in motion)—In Type II, problems begin to show up on the skin. This client is in his or her 30s or 40s. Early signs of sun damage are apparent, such as senile lentigines and keratoses that are on the skin but not yet visible. Smile lines appear at this stage. Not only nasolabial (those lines from the nose to the mouth) but also a secondary set of lines may be present during a smile parallel to the nasolabial line. At this age, foundation is worn and acne scarring is more obvious.
- Type III (advanced, wrinkles at rest)—This client is in his or her 50s and has advanced photoaging. Many dyschromias, telangiectasias, and visible keratoses exist. The wrinkles are present even when the face is at rest. Acne scarring is deep and not covered by makeup, and makeup is used extensively.
- Type IV (severe, only wrinkles)—The client is in his or her 60s, 70s, and beyond. The skin is defined as *sallow and gray with many wrinkles;* acne scarring is also part of this category. Previous skin cancers are also specific to this class. It is stated in this category that makeup cannot be worn, because it cakes or cracks.

Now that you understand the specifics of the categories, some examples will be helpful. A 40-year-old woman who exhibits yellow, graying skin with actinic keratoses, has not had any skin cancers, and wears little or no makeup would be classified as Type III. The overwhelming descriptor that puts her into the Type III would be the lack of skin cancers.

A second example is a 35-year-old woman with severe acne scars and visible dyschromias; she wears heavy makeup and has not had any keratoses or skin cancers. This is a tough one. Does she belong in Type II, Type III, or Type IV? If you let the acne scars be the descriptor, then she belongs in Type IV; if you let the solar damage drive the descriptor, she would be a Type II. Choose the overriding characteristic and use it to determine the classification.

Rubin Classification

The second system that is used to classify aging is the Rubin classification. The Rubin classification has simplified the Glogau and addresses only photoaging. This classification has only three levels. The specific categories that are addressed in this classification include alterations in pigmentation, texture, the presence of keratoses, and wrinkling (Table 4–8).

Table 4–8 The Rubin Method of Photodamage Classification

Level	Clinical Signs	Abnormalities
Level one (least severe)	Alterations in the epidermis only	Pigmentation and texture (freckles, lentigines, a dull rough texture because of increased thickness of the stratum corneum)
Level two (more severe)	Epidermis Papillary dermis	Same as those with level-one damage; however, pigmentary and texture charges are more marked. In addition, clients may have actinic keratoses, liver spotting, and definite increase in wrinkling
Level three (most severe)	Epidermis Papillary dermis Reticular dermis	Same as those with level-one and level-two damage; in addition, a thick leathery appearance and feel, a yellowish tint, and a pebbly texture and open comedones

Dr. Mark Rubin has been lecturing on cosmetic dermatology and skin rejuvenation at the University of California at San Diego for over 13 years. In addition, he conducts workshops on matters such as cosmetic peeling for physicians around the country. He has personally trained over 700 doctors from several countries on his techniques for skin rejuvenation. Dr. Rubin's work has been published in both books and medical journals. Currently he is conducting research at the Lasky Clinic in Beverly Hills on the subjects of chemical peels and laser resurfacing. He is also a diplomat of the American Board of Dermatology and the National Board of Medical Examiners.

Pigment

Pigment is evaluated in all three categories of the Rubin classification. You know that, as the skin ages, changes in pigment occur. What you will be looking at in the Rubin classification is the pigment changes that are related to solar damage as opposed to those created, for example, by pregnancy. Included in the analysis of the pigment are freckles and lentigines. Sometimes, if the client is older, the lentigines will be referred to as *senile lentigines*.

Texture

Texture is a strong marker for the condition of the skin. Evaluation using adjectives such as *dull, rough, leathery,* and *pebbly* help you to place the client in the correct category.

Wrinkling

You now know that wrinkling may be static or dynamic, as well as fine, moderate, or coarse. The wrinkling in the Rubin classification is not this detailed. The classification simply acknowledges that wrinkles exist and the location of the wrinkles. It will be important for you to take your analysis one step further and define the wrinkles that fall into more detailed categories.

Using the Rubin Classification

The Rubin classification is extraordinarily easy to use. With only three specific definitions, clients easily fall into a specific category. Remember, this classification relates only to extrinsic aging patterns.

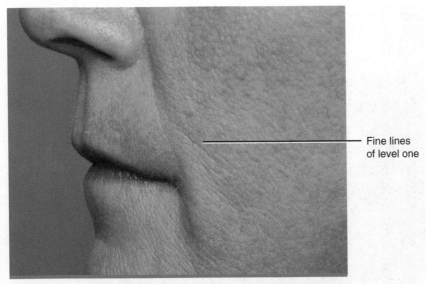

Fine lines
of level one

Figure 4–9 Rubin classification for aging level one (see Table 4–8 on page 109).

You will need to create an intrinsic aging analysis if you use this classification.

- Level One—Level one is defined as *least severe* solar damage. It represents those who have a few freckles, perhaps some lentigines, and the beginning of a thicker stratum corneum. Those in level one rarely have wrinkles; if they do, it is fine static wrinkling. We do not define a chronologic age for these clients, because this client can be 20 years old or 45 years old depending on sun exposure (Figure 4–9).
- Level Two—Level two is defined as *more severe* solar damage. In addition to freckles and lentigines, a marked change and advancement of the irregularity of the color of the skin exists. The stratum corneum is thicker and more irregular. More wrinkles, usually around the eyes and in the nasolabial fold (smile line), are seen. Additionally, Dr. Rubin feels the skin will begin to look *crinkled* at this level (Figure 4–10).
- Level Three—Level three is defined as *most severe* solar damage. In this category the skin is wrinkled at rest, many dyschromias exist, and the skin is thick and leathery in appearance and to the touch. The skin has the yellow, dull, sometimes-gray color that clients complain looks "dirty." The histologic changes in this category penetrate to the reticular dermis. This level of solar damage also has some open comedones, making the surface even more irregular (Figure 4–11).

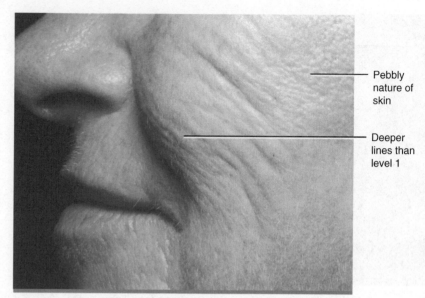

Pebbly nature of skin

Deeper lines than level 1

Figure 4–10 Rubin classification for aging level two (see Table 4–8 on page 109).

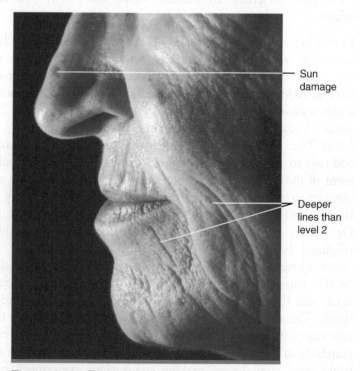

Sun damage

Deeper lines than level 2

Figure 4–11 Rubin classification for aging level three (see Table 4–8 on page 109).

▪ PUTTING IT ALL TOGETHER

On the surface, skin typing and analysis seem straightforward and easy to do. Although the categories are clear and the idea of using the definitions to categorize clients seems simple, it is not as easy as you may think.

Examples

How do you put the Fitzpatrick Typing scale and one of the aging classifications together to have an understanding of the skin? To understand this process, consider the following:

- Example #1 (Figure 4–12)—Melinda is a 35-year-old woman. She was raised in Northern California, but spent her college years in New York City. Melinda loved to sun with her girlfriends, usually applying Hawaiian tanning oil to her face with a sun protection factor of four (SPF 4). She thought SPF 4 was enough protection to prevent damage from the sun. She comes to your office complaining of solar damage that is presenting as freckles and some very fine lines, especially around the eyes. The texture of her skin is rough and dry, but she has never had acne. She wears quite a bit of makeup, including foundation, blush, eye, and lip color. She has white skin. Her eye color is light blue, and she has blond hair. Her mother is of English heritage, but her father has brown hair and eyes and is German. She burns in the sun on the first exposure, usually in about 20 minutes. What is the Fitzpatrick skin type? What Glogau classification is she? What Rubin classification is she? Is she a candidate for microdermabrasion?

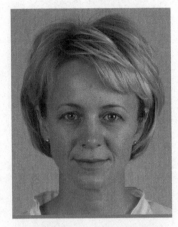

Figure 4–12 Example #1— Case study analysis. Melinda is a 35-year-old woman.

- Example #2 (Figure 4–13)—Joan is a 55-year-old retired woman. She and her husband of 30 years love to golf. Joan was raised in Dallas and went to college in Southern California. She loves the sun and likes to be tan. Joan used baby oil on her face and chest with aluminum foil as a reflector to ensure a tan. Joan had a facelift five years ago. She comes to the office today complaining of the texture of her skin. She would like her skin to be smoother, just like her new granddaughter. Joan's skin is white; she has light brown hair and light brown eyes. Her parents were Italian. She wears moderate makeup, eye color, lip color, and blush. Her skin is solar damaged; she has a pebbly texture and many lines (both static and dynamic) that are moderately deep. She had acne as a teenager, and some scars remain on her cheeks. She will only turn pink when she is in the sun without SPF, then she will tan right away. What is the Fitzpatrick skin type? What is the Glogau classification? What is the Rubin classification? Is she a candidate for microdermabrasion?

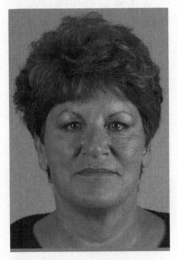

Figure 4–13 Example #2— Case study analysis. Joan is a 55-year-old woman.

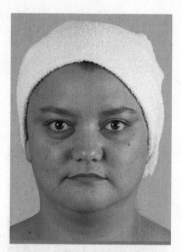

Figure 4–14 Example #3—Case study analysis. Phyllis is a 48-year-old woman.

> Clients in the *deeper aging categories* (level two and above) have problems that are, for the most part, not going to be *solved* by microdermabrasion. Your choice to treat these clients will come with the caveat of realistic expectations.

- Example #3 (Figure 4–14)—Phyllis is a 48-year-old widow. She is living alone in New York City, where she is a police officer. She is outdoors every day. She is a native New Yorker who played in the sun during the summer but never sat in the sun. Phyllis has dark brown skin, her hair is naturally black, and her eyes are brown. She was adopted and never knew her birth parents. She wears no makeup. Her skin is oily, thick, and has broken out since she was a teenager. She has scarring because of the breakouts. She never burns and never wears an SPF. She would like to improve her breakouts and make the skin a little bit smoother. What is the Fitzpatrick skin type? What is the Glogau classification? What is the Rubin classification? Is she a candidate for microdermabrasion?

CONCLUSION

Now you understand the method by which all medical professionals collect information about the skin's color and aging. Your own analysis will help you to choose your clients wisely. The skin color analysis tells you who will tolerate moderate treatments, who will tolerate aggressive treatments, which clients tan, and how much time they normally spend in the sun (an important part of the compliance component of medical skin care treatments). Clients in the deeper aging categories (level two and above) have problems that are, for the most part, not going to be solved by microdermabrasion. Your choice to treat these clients will come with the caveat of realistic expectations. When you meld the two classifications (skin color analysis and aging analysis), you can select your clients with ease, knowing that you have an understanding of the predictable outcome.

Top 10 Tips to Take to the Spa

1. The Fitzpatrick Skin Typing process is a commonly accepted method of predicting the skin's response to UV light.

2. The Fitzpatrick Skin Typing process can predict the skin's response to chemical peeling, laser treatments, and microdermabrasion.

3. The Fitzpatrick Skin Typing method should be used on every client seen to ensure the proper treatment plan has been selected.

4. The aesthetician must inquire about the client's ethnic history and sun exposure history to find the right Fitzpatrick assignment.

5. Eye color and natural hair color are indicators for Fitzpatrick assignment.

6. A Glogau classification or a Rubin classification is necessary to complete client analysis.

7. Melding an aging analysis and a skin-typing assignment will determine who is best suited for microdermabrasion treatments. Usually skin types I, II, and III have the best results with microdermabrasion.

8. The Rubin classification is easier to use than the Glogau classification.

9. Generally, most skin types are *mixed* and require study to ascertain the correct typing.

10. Asking questions about childhood sunburns will help determine the accurate skin type.

Chapter Review Questions

1. Why do you determine skin type before doing microdermabrasion? Why do you do an aging analysis before microdermabrasion?

2. How do you identify the skin type of someone who is tanned?

3. How do you identify the skin type of someone with colored hair?

4. How do variables in individual skin type affect microdermabrasion treatments?

5. Explain the difference between skin condition, type, and analysis.

6. Discuss a few of the different types of skin typing and describe the situations in which they might be appropriate to use.

7. Why might Fitzpatrick Skin Typing be the preeminent skin typing method for microdermabrasion?

8. True or False: The Glogau Skin Typing method is used to evaluate skin type for suitability for microdermabrasion.

9. Describe the different levels of Fitzpatrick Skin Type. Which are most suitable for microdermabrasion treatment?

10. Why is important to discuss genetic skin considerations with the client?

11. What is the single most important consideration when it comes to skin typing? How might you ascertain this information from your clients?

12. What are some of the symptoms of solar aging?

13. True or False: The most common types of irregular pigment are those associated with sun damage.

14. Describe the different levels within the Glogau Classification Method. Which are most responsive to microdermabrasion treatments?

15. What are keratoses? What types are there?

16. Describe the Rubin Classification Types. Which ones will benefit the most from microdermabrasion?

17. A client comes into your spa. She is a 61-year-old female with Fitzpatrick Type II skin, graying blond hair, and deep wrinkling, Rubin level two. Her skin is fair, and pigment is somewhat even considering her age and her moderate sun exposure when she was younger. A friend who has regular microdermabrasion treatments raves about the results, and she is convinced the treatment can take ten years off her appearance. How would you deal with this client?

Chapter References

1. Rubin, M. (1995). *Manual of chemical peels*. Philadelphia: Lippincott, Williams & Wilkins.
2. *Fitzpatrick Skin Typing Chart* (Part 1—Genetic Disposition). (2005). Used with the permission of the Medical Procedure Center, P.C., and adapted from multiple sources.
3. *Fitzpatrick Skin Typing Chart* (Part 2—Reaction to Sun Exposure). (2004). Used with the permission of the Medical Procedure Center, P.C., and adapted from multiple sources.
4. *Fitzpatrick Skin Typing Chart* (Part 3—Tanning Habits). (2004). Used with the permission of the Medical Procedure Center, P.C., and adapted from multiple sources.
5. *Fitzpatrick Skin Typing Chart* (Part 4—Scoring). (2004). Used with the permission of the Medical Procedure Center, P.C., and adapted from multiple sources.
6. *Fitzpatrick Skin Typing Chart* (Part 5—Your Fitzpatrick Skin Type). (2004). Used with the permission of the Medical Procedure Center, P.C., and adapted from multiple sources.

Fundamentals of Skin Care

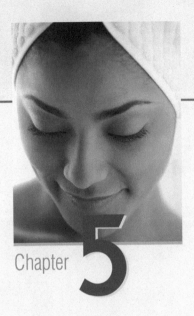

Chapter 5

Key Terms

acetic acid
acid mantle
acidic
alkaline
alpha hydroxy acids
    (AHAs)
anthranilates
antimicrobials
ascorbyl palmitate
azelaic acid
benzophenones
camphors
cinnamates
citric acid
d-alpha tocopherol
detergents
dibenzoylmethanes
Eldopaque®
emollients
erythema
ester
free radicals

gel solution
glycolic acid
humectants
hydroquinone
kojic acid
l-ascorbic acid
lactic acid
magnesium ascorbyl
    phosphate
malic acid
Melquin®
moisturizers
neutral
nicotinamide
para-aminobenzoic
    acid (PABA)
Parsol 1789®
photodamage
potential of hydrogen
    (pH)
preservative
Renova

Retin A® (tretinoin)
Retin A
    Microsphere®
retinols
retinyl palmitate
salicylates
selenium
sodium lauryl
    isethionate
sodium lauryl sulfate
sun protection factor
    (SPF)
sunscreens
surfactants
tartaric acid
titanium dioxide
tyrosine
ubiquinone (Co-Q$_{10}$)
vitamin B
vitamin C
vitamin E
zinc oxide

Learning Objectives

After completing this chapter you should be able to:

1. Discuss the importance of cosmeceuticals.
2. Identify the significance of moisturizers and cleansers.
3. Discuss the use and importance of moisturizers and cleansers.
4. Describe the use and importance of vitamin C.
5. Discuss the use and importance of sunscreens.
6. Discuss the use and importance of hydroquinone.
7. Discuss the use and importance of retinoids.

INTRODUCTION

Although the focus of this text is microdermabrasion, the treatment does not happen independently. A good microdermabrasion treatment program requires three components: (1) the pretreatment plan, (2) the clinical treatment, and (3) the post-care plan. The three components are equally necessary, and the outcome can be compromised if any one of the three is not followed through.

The products used in the at-home segment (pretreatment and post-treatment) of the microdermabrasion program include cosmeceuticals, quality **sunscreens**, **moisturizers**, cleansers, and, in a medical environment, prescription products. As a skin-care professional you already have knowledge of the principles and value of quality sunscreens. In addition, although cleansers and moisturizers seem to be elementary subjects, they really will influence the success or failure of a program more than we once understood. Prescriptions are necessities in many medical skin programs, and this concept may be new to you. Furthermore, prescriptions may not be available to all aestheticians and clients. This will depend on the particular spa environment. Typically, only aestheticians who work in a medi-spa, supervised by a medical doctor, may recommend prescription-strength remedies to their clients. Finally, cosmeceuticals are a type of product that you should understand and know how to represent to your client. Cosmeceuticals will be discussed in greater detail in this chapter. This chapter will address medical skin care products that are absolutely necessary to augment the result of the procedure, and products that will make a noticeable difference when used properly, or improperly.

sunscreens
Any agent that protects the skin from harmful UVA and UVB light, helping to protect skin from photodamage including skin cancers and dyschromia; blocks rays either by physical or chemical means.

moisturizers
Agent that replenishes moisture to the skin.

▪ COSMECEUTICALS

The Food and Drug Administration (FDA) was created in 1938 to review products and keep the citizens of our country safe. The product review fell into two categories: (1) the drug category, and (2) the cosmetic category. Cosmetics, according to the FDA, are "intended for beautifying and promoting attractiveness."[1] A drug, on the other hand, is defined as a "substance used in the diagnosis, cure, treatment or prevention of disease, *intended to affect the structure and function of the body*."[2] While this simply defines drugs and cosmetics, the definitions are rather antiquated, and leave a vast gray area.

Dr. Albert Kligman, a professor emeritus at the University of Pennsylvania's school of dermatology, agreed. He thought that the two definitions were blurred. He theorized that drugs and cosmetics overlapped quite a bit. According to Dr. Kligman, it is not the ingredients in the product, but the claims made by the product's manufacturer that differentiate drugs from cosmetics.

At a meeting of the Society of Cosmetic Chemists in 1980, Dr. Kligman introduced a thought-provoking question: "Are there any ingredients that we apply to the skin that *do not* affect its structure?" The idea and the subsequent term, *cosmeceutical*, caused discussion and polarization that continues today. He meant the term to include those products that do more than decorate or camouflage but less than a drug would do.[3] To prove his point that all ingredients penetrate the skin, Dr. Kligman did a small yet meaningful experiment. He applied wet cotton to the skin and used a dressing to hold it in place. By the end of the second day, the water had begun to cause an inflammatory response in the dermis. Thus, even water can penetrate the skin, supporting the argument that even the most basic of elements can change the surface of the skin: hence, the term *cosmeceuticals*. This experiment and the ensuing argument had, and still has, great consequences for the aesthetics industry.

The FDA has not updated the cosmetic or drug categories, and the agency has no intention of making changes any time soon. Although this is a good thing for cosmetic companies and their products, it does leave room for interpretation as to what constitutes drugs and what constitutes cosmetics. The FDA does not recognize cosmeceuticals; however, it is important for skin-care professionals to be aware of the term and what it means. Many interpretations exist. To be purists about both the definition and the potential of products on the skin, all skin-care products should be identified as cosmeceuticals (because even a moisturizer will change the barrier effect of the skin). The ways in which products are used define the new reality. In many ways, national economics drive the unwillingness of the FDA to change the current laws as defined in 1938. Chaos would certainly follow if such significant changes were implemented. For example, imagine the uproar if body lotion were to be reclassified as a drug.

What ought to be achieved with this definition is a categorization of *more active* products versus *less active* products, such as cleansers and moisturizers. By using the term *cosmeceuticals,* products can differentiated and a sense of value for both the aesthetician and the client can be created. Among the products classified in this category are **alpha hydroxy acids (AHAs)**, **vitamin C**, and **retinols**. The aforementioned products are not prescriptions but do have scientifically known effects on the skin and its layers.

Using Cosmeceuticals

Cosmeceuticals are found in salons, on cable shopping networks, and on retail shelves in varying percentages and **potential of hydrogen (pH)**, making their use (and result) somewhat unpredictable for the average consumer. Complicating matters even more, most consumers are unaware of the degree to which these products affect their skin. The above-mentioned outlets have less of an opportunity to provide the information necessary to help the client learn to use the product properly. Using cosmeceuticals is a responsibility. Education of the staff and the client, and ethical marketing, are key points to the success of cosmeceuticals in the spa.

As discussed, intended use defines the category of the product. Marketing should not be misleading and should stay within the category. Therefore, using phrases such as "appears to" or "will seem to" are important marketing terms that do not overstep the bounds of the FDA definitions. Abuse of marketing terms always get the attention of the FDA.

Medical Office and Cosmeceuticals

In the medical world of skin care, cosmeceuticals are a staple in the product cabinet. The ingredients are well-recognized by aestheticians and clients as *active* but not *medicinal*. Choosing the cosmeceutical products for a medical office is a daunting task. Many available product lines are directed specifically at medical offices. The basic products that should be in the cosmeceutical armamentarium of the medical office include active cleansers, moisturizers, and vitamin C.

Salon and Spa Cosmeceuticals Use

The spa world has access to cosmeceuticals just like the medical spa, but the vendors may be different. The spa has an increased responsibility to

---

Education is an ongoing responsibility of the spa. New employees should be well educated about the product that is available to sell. In turn, employees should be capable of educating clients, recognizing problems and anticipating results.

To be purists about both the definition and the potential of products on the skin, all skin-care products should be identified as cosmeceuticals, because even a moisturizer will change the barrier effect of the skin.

---

alpha hydroxy acids (AHAs)
Mild organic acids used in cosmeceutical products; AHAs "unglue" cells in the epidermis, allowing keratinocytes to be shed at the stratum granulosum and providing skin with a healthier texture.

vitamin C
Antioxidant that is a necessary factor for the formation of collagen in connective tissue and maintenance of integrity of intercellular cement.

retinols
Vitamin A derivatives that must first convert to retinoic acid before being useful to the skin.

potential of hydrogen (pH)
Scale by which a material is characterized as being acidic (pH less than 7.0), alkaline (greater than 7.0), or neutral (7.0).

Table 5–1 Inventory of Cosmeceutical Products for the Medical
Spa and Luxury Spa

Cleansers (with alpha hydroxy acids [AHAs])
AHAs (glycolic and lactic)
Salicylic acids
Vitamin C
Power moisturizers

be mindful of these products and dispense them carefully. The public may perceive that the products they purchase from the spa are weaker than those from the medical office, but this is simply not true. Furthermore, the client may believe that because the products are not those found in the medical setting, he or she will not be at risk for potential complications. Again, simply not true. Because the luxury spa may not have a physician on staff, it will be necessary to choose products that are higher in pH than the ones found in the medical spa. This is just common sense to protect the spa from liabilities. The product line chosen by the salon or spa should include the same basic components as the medical spa: cleansers, AHAs, vitamin C, and *power* moisturizers (Table 5–1).

CLEANSERS

A good cleanser will have an immediate, noticeable effect on the skin. To understand what makes a *good* cleanser, one should begin with pH, which defines any good cleanser or soap (Table 5–2). A basic rule of

Table 5–2 Common Hand and Bath Soaps[5]

Soap	pH Range
Camay®	9.2–9.7
Dial®	9.2–9.7
Dove®	6.8–7.2
Irish Spring®	9.2–9.7
Ivory®	9.2–9.7
Lever 2000®	8.8–9.2
Palmolive®	9.8–10.2
Zest®	9.8–10.2

Try to stock at least three cleansers: one with glycolic acid for normal and combination skin, one with salicylic acid for oily and acne-prone skin, and one that is void of active ingredients. When considering the treatment products, have a broad selection including glycolic acids in varying percentages and vehicles (creams, solutions, serums), lactic acid in varying percentages and vehicles, and a salicylic acid toner. When evaluating vitamin C, carry two types of vitamin C (one in an *l*-ascorbic form and one in a magnesium ascorbyl phosphate or ascorbyl palmitate form). Finally, moisturizers need to contain antioxidants, usually green tea, selenium, or vitamin E.

The importance of cosmeceuticals in a medical plan cannot be overstated Their effect on the skin is unlike the prescriptions available but, when combined, their sum is greater than the individual parts.

glycolic acid
Alpha hydroxy acid derived from sugar cane; has a small molecular size that allows for easier penetration into the skin.

lactic acid
Alpha hydroxy acid derived from milk.

magnesium ascorbyl phosphate
Water-soluble and fat-soluble form of vitamin C; it is a vitamin C ester.

ascorbyl palmitate
Fat-soluble form of ascorbic acid.

selenium
Chemical agent resembling sulfur; helps protect the skin from solar-induced skin cancers.

vitamin E
Antioxidant that has been shown to inactivate free radicals; the exact mechanism that controls this function is unknown.

alkaline
Anything that has a pH greater than 7.0.

sodium lauryl isethionate
Similar to sodium lauryl sulfate but not as irritating; less effective as an emulsifier.

acidic
Anything that has a pH less than 7.0.

acid mantle
Thin coating on the stratum corneum that is intended to protect the skin from infection and has a pH of 4 to 6.5; frequent use of products that are too alkaline puts the skin at risk for infection.

detergents
Synthetic cleansing agent that acts as a wetting agent and emulsifier.

surfactants
Surface-active agent that lowers surface tension.

antimicrobials
Agent that halts or prevents the development of microorganisms.

thumb is that the more alkaline (pH higher than 7.0), the more drying the product will be to the skin. Because the normal pH of the skin is between 4.5 and 6.5,[4] using a more alkaline cleanser or body soap is likely to make the skin feel tight and dry. A moisturizing bar such as Dove, which contains sodium lauryl isethionate, will have a pH of 5 to 7. This pH is still not quite acidic enough to prevent disruption of the acid mantle.

It can safely be assumed that over-the-counter (OTC) soaps are more alkaline and that cleansers are more acidic. In addition, that dry tight feeling left by soap is not an indication of cleanliness, but rather a stripping of the acid mantle of the stratum corneum. This is a point of education with your clients, especially the oily or acne-prone client.

The second important component of cleansers is the actual ability to cleanse the skin. Cleansing is made possible by a variety of substances including detergents, surfactants, antimicrobials, emollients, moisturizers, humectants, and preservatives. Examples of common ingredients found in cleansers are sodium lauryl sulfate and diethanolalamine (DEA), cocamidopropyl betaine, isohexadecane. These ingredients all remove oils, dirt, and makeup, and have been used for many years without complications to humans. These ingredients work and are safe for use around the eyes and mouth.

Acid Mantle: Our Protection Against Infection

The acid mantle is a thin coating on the stratum corneum that measures 4 to 6.5 pH. The purpose of this acid cover or mantle is to protect the skin from bacteria and fungal infections. A constant disruption in the acid mantle can cause the skin to be at risk for infection. It is important to select moisturizers and cleansers that avoid putting the skin at risk. Most soaps are alkaline. It can take the skin up to 36 hours to recover from a cleansing with an alkaline cleanser. The products selected for clients should be neutral or slightly acid-based to keep the skin from excess dryness and risk of infection.

The choice of a cleanser for your client is based on the two important facts already covered: (1) pH and (2) the ability to cleanse. However, one cleanser is not right for all skin types or conditions, so the aesthetician must evaluate the skin and choose a cleanser carefully (Table 5–3). For example, oily skin requires salicylic in the cleanser,

Table 5-3 Common Cleansers and Moisturizers in the Medical Office

Manufacturer	Product	pH Range
Hymed®	Hymed liquid soap	5.5–5.9
	Hymed facial cleanser	4.3–5.7
	Super-hydrating lotion	5.55–6.6
La Roche®	Purifying cleanser	5.25–5.8
	Hydroactive emulsion	5.5–6.5
Jan Marini®	Glycolic cleanser	3.0–3.4
	BioCleanser	4.8–5.2
	All moisturizers	neutral
Niadyne®	Facial cleanser	6.8–7.2
	Moisturizer	7.1–7.4
Skinceuticals®	Normal to dry cleanser	4–6
	Oily/combination	4–6
	Moisturizer	7.1–7.7
IS Clinical®	All-skin cleanser	6.0–6.2
	Moisturizer	6.0–7.0
Dermalogica®	Cleanser	4.5–5.5
	Moisturizer	4.5–5.5
Neostrada®	Cleanser	3.8–4.2
	Antibacterial cleanser	3.8–4.2
	Daily moisturizers	8–15
MD Formulations®	Oily/combination	3.5–3.9
	Dry/normal	3.5–3.9
Murad®	Refreshing cleanser	5.5–6.1
	Clarifying cleanser	3.8–4.5

emollients
Product that has a softening or soothing effect on the skin.

humectants
Moisturizing agent.

preservative
Agent used to prevent spoilage.

sodium lauryl sulfate
Common ingredient in household detergents and soaps; most commonly used as an emulsifier.

neutral
Having a pH that is exactly 7.0; neither acidic nor alkaline.

If the client insists on the use of washcloths, chamois, or sponges, it is important to teach him or her how to clean the *implement* after each use. If possible, these implements should be considered single-use items. Once finished with the facial cleansing routine, the sponge, washcloth, or chamois should be tossed into the washing machine. That said, disposable sponges are a wise recommendation. If the sponge is disposable, throw it away. Do not try to get more than one use out of it. Finally, if a client chooses to use a facial-cleansing implement, a tendency exists to pull harder, push harder, and generally be rougher on the skin than one would be with just the fingertips.

whereas dry skin needs to be cleansed gently, without AHAs. By making a careful evaluation of the client's skin type and skin condition, you can select the appropriate cleansing product.

Client Education for Cleansers

Most individuals are aware of how to use cleansers and moisturizers; however, even the simplest task can sometimes be overwhelming when starting a new program. Therefore, explain how to use each product, beginning with the cleanser.

Cleansers should be used with the fingertips (massaged into a wet face, splashed off, patted dry). Washcloths, sponges, and facial chamois have several drawbacks and are not recommended. First, they can harbor bacteria and cause breakouts. Second, washcloths often do not rinse clean of the laundry detergent. This can be noted by the suds or film of suds in the sink when the washcloth is filled with water before use. When using a washcloth under these circumstances, you are adding detergent (laundry detergent) to the facial cleanser.

Exfoliation

Exfoliation is an important part of the cleansing routine, especially when using cosmeceuticals and prescriptions. Products such as AHAs and Retin A® (tretinoin) have a tendency to slough the skin and compact the stratum corneum. The result of this action on the skin is peeling, commonly called *facial dandruff*. Clients will often require assistance with cleansing this peeling with as little irritation and injury to the skin as possible (Table 5–4).

Cleansers for Normal Skin

Normal skin requires a cleanser that will dissolve the makeup and oils from the face and neck. It does not generally need to be augmented with AHAs. The cleanser stocked at your medical spa or luxury spa should be a milky cleanser, preferably with isohexadecane.

Cleansers for Oily Skin

Oily skin cleansers need to be prepared to treat acne-prone skin as well. These cleansers should include salicylic acid. Salicylic acid will digest

Retin A® (tretinoin)
Keratolytic agent used to treat acne and reverse photodamage.

Table 5–4 Cleansers for Specific Skin Types

Normal Skin	Mild cleanser containing isohexadecane
Oily Skin	Cleanser should contain salicylic acid
Dry Skin	Cleanser should contain moisturizers such as glycerin or lactic acid
Combination Skin	Cleanser should contain glycolic acid
Sensitive Skin	Cleanser should contain moisturizers such as glycerin but no AHAs

debris on the surface of the skin. This is extraordinarily helpful for those oily-skinned individuals who break out regularly.

Cleansers for Dry Skin

Cleansers for dry skin should focus on ingredients that improve the hydration of the stratum corneum such as glycerin or lactic acid. These cleansers should be creamy in nature.

Cleansers for Combination Skin

A cleanser for combination skin is often the most difficult to choose. If areas of the skin are vastly different (e.g., the cheeks are much drier than the T-zone), an inappropriate cleanser could cause the dry areas to become drier and perhaps sensitive. Combination skin should really be considered normal, with a T-zone of larger pores and slightly more sebum activity. Use a cleanser with glycolic acid for this skin type.

Cleansers for Sensitive Skin

Cleansers for sensitive skin usually are fragrance-free, color-free, and do not have any AHAs or *bioactive* ingredients. Sensitive skin is also often dry, so similar choices for these skin conditions should be suitable.

ALPHA HYDROXY ACIDS

AHAs are so much more than they were in the 1990s when the application was a simple **gel solution**, the purpose of which was still under investigation. More is known about these acids today, and their use in the skin-care industry is nearly universal in cleansers, moisturizers, and treatment products. For example, AHAs may change the condition of the lipid barrier of the skin, allowing a faster penetration of products. This is so important. Think about it—a product that will help the absorption of Retin A or moisturizers. In fact, some believe that AHAs help to improve dry skin. It helps you to understand that a program without AHAs is basically useless or at the very least elementary (Tables 5–5 and 5–6).

AHAs have gained and sustained popularity in cosmetic products over the past 19 years because of their efficacy, safety, and ease of use. In the beginning, the public had uneasiness about *acids* on the face, and some clients were truly frightened of the idea of acids being applied to their skin. Although most people think of acids as strong and dangerous, two

gel solution
Semisolid material that is easily absorbed in the skin without the irritation associated with other cream-based solutions.

Table 5–5 Alpha Hydroxy Acids for Specific Skin Types

Normal skin	AHAs should be 12%–18%, and pH should be in the 3.0–3.5 range
Oily skin	AHAs (preferably salicylic) 10%–12% and a higher pH, around 3.8
Dry skin	AHAs (preferably lactic acid) should be eased into program with 8%–10% and a higher pH, about 4.0–4.3
Combination skin	AHAs should be 12%–18% gels or serums and pH should be in the 2.8–3.5 range
Sensitive skin	AHAs (preferably lactic acid) should be eased into program with 8%–10% and a higher pH, about 4.0–4.3

Table 5–6 Alpha Hydroxy Acids for Specific Skin Types

Skin Type	Alpha Hydroxy Acids (AHAs)	pH Range
Normal skin	12%–18%	2.8–3.5
Oily skin	Preferably salicylic 10%–12%	About 3.8
Dry skin	Preferably lactic acid should be eased into program with 8%–10%	About 4.0–4.3
Combination skin	12%–18% gels or serums	2.8–3.5
Sensitive skin	Preferably lactic acid should be eased into program with 8%–10%	About 4.0–4.3

AHAs are fruit acids or organic acids. They are derived from products such as sugar cane (glycolic acid), apples (**malic acid**), grapes (**tartaric acid**), citric fruit (**citric acid**) and milk (lactic acid).

acetic acid
Mild organic acid derived from vinegar.

malic acid
Alpha hydroxy acid derived from apples.

tartaric acid
Alpha hydroxy acid derived from grapes.

citric acid
Alpha hydroxy acid derived from citrus fruit, such as oranges and grapefruit.

types of acids exist: (1) organic or fruit acids and (2) mineral acids. Mineral acids are very strong and can be dangerous; they include hydrochloric acid and sulfuric acid. The idea of these acids being put on the skin is a scary thought. Organic acids, on the other hand, are usually very mild and are commonly found in everyday life. Examples of organic acids are glycolic acid, lactic acid, or even **acetic acid** (vinegar).

Glycolic acids are often selected for use in cosmetics because of their small molecular size and easy penetration into the skin. It is now known that AHAs work on both the dermis and the epidermis. In the epidermis, the AHA "unglues" cells and allows the shedding of keratinocytes at the stratum granulosum.[6] In the dermis, AHAs work by increasing the ground substance and boosting collagen remodeling. Clinically, this phenomenon is observed as an initial dryness followed by a plumpness of the skin.

Aside from the particular AHA (glycolic versus lactic), two other important considerations exist when selecting an AHA: (1) pH and (2) percentage. If the pH is low and the percentage is high, there will be greater bioavailability of the acid. This phenomenon allows the skin to absorb the AHA quickly and efficiently. The pH and the percentage work together, and the proper balance is critical to the overall success the product will have on the skin. The pH range should be approximately 3.0 to 4.0, and the percentage should be 12 to 18 percent for the best result.

Client Education for Alpha Hydroxy Acids

The FDA evaluated AHA safety in 1997. The information that came from this evaluation gave specific recommendations about the percentages of glycolic appropriate for OTC use compared with salon or spa use. Additionally, the FDA spoke to the importance of using sunscreen when using AHAs.

Alpha Hydroxy Acids for Normal Skin

Normal skin can tolerate just about any type of glycolic acid: cream, solution, gel, or serum (a serum or gel, if possible). The pH of the solution should be in the range of 3.0 to 3.5. The percentage of AHA should be 12 to 18 percent.

Alpha Hydroxy Acids for Oily Skin

Oily-skinned clients often break out. The glycolic for these clients needs to be potentially less irritating: a 3.8 pH and a moderate percentage such as 10 to 12 percent. When the client is breaking out, a salicylic acid (which is not an AHA) is preferable over glycolic, although both can work well. The salicylic at 10 to 12 percent with a pH of 3.8 seems to do a better job at unroofing the comedones and clearing the debris on the surface of the skin. Use a solution over a gel, cream, or serum in this case. Clients with oily skin will respond better to a solution.

Alpha Hydroxy Acids for Dry Skin

Dry skin requires a slow start with AHAs because they will sting and cause erythema and irritation. For glycolic, choose a product that is high

Show clients the dose you want them to use. For example, tell clients to use a pea-sized amount, and then squirt this amount onto the back of your hand so they can see what you mean. Then lift this amount up and use the fingertips of both hands to apply it to the face. The leftover amount should be massaged into the backs of the hands. Let them know *this is a medicine, not a moisturizer.* If the skin is feeling dry, apply a little bit more moisturizer or evaluate the moisturizer being used; do not use more glycolic cream. Remind clients that it is okay for the AHA to tingle or even sting a little. AHA with a pH of 3.0 or less will usually sting or burn, especially when used by the beginner client. This sting or burn should subside in about 60 to 90 seconds; if not, the client should splash it off. Initially, the stinging might happen every day, but if the client uses the product regularly as advised, the stinging will subside over time. If it does not get easier and the client experiences persistent erythema, change the product to a higher pH product. These problems often have less to do with the

Continued

Client education about AHAs should focus on the application and use of the product. Specifically, the client needs to understand that *overuse* will cause irritation, erythema, and ultimately frustration. This educational process is best accomplished by a demonstration on the proper use of the product followed by written instructions.

erythema
Spot on the skin showing diffused redness caused by capillary congestion.

free radicals
Atoms with an unpaired electron.

Oral vitamin C, whether from food or supplements, is not adequate to perform the antioxidant tasks necessary to improve the skin. Oral vitamin C does not make it to the dermis before it is either used up or expired. It is recommended that all therapeutic programs include a topical vitamin C.

in pH (4.0 up to 4.3) and low in percentage, perhaps 8 to 10 percent. You can ease up the dose as the client is able to tolerate the product. Lactic acid is recommended for dry skin. Clients will tolerate it without as much irritation or erythema. If possible, then choose a product, regardless of your AHA choice, that is in a cream or gel form.

Alpha Hydroxy Acids for Combination Skin

The best choice for combination skin is glycolic gels or serums. This skin condition will respond best to these delivery vehicles. The percentages and pH are very much the same as the normal skin applications.

Alpha Hydroxy Acids for Sensitive Skin

AHAs may be difficult for sensitive skin types to tolerate. A low percentage and a high pH are the best choice. Like dry skin, lactic acid may be better tolerated than glycolic acid for sensitive skin. If you have the flexibility to start with a high pH and low percentage lactic acid, that is great; begin there on an every-other-day basis. Evaluate the skin in one week to determine if the application can be increased to daily. If so, instruct the client accordingly. If not, just stay at every other day. The client will benefit even at this rate.

VITAMIN C

Free radicals cause damage to cells, forcing the aging process into an accelerated pace. Free radical damage occurs when atoms or groups of atoms have an odd (unpaired) number of *electrons*. Smoking, air pollution, and the sun all stimulate free radical damage to the skin. Simply by exposing your skin to the sun, the level of vitamin C in the skin drops by 30 percent[7] and, subsequently, free radicals are formed. *Antioxidants* couple with free radicals to neutralize the unpaired electron. Vitamin C is recognized for its strong antioxidant properties and *photoprotective* properties,[8] although it is *never* recommended that vitamin C be substituted for sunscreen (Table 5–7).

Because topical vitamin C has become a fundamental part of a skin-care program, there has been controversy over how much and what type is the best. The answer to this question, much like other subjects within skin care, varies based on the available data and the aesthetician's interpretation of that data. The questions to be asked include: should

Table 5–7 Vitamin C for Specific Skin Types

Skin Type	Vitamin C Preference	pH Range
Normal skin	Both ester and *l*-ascorbic (10% to start)	3.6–3.8
Oily skin	*l*-ascorbic 12%–15%	3.6–3.8
Dry skin	Ester in an emollient delivery vehicle	4.0–4.3
Combination skin	Both ester and *l*-ascorbic (10% to start) in a serum or cream delivery vehicle	3.0–3.5
Sensitive skin	Ester	4.0–4.3

the topical vitamin C be an **ester** or *l*-**ascorbic acid**? A cream or a gel? A separate application or combined with a moisturizer? The debate begins by answering these questions.

ester
Water- and fat-soluble.

l-ascorbic acid
Water-soluble vitamin C.

Client Education for Vitamin C

Because vitamin C is an extra step in the program, some clients are reluctant to add the product as a separate component of the program. However, because of its strong antioxidant value, every client should be on topical vitamin C. Two reasons make it advisable to wait until the second or third week to add this step into the program: First, vitamin C can be irritating; when the program starts with AHA and Retin A, it may be too much for the client to tolerate. Second, clients should "get into the swing" of a new program and find success with the multisteps before you throw something else into the mix. For this reason, you may want to add vitamin C into the morning routine after the AHA.

Topical vitamin C comes in two varieties: (1) *l*-ascorbic (water-soluble) and (2) esters (water- and fat-soluble). The esters and *l*-ascorbic are distinctly different. Originally identified at Duke University, *l*-ascorbic acid penetrates quickly and is used by the skin immediately. However, it deteriorates quickly through oxidation if it is in a light-colored container that is exposed to air each time the client uses the product. This is why you will often see vitamin C in a dark-brown bottle or an airless container. Vitamin C esters are ascorbyl palmitate and magnesium ascorbyl phosphate. They have a longer shelf life and are *time released* on the skin. The time-released phenomenon is due to the ester waiting for the skin to convert the product into usable vitamin C. Esters have a more even absorption compared with the blast of *l*-ascorbic. Esters are also less irritating. The pH is important with vitamin C: 3.5 pH or lower creates the best environment for the product to absorb.

It is important to understand about percentages when dealing with vitamin C, because clients will always ask. If the product you are using is *l*-ascorbic, a percentage can be determined. If, on the other hand, you are using an ester, a percentage cannot be determined. Because the esters are a precursor to the actual vitamin C, the actual percentage cannot be determined.

The *most important* thing for a client to know about vitamin C is its antioxidant powers. Another important fact for the client to know is that the skin, like the body, can only take as much vitamin C as it can absorb. The remaining amount will sit on the surface of the skin without being absorbed, so more is not always better.

Vitamin C for Normal Skin

Normal skin can tolerate both the esters and the *l*-ascorbic acid. If you can find the product in a serum or a cream, it will be best for this skin type. Keep the pH around 3.6 to 3.8; if you are using an *l*-ascorbic, you will be able to ascertain a percentage. Around 10 percent would be a good place to start.

Vitamin C for Oily Skin

Vitamin C for oily skin should be in a serum or solution form. This client may find creams and gels too sticky. Solutions penetrate quickly and do not make the client with oily skin concerned about extra creams and potential breakouts. Once again, keep the pH around 3.6 to 3.8. This client will tolerate *l*-ascorbic acid 12 to 15 percent and *l*-ascorbic should be the preferential choice over the ester group.

Vitamin C for Dry Skin

Vitamin C can be especially irritating to dry skin. Therefore, an ester is the best choice for these skin types. Look for a cream or gel that has a higher pH and an emollient vehicle.

Vitamin C for Combination Skin

Vitamin C for combination skin is similar to that for normal skin. Either *l*-ascorbic 10 percent or esters will work just fine. The vehicle should be a serum or a cream. Be sure the pH is not too low because this will cause irritation.

Vitamin C for Sensitive Skin

Although vitamin C is a wonderful antioxidant and increases the photo-protection of the skin, sensitive-skinned clients may not be able to tolerate this product. The client may find the product, regardless of whether it is an ester or *l*-ascorbic, simply too irritating. If you are going to try a sensitive-skinned client on vitamin C, stay away from the *l*-ascorbic and start by trying a mild ester. The client will have the greatest opportunity for success with an ester with a higher pH. In addition, try a multivitamin moisturizer that contains vitamin C for this skin type, as it may be better tolerated.

▪ MOISTURIZERS

It is hard to get a consensus when defining dry skin. To say the skin lacks water is far too simple a definition for this very complex problem. Some physicians describe dry skin using multifaceted definitions that use the concepts of transepidermal water loss (TEWL) or natural moisturizing factor (NMF). Others define dry skin by the simple appearance of the skin (rough, red, flaky, tender, and so forth).

Dry skin can have a variety of causes. Once again, little consensus exists on the *cause* of dry skin. It can, however, be agreed that there are several *factors* that cause dry skin, among them, the lack of humidity in the air, extremes of temperature, diseases of the skin, and systemic diseases that *secondarily* cause dry skin. Dry skin can also be created by one's environment through exposure to chemicals that can react on the skin.

It is now understood (from Dr. Kligman's experiment) that a simple occlusive dressing with water (a wet gauze applied to the skin with an airtight dressing over it) will affect the stratum corneum. Therefore, it could be said that it is easy to moisturize the skin. This is not necessarily true. Two types of products are applied to the skin for the purpose of moisturizing: (1) a humectant and (2) a lubricant. In this text a moisturizer will be defined as a *humectant*, and an emollient will be defined as a *lubricant*.

As discussed, a moisturizer is a product that penetrates the skin and increases the water content (hydration) of the stratum corneum. Lubricants, on the other hand, do not have the ability to attract water but are more likely to seal in what water is available in the stratum corneum. The products most often used in lubricants include petrolatum, beeswax, lanolin, and perhaps some oils. In reality, the very best moisturizers are probably a combination of humectants and lubricants.

When a moisturizer is applied to the skin, a change in the appearance and feeling of the skin is noticeable. When using a moisturizer (instead of an emollient), this change is strictly related to the number and blend of humectants in the moisturizer itself and their effect on the skin. Remember that NMF is a blend of *natural* humectants found in the skin. The content of NMF in the skin is directly related to the hydration or water content of the stratum corneum. Lubricants, by comparison, increase the water content of the stratum corneum by simple occlusion, reducing the water loss by use of a sealant.

Composition of Natural Moisturizing[9]

PERCENTAGE OF NATURAL MOISTURIZING FACTOR (NMF)

Amino acids—40%

Pyrrolidone carboxylic acid—12%

Lactate—12%

Urea—7.0%

Na, Ca, K, Mg, phosphate, chloride—18.5%

NH_3, uric acid, glucosamine, creatinine—1.5%

Remainder unidentified

Na, Sodium; *Ca*, calcium; *K*, potassium; *Mg*, magnesium; *NH₃*, ammonia

Creating the perfect moisturizer is not as simple as understanding the composition of NMF and replacing the missing and depleted components to the skin. In fact, water-binding capacities, penetration, and the degree of solvency all play a role. In addition to the simple issues of moisturizing the skin, also include other additives to the moisturizers such as vitamins, antioxidants, and sunscreens. So how do you choose the perfect moisturizer? In addition, is your *favorite* moisturizer the right moisturizer for everyone?

More than Just for Moisturizing

Understandably, consumers can become overwhelmed with the choices that are presented to them in a department store or supermarket. Often they are uninformed about their own skin and which of the many products will best suit them. Frequently it is the *power punch* in the moisturizer that makes the client buy rather than the chemistry of the moisturizer—and why not? Vitamins and antioxidants are far more interesting and simple to understand than the effects of *urea* and *lactate* on the skin.

Several power punches to moisturizers should be discussed, including vitamin E, selenium, nicotinamide, and ubiquinone (Co-Q$_{10}$).

Vitamin E is also called *d-alpha tocopherol*. Vitamin E has been shown to have two important benefits for the skin: (1) protecting cellular membranes and (2) inactivating free radicals.[10] Vitamin E has long been considered a good topical for healing scars; this is not true, and vitamin E usage should be limited to its known benefits. It should be used in a cream form.

Selenium has also been shown to be a powerful antioxidant for the skin. Selenium helps to protect the skin from solar-induced skin cancers. However, it functions best when combined with vitamin E.

Niacinamide, or vitamin B, is often found in moisturizers. Niacinamide has been shown to be successful in the treatment of chronologic aging by decreasing the TEWL of the stratum corneum.[11] Studies also point to efficacy in the treatment of acne.

Co-Q$_{10}$ can be found both as a separate product serum and as part of the moisturizer. Little available documentation exists concerning the action of ubiquinone on the skin. However, the few studies that are available are promising. Co-Q$_{10}$, or ubiquinone, is a cellular antioxidant. It is found in almost all body tissues, including the skin. A recent study demonstrated a 27-percent reduction of periorbital wrinkles with the application of ubiquinone.

Topical antioxidants are unique and identifiable as free-radical scavengers. A moisturizer that contains all or most of these antioxidants is the most effective moisturizer.

nicotinamide
Member of the vitamin-B complex that has been shown to decrease TEWL.

ubiquinone (Co-Q$_{10}$)
Lipid-soluble cellular antioxidant present in virtually all cells.

d-alpha tocopherol
Vitamin E.

vitamin B
See *nicotinamide*.

Client Education for Moisturizers

With regard to selecting moisturizers for clients, the status of the client's skin, the effect of AHAs and Retin A, and the end point you are trying to achieve all need to be considered. It is important for the client to understand some of the basics about moisturizers and to be able to appreciate that the moisturizer you select for him or her has been selected for a specific reason. As we have discussed, the aesthetician must ensure that clients understand two things about the moisturizing process: (1) the difference between moisturizing and lubricating and (2) the importance of antioxidants in the moisturizer. Moisturizing is not as simple as spreading a cream on the face.

Sunscreens and Moisturizers

One final concept must be addressed when speaking of moisturizers: the concept of moisturizers mixed with sunscreens (Table 5–8). It is

Table 5–8 Moisturizers for Specific Skin Types

Skin Type	Moisturizers Containing:
Normal skin	Glycerin, hyaluronic acid, and lactic acid
Oily skin	Water as main ingredient and glycerin
Dry skin	Urea, lactic acid, hyaluronic acid
Combination skin	Glycerin, hyaluronic acid, and lactic acid
Sensitive skin	Hyaluronic acid, no lactic acid

possible that as many opinions are heard on this subject as there are moisturizers and sunscreens. Clients like this blend, because it is one fewer step in the routine. Some aestheticians dislike this combination, because they feel that these products are not as moisturizing as they would be without the sunscreen component. In reality, produced with plenty of humectants, these products should work just fine and are a great way to simplify a program. Additionally, this may be the only way you are able to get a client to wear sunscreen.

Moisturizers for Normal Skin

Moisturizers for normal skin should include glycerin, lactic acid, and hyaluronic acid. The proper combination of these ingredients will keep the skin moisturized and soft.

Moisturizers for Dry Skin

Dry skin is, of course, the litmus test for a moisturizer. The best ingredients seem to be urea, lactic acid, and hyaluronic acid. If you can find a moisturizer that also contains lubricants, this will be helpful to the client. Perhaps the moisturizer might also have glycerin. However, dry skin can also be sensitive, and aggressive mixtures of these products can also cause irritation.

Moisturizers for Oily Skin

Even though the skin is oily, it still needs spot treatment for dry areas. The oily areas do not really need full moisturizing. However, under the eyes and cheeks will need regular treatment.

Moisturizers for Combination Skin

Combination skin can be treated much like normal skin, although it is best to avoid treating the oilier areas with moisturizer unless they feel dry. The general rule is to apply the moisturizer only to the needed areas.

Moisturizers for Sensitive Skin

The best moisturizers for sensitive skin are simple moisturizers that will not cause any potential rash or allergy. Look for a product that is simple and contains glycerin.

▪ SUNSCREENS

Sunscreens are used for the purpose of protecting the skin from **photodamage** resulting from ultraviolet (ultraviolet A [UVA] and ultraviolet B [UVB]) light. This protection helps reduce photoaging and all of the associated problems such as collagen depletion, dyschromias, and skin cancers. Sunscreens come in two varieties: (1) chemical sunscreens and (2) physical sunscreens (Table 5–9). The description of sun*block,* once used to describe these products, has evolved as the FDA

photodamage
Damage caused by repeated and unprotected sun exposure over time; also called *solar damage.*

Table 5–9 Sunscreens for Specific Skin Types

Skin Type	Blocking Components	Application
Normal skin	Combination of chemical and physical (any SPF)	After moisturizer but before makeup
Oily skin	Chemical (at least SPF 15)	Will require behavior modification, because most will cause breakouts
Dry skin	Chemical (with a lower SPF)	Reapply often, because SPF will be lower
Combination skin	Combination of chemical and physical (any SPF)	After moisturizer but before makeup
Sensitive skin	Physical (at least SPF 15)	Reapply often, because physical blockers come off more easily

para-aminobenzoic acid (PABA)

Cousin of the B complex that is found in animals; most common use is as an effective sunscreen.

salicylates

Salt derivative of salicylic acid that is used as a chemical agent in sunscreens.

benzophenones

Chemical absorbers that respond to UV light by generating a free radical capable of rapid polymerization.

cinnamates

Derivative of cinnaminic acid that is useful for protection against low levels of UVB rays; makes sunscreens waterproof.

dibenzoylmethanes

UVA ray absorber.

camphors

Used topically as an anti-itch agent; derived as a gum from evergreens native to China and Japan.

anthranilates

Weak UVB filters that mainly absorb in the near-UVA portion of the spectrum.

Parsol 1789®

Preferred sunscreen ingredient that protects against photodamage and premature aging of the skin from exposure to UVA light.

zinc oxide

Physical sunscreen that scatters and reflects light rather than absorbing or filtering it.

titanium dioxide

Physical sunscreen that scatters light rather than absorbing or filtering it.

has pushed the industry to use the description sun*screen,* recognizing that *block* is a misnomer.

Each of the chemical ingredients found in sunscreen is effective at certain light wave lengths. Chemical sunscreens absorb UV light. To make sunscreens most effective, manufacturers usually combine zinc oxide or titanium dioxide with the chemical. The chemicals used in sunscreen include **para-aminobenzoic acid (PABA)**, PABA derivatives, **salicylates, benzophenones, cinnamates, dibenzoylmethanes, camphors, anthranilates,** and other miscellaneous chemicals.[12]

Parsol 1789® is avobenzone dibenzoylmethane.[13] Parsol 1789 has become a popular and preferred chemical ingredient because of its effectiveness. In the past, Parsol was felt to destabilize in the bottle, but newer preservatives have solved this problem. If a waterproof sunscreen is the product of choice, be sure your sunscreen includes a cinnamate.

Cinnamates are insoluble in water and are the best product for waterproof sunscreens. Physical blocks such as **zinc oxide** or **titanium dioxide** work by scattering and reflecting the light rather than absorbing the light. Many may remember zinc oxide as the white stuff parents used to put on their children at the pool or at the beach.

Client Education for Sunscreen

Sunscreen is the most important product that you will talk about with your client. With solar-induced skin cancers increasing at an alarming rate, it is incumbent on the aesthetician to discuss with the client the importance of sunscreen. Additionally, as you add AHAs, Retin A, and bleaching agents to your clients' programs, you put their skin at greater risk of sunburn when exposed. Simply put, sunscreen must be worn. So whether it is in a moisturizer or a separate step, add it to programs and be disciplined about the use. Clients should wear at least a 20 if not a 25 SPF daily. Because SPF is a difficult concept to understand, the FDA is changing the rating for sunscreens to more understandable labels: *minimum, moderate,* or *high* sun protection.

Beyond just adding sunscreen to the skin care program, clients need to learn to use adequate amounts of sunscreen. Unfortunately, most clients seem to apply sunscreen minimally with only a small film. The FDA recommends that sunscreen application should be 2 mg/cm^2. This is approximately 1 oz for the entire body.[14] In addition, the sunscreen should be applied at least 30 minutes before sun exposure to ensure the chemicals have had the opportunity to bind to the stratum corneum.

Sunscreen for Normal Skin

Sunscreen for normal skin should be a combination of both chemical and physical components. Sunscreen should be applied after moisturizer and before makeup.

Sunscreen for Dry Skin

Individuals with dry skin often have trouble if the sunscreen is too heavily composed of physical blocking agents such as zinc oxide and titanium dioxide. These products can be drying to the skin, even though they are occlusive. A chemical block of lower SPF will be the most useful for dry skin. Clients should be instructed to reapply often so that they do not burn.

> An SPF of at least 20 and preferably 25 should be worn every day. Sunscreen in makeup foundation is not adequate, because it is usually only around SPF 8. For those clients who have not used sunscreen before, this recommendation will be a change. Some clients are annoyed by the way sunscreen floats on the skin and is greasy. A moisturizer with a sunscreen better serves these clients, because it is usually less noticeable under these circumstances.

> **Sun protection factor (SPF)** determines the amount of time you can be in the sun with protection from a sunscreen before you burn. For example, if your skin normally burns in 30 minutes without SPF, applying an SPF 15 theoretically gives you 450 minutes or 7½ hours of safety.

sun protection factor (SPF)
Determines the amount of time an individual can be in the sun with protection from a sunscreen before burning. SPF is difficult to understand and varies from one individual to the next, depending on skin type.

Sunscreen for Oily Skin

People with oily skin have a lot of trouble with sunscreens, because the product itself can be oily. It is a behavior modification for these people (one that is not easy, especially if they are breaking out).

Sunscreen for Combination Skin

Combination skin should be treated like dry skin in terms of sunscreen choices. A product with a combination of physical blocking agents and chemical agents is the best choice.

Sunscreen for Sensitive Skin

Sensitive skin is the most difficult to treat with sunscreen. Usually the physical blocks are best, although some milder chemical blocks will also work.

▪ HYDROQUINONE

hydroquinone
Safe, topical bleaching agent that inhibits the production of tyrosine within melanocytes; topical agent used to decrease the hyperpigmentation on the skin.

tyrosine
Enzyme that produces melanin in melanocytes, overproduction of melanin is associated with hyperpigmentation.

Melquin®
Three-percent concentration of hydroquinone; bleaching agent used to treat hyperpigmentation.

Eldopaque®
Four-percent concentration of hydroquinone; bleaching agent used to treat hyperpigmentation.

Hydroquinone is a commonly used bleaching agent in the medical spa, available only by a physician's prescription. It is found naturally in bearberry, cranberry, cowberry, and some varieties of pears. Hydroquinone easily oxidizes (a chemical reaction that occurs when it is combined with oxygen) when exposed to the air and alkaline solutions. Hydroquinone works on melanocytes by inhibiting the production of **tyrosine**, the enzyme that produces melanin at the melanocytes. The overproduction of melanin is associated with melasma and other types of hyperpigmentation. Commercially produced hydroquinone comes in 2 percent (OTC form), 3 percent (**Melquin®**) and 4 percent (**Eldopaque®**) (Table 5–10).

Hydroquinone has been at the center of some on-again-off-again controversies regarding safety, efficacy, and applicability for certain skin types. The most noted authority on hydroquinone is Dr. Zen Obagi. His experience in hydroquinone use for all skin types has created a wealth of scientific data. Dr. Obagi believes that hydroquinone is an essential step in a medically indicated program targeting hyperpigmented skin. The use of hydroquinone is often mixed with Retin A or AHA, a process he refers to as *blending*.[15] Whether the process is bleaching,[16] the single application of hydroquinone, or blending, the use of hydroquinone is essential to treat hyperpigmentation. Hydroquinone is the safest depigmenting agent available, and adverse effects with the use of hydroquinone are rarely seen. In the rare case they are noted, it is usually after years of use.[17] Dr. Obagi states that this contrasts with depigmenting agents used in the past, such as mercurial compounds,

Table 5–10 Hydroquinone for Specific Skin Types

Skin Type	Dose	Possible Reactions
Normal skin	6%–8% every evening	Pigment should disappear quickly with minimal reactions
Oily skin	4% every evening	May result in post-inflammatory hyperpigmentation
Dry skin	3%–5% every other evening	Irritation possible
Combination skin	6%–8% cream in combination with Retin A	Pigment should disappear quickly with minimal reactions
Sensitive skin	3%–4% every other evening	Irritation possible

which caused kidney damage, and monobenzone, which caused permanent melanocyte destruction."[18]

Kojic acid is a bleaching agent that is often used in combination with hydroquinone. Kojic acid is derived from bacteria on Japanese mushrooms and is more effective when used with hydroquinone and other therapeutic products. Kojic acid is usually used in 2 percent solutions.

Azelaic acid is an antibacterial usually used for acne treatments, but has also been shown to decrease discolorations. Used at 15 to 20 percent, this product can be as efficacious as hydroquinone without the potential for irritation.[19] Like hydroquinone at higher percentages, azelaic acid is a prescription medication. When used for significant post-inflammatory hyperpigmentation, it should be used in the morning with AHAs and vitamin C (and hydroquinone should be used in the evening with Retin A). This approach will give the program a real bump and improve the dyschromias more rapidly.

When a bleaching agent is discontinued, a chance exists that the pigment will reappear, especially if the client does not consistently use sunscreen. To solve hyperpigmentation, bleaching agents should be used as *part* of a program.

Client Education for Hydroquinone

Hydroquinone can be irritating to the skin at higher percentages. Sometimes, it can actually be the source of irritation rather than the usual suspected culprits, Retin A or AHA. This is especially true if the percentage you have suggested is over 6 percent.

Hyperpigmentation can occur when using hydroquinone. This can happen if the client fails to wear sunscreen, thinking that the hydroquinone is taking care of the problem (which is simply not true). Therefore, clients must be made aware of the importance of using a sunscreen as a condition of treatment. In addition, the client should be educated on how pigment occurs, so he or she can work *with* you to solve the problem. The phenomenon of post-inflammatory hyperpigmentation should also be considered. For those skin types that are very sensitive to post-inflammatory hyperpigmentation, the hydroquinone irritation or irritation from any therapeutic product can increase rather than decrease the pigment. The key to avoiding this is twofold. Keep the product percentages mild and the application minimal. Next, include some topical steroid with the application of the hydroquinone. An over-the-counter brand should suffice, but sometimes a prescription is required. This will make all the difference in the program. The client obviously cannot use the steroid indefinitely, but it is useful to start on the program. Consult with your physician before implementing this step.

kojic acid
Bleaching agent derived from bacteria on a Japanese mushroom; usually used in conjunction with hydroquinone.

azelaic acid
Antibacterial agent that is usually used for acne treatment and has shown promise in minimizing dyschromia; kills the bacteria that infect pores.

All bleaching agents are temporary solutions for the problem of hyperpigmentation.

> A delayed redness associated with hydroquinone use may appear the afternoon after the previous evening's use. There may be two reasons this is happening: (1) quantity or (2) frequency. First, the client may be using too much. Remind the client that a pea-sized amount is all that is needed. It is a medicine, not a moisturizer. Second, using it every night may be too often. Evaluating quantity and frequency is the best way to determine the cause of the problem.

Hydroquinone for Normal Skin

Normal skin can tolerate a hydroquinone cream of approximately 6 to 8 percent. When used every evening as a step in a therapeutic program (including the clinical program of microdermabrasion), the pigment will disappear rather quickly.

Hydroquinone for Dry Skin

Dry skin is always at risk for irritation. Start this individual at a lower dose (3 to 5 percent) and begin every other night.

Hydroquinone for Oily Skin

Some oily, acne-prone skin may have a tendency toward post-inflammatory hyperpigmentation, depending on the skin type. Use a gel solution for these clients. Usually, 4 percent once nightly will improve the skin coloration. Gel solutions sometimes oxidize more quickly than creams, especially if they are made for you by a pharmacy. Be sure to alert your client that when the product turns yellow, it is time to replace the tube or bottle.

Hydroquinone for Combination Skin

Once again, treat combination skin as you would normal skin. Use less of the hydroquinone in the T-zone (the T-zone is usually less pigmented). Use a cream of 5 to 8 percent every night with Retin A.

Hydroquinone for Sensitive Skin

Sensitive skin may not be able to tolerate hydroquinone. It is a good idea to start with a lower percentage and apply every other night. If the client can tolerate this application, move the applications to every night.

▪ RETINOIDS

Retinoids act by normalizing growth and differentiation in the keratinocytes. Retinoids are vitamin A. Retin A (tretinoin) is truly the gold standard of skin care products. The use of tretinoin, retinol, or other topical vitamin A formulations has been shown to have positive effects on the skin (Table 5–11).

Retin A is a must-have product to help reverse the aging process, specifically photoaging. The groundbreaking work with Retin A on aging was done by Dr. Albert Kligman in the 1980s, when a group of middle-aged women being treated for acne noticed an improvement in their fine lines and wrinkles. This observation set in motion the first clinical study, which became the basis for understanding the benefits of Retin A for aging skin. Tretinoin, interestingly, works not only on the appearance of photoaged skin but also on the pathology of photoaged skin. Clinical improvement of the skin, such as reduction in fine lines, hyperpigmentation, and lentigines, can be seen in as little as one month. Stopping the product can cause a reversal of the result. Some practitioners believe that Retin A can provide a superior result to superficial chemical peels,[20] but combining therapies is the best approach (Table 5–12).

Retin A is a prescription medication. However, vitamin A derivatives such as retinol and **retinyl palmitate** are available over the counter. The difference between Retin A and retinol or retinyl palmitate is that the latter two must convert to retinoic acid to become useful on the skin.

retinyl palmitate
Vitamin A derivative that must first convert to retinoic acid before it can be useful to the skin; also thought to be useful for collagen synthesis.

Client Education for Retinoids

All retinoids can be potentially irritating. Overdosing clients on these products is not in anyone's best interest. The redness, flakiness, and tender skin that present when the product is overused make clients

Table 5–11 Retinoids for Specific Skin Types

Skin Type	Dose
Normal skin	0.05% Retin A (0.025% for thinner skin) cream or Renova®
Oily skin	Differin®
Dry skin	0.02% Renova every second or third night
Combination skin	Retin A 0.05% cream for aging or 0.025% gel for breakouts
Sensitive skin	OTC retinol or Renova 0.02%

Table 5–12 Retin A Strength and Delivery

Retin A micro	0.1%
Retin A cream	0.025%
Retin A cream	0.05%
Retin A cream	0.1%
Retin A gel	0.01%
Retin A gel	0.025%
Retin A liquid	0.05%
Renova	0.02%
Renova	0.05%

reluctant to carry on a program. Clients need not look like raw meat to use these products. These products are *medicines, not moisturizers;* instruct your clients accordingly. Use a pea-sized amount on the back of the hand (you can mix in the hydroquinone for a single application). Spread the entire amount over the face and neck. Any extra is massaged into the back of the hands.

Like hydroquinone and AHAs, these products can cause irritation and erythema. The investigative process remains the same; *quantity* or *frequency*. Clients are likely to be using too much product because it is difficult to get a pea-sized amount around the face and neck. Mixing it with the hydroquinone helps, but if they need more volume, add a dab of moisturizer. If this solution does not decrease the symptoms, the problem is frequency. Some practitioners believe that clients should "tough it out" and get through the initial process of flakiness and irritation. However, decreasing the product to every other day is not a problem. Ultimately, the goal is for the client to tolerate the treatment and for the treatment to be successful. The last option is to change the product strength or carrier vehicle. Specifically, the carrier vehicle in the case of Retin A could be a change to **Renova** or to **Retin A Microsphere®** to assist with penetration. These products are more moisturizing and have a gentler penetration process.

Retinoids for Normal Skin

Retin A should be a common denominator in the skin-care program. If the skin is thin, it is better to start with a low dose such as

Renova
Tretinoin that is meant specifically for aging; recommended for clients with drier skin.

Retin A Microsphere®
A gentler Retin A, based on an advanced delivery system.

0.025 percent cream or Renova. This will help the skin to peel less, while building the dermis. The average dose is 0.05 percent in Retin A cream or Renova every night.

Retinoids for Dry Skin

At first glance it may seem that adding Retin A to the dry-skinned individual's program may not be the smartest move, because the skin may get drier and peel. It can be added to the program in a low dose if this client will tolerate the product. Try 0.02 percent Renova every other or every third night, working up to every night over the course of a month.

Retinoids for Oily Skin

Tretinoin choices for oily and acne-prone skin pose a more complex problem. Sometimes the acne needs to be treated first. Consider Differin for this client. It is a retinoid and will clear the acne and improve the aging issues at the same time.

Retinoids for Combination Skin

Retinoids for combination skin should be directed at the most significant problem, whether it is aging or breakouts. Select the product based on the overwhelmingly obvious problem. If it is aging, go with Retin A (not Renova) in the 0.05 percent cream. If the more obvious problem is breakouts, go with Retin A 0.02 percent gel.

Retinoids for Sensitive Skin

Retinoids can play havoc with sensitive skin. The best approach is to try an OTC retinol cream and see if the client can adjust to this product. Then, as the skin becomes more accustomed to the product, begin to build into the prescriptions, starting with Renova 0.02 percent.

▪ CONCLUSION

Product technology is exploding; every day you see a new product with a "super molecule" or some type of technology that improves performance over its predecessors. Some of the newest product technology is coming in the form of growth hormones, peptides, and idebenone, a molecule similar to Co-Q$_{10}$. Since products are necessary for cleansing, moisturizing, and protecting, the value of daily cosmeceuticals cannot be underestimated and you will continue to see advances that improve the products that are used on the skin. Each medical spa should have a protocol about dispensing and monitoring clients using cosmeceuticals and topical prescription products. As an aesthetician, it is your responsibility to dispense these products with knowledge and care. Each product should have a separate informational sheet (telling what the product does) and an instructional sheet (telling how to use the product). The success of the program depends on these simple steps.

▶ ▷ ▷ Top 10 Tips to Take to the Spa

1. The pH of products will make products more intense (lower pH) or less intense (higher pH).

2. A cleanser with a lower pH will keep the skin from becoming too dry. Bath soaps usually have a more alkaline pH.

3. Using a washcloth or facial chamois can cause the skin to be drier because of the laundry detergent residue left in these implements.

4. Hydroquinone, Retin A, or Renova are necessary to consider the program therapeutic.

5. Vitamin C is manufactured either as an ester (fat- and water-soluble) or as l-ascorbic (water-soluble only).

6. Hydroquinone alone will not solve a pigment problem. Sunscreen is necessary to eliminate solar stimulation of the melanin.

7. Products can cause irritation if they are overused; remember the principles of quantity and frequency.

8. Retin A is vitamin A and is the gold standard for therapeutic programs.

9. A sunscreen of at least SPF 15 (preferably SPF 20) should be worn every day to protect the skin from solar damage.

10. Moisturizers come in two types: humectant (moisturizing) and emollient (lubricating).

Chapter Review Questions

1. What are the three components of a successful microdermabrasion outcome?

2. Define cosmeceuticals. What are they, and what separates them from cosmetics and pharmaceutical-grade products?

3. What is the FDA? What role do they play in the aesthetics industry?

4. List three cosmeceuticals you may use in your practice, and explain their action.

5. Explain what pH is, and why it is an important function of product recommendation. What is the normal pH level for human skin?

6. Are the products found in a medical spa more active or effective than those found in a salon or day spa?

7. What types of cleansers ought to be stocked in a spa? For which skin conditions are these recommended? What do you need to tell your clients about cleansers?

8. What is a cleanser? What constitutes a good cleanser?

9. Explain the function of the acid mantle, and how it relates to the cleanser choice.

10. What are some of the common ingredients found in cleansers? What do they do?

11. Why is exfoliation an important component of the microdermabrasion pretreatment program?

12. What are the considerations for cleansers with regard to skin condition?

13. What are AHAs? What are the considerations for AHAs with regard to skin condition?

14. What are the more common AHAs found in the spa environment?

15. What is vitamin C? Free radicals? What are the considerations for vitamin C with regard to skin condition?

16. What are some of the common additives to moisturizers? What do they do?

17. What are moisturizers? What are the considerations for moisturizers with regard to skin condition?

18. Why is it suggested that you recommend that your clients use a moisturizer with a sunscreen component?

19. What are some of the common ingredients used in sunscreens? Which would you recommend to your clients as part of a microdermabrasion regimen based on their skin condition?

20. What are some of the products used to treat pigment disorders? What might you need to consider with regard to skin condition?

21. What are retinoids? What might you need to consider with regard to skin condition?

Chapter References

1. Elsner, P. & Maibach, H. L. (Eds.). (2000). *Cosmeceuticals: Drugs vs. cosmetics*. New York: Marcel Dekker, Inc
2. Elsner, P. & Maibach, H. L. (Eds.). (2000). *Cosmeceuticals: Drugs vs. cosmetics*. New York: Marcel Dekker, Inc
3. Murphy, R. (2003, March). *Cosmeceuticals: Can science support the claims?* [Online]. Available: http://www.skinandaging.com/sa
4. Draelos, Z. (2002, January 7). *Skin hair and cleansers*. [Online]. Available: http://www.emedicine.com
5. Yosipovitch, G. (2003, March). *The importance of skin pH. Skin & Aging* [Online]. Available: http://www.skinandaging.com/sa
6. Rubin, M. (1995). *Manual of chemical peels: Superficial and medium depth*. Philadelphia: Lippincott, Williams & Wilkins.
7. American Academy of Dermatology. (2002, February 25). *Vitamins to protect against and reverse aging: The truths vs. the tall tales*. [Online]. Available: http://www.aad.org
8. American Fitness. (1998, November). *CNo wrinkles*. [Online]. Available: http://www.findarticles.com
9. Elsner, P. & Maibach, H. L. (Eds.). (2000). *Cosmeceuticals: Drugs vs. cosmetics*. New York: Marcel Dekker, Inc
10. American Academy of Dermatology. (2002, February 25). *Vitamins to protect against and reverse aging: The truths vs. the tall tales*. [Online]. Available: http://www.aad.org
11. Chui, A. & Kimball, A. B. (2003, November 17). Topical vitamins, minerals, and botanical ingredients as modulators of environmental and chronological skin damage. *British Journal of Dermatology, 149*(4), 681–691.
12. Bennett, M. & Petrazzuoli, M. (2001, July). What patients should know about sunscreen. *Skin & Aging* [Online]. Available: http://www.skinandaging.com/sa
13. Bennett, M. & Petrazzuoli, M. (2001, July). What patients should know about sunscreen. *Skin & Aging*. [Online]. Available: http://www.skinandaging.com/sa
14. Bennett, M. & Petrazzuoli, M. (2001, July). What patients should know about sunscreen. *Skin & Aging*. [Online]. Available: http://www.skinandaging.com/sa
15. Obagi, Z. (2000). *Skin health restoration and rejuvenation*. New York: Springer-Verlag, New York, Inc

16. Obagi, Z. (2000). *Skin health restoration and rejuvenation.* New York: Springer-Verlag, New York, Inc

17. Obagi, Z. (2000). *Skin health restoration and rejuvenation.* New York: Springer-Verlag, New York, Inc

18. Obagi, Z. (2000). *Skin health restoration and rejuvenation.* New York: Springer-Verlag, New York, Inc

19. Breathnach, A. S. (1996, January). Melanin hyperpigmentation of skin: Melasma, topical treatment with azelaic acid, and other therapies. *Cutis, 57*(Suppl. 1), 36–45.

20. Rolewski, S. L. (2003, December 5). *Clinical review: Topical retinoids* [Online]. Available: http://www.medscape.com

ADDITIONAL RESOURCES

http://www.cunliffe-awards.org

Consultations

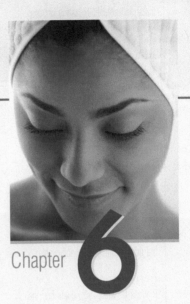

Chapter 6

Key Terms

body dysmorphic
   disorder (BDD)
client information
   sheet
consultation
differentiate

health history sheet
image businesses
impressions
perception
photographs
realistic expectations

skin history sheet
unrealistic
   expectations
Wood's lamp

Learning Objectives

After completing this chapter you should be able to:

1. Understand the importance of knowing the client's history.

2. Determine if your clients have reasonable expectations for treatment and how to re-educate them in the event they do not.

3. Understand how to conduct a thorough analysis of your clients and their individual circumstances.

4. Learn what is involved in taking client photographs and the value of doing so.

5. Evaluate clients for a home care and treatment program.

INTRODUCTION

impressions
Initial and potentially lasting opinions or judgments of a person, place, or thing.

image businesses
Type of business in which the way the public views the company is based largely upon how things look, or how they are perceived, more than actual performance.

consultation
Initial visit with a professional during which the client and the professional both investigate whether a specific treatment or service is warranted and if the desired outcome is achievable.

perception
Process by which individuals use their senses to make decisions or gather information.

differentiate
To make something stand out or be unique compared with something that would otherwise be similar.

In most businesses, particularly in the medical and luxury spa business, your success will be driven by the impressions people have of you and the aesthetic industry, because they are image businesses. The first impression a new client has of your office and your expertise is based in part on the cleanliness of the office, the knowledge and friendliness of the staff, and, last but certainly not least, your appearance. In the consultation or treatment room, clients' ability to listen and hear pertinent information is affected by how comfortable they feel. That *comfort zone* includes how "medicinal" the room appears (this can be intimidating), the seating arrangement, and your professionalism. Professionalism relates to your appearance, knowledge, and command of the language. Mastering the skills of friendliness, cleanliness, comfort, professionalism, and communication can affect the client's first and lasting impressions. Furthermore, the perception the client has of you is one that extends to your ancillary staff, merchandise partners, and the overseeing physician and his or her partners. The impression the client has of you and the facility will determine trust, which is the foundation of any relationship.

The office consultation is the first face-to-face meeting with the client. It is the first and best opportunity to make a positive impression and create a lasting relationship. Many times, the client's decision to buy is made by the time he or she is escorted to the treatment room. More so than in most other businesses, a bad day can have serious consequences for your long-term success. Therefore, it is important to create a good first impression when meeting new clients for the first time.

The aesthetician and client share a mutual objective: improving the client's appearance. The client came to you because he or she has a *need* to look better. You are in your position because through your education and experience you can *fulfill* that need. This is an important fact when it comes to relationship building and creating good first impressions. Communicate this fact to the client, and he or she will certainly feel more comfortable.

Many aestheticians follow a consultative process that is modeled from physicians or processes that they learned in school or at other jobs. As a professional providing skin consultations, you must differentiate yourself from others to be successful. Differentiation is "to form or mark differently from other things; distinguish."[1]

Differentiation does not necessarily involve creating comfortable seating areas with televisions, beverages, and literature. These niceties are really in-house marketing and have little to do with the care you give your clients. While creating an environment of comfort and luxury are nice, and do affect the client's impression of your spa business, it will not set your spa apart from any other spa in the region. Differentiation means a *change* in the process. A notable difference in care will have an equally notable difference in the client's perception.

▪ OFFICE CONSULTATION

On the surface, the objective of the consultation is to determine the client's candidacy for a particular procedure (for example, microderm-abrasion). However, this objective includes little or no concern for the client's concerns or fears, only concern for collecting information. Instead, the focus of the consultation should be to build a relationship. For a consultative process to be mutually successful, the client must be able to communicate his or her fears, concerns, and objectives for the treatment in a safe and trusting environment. Many individuals are nervous when seeking your services. They have concerns of vanity, cost, pain, and scarring. Think of the consultation process as a *scavenger hunt* for information, and remember that no scavenger hunt is ever the same. Therefore no consultation will ever be the same.

The consultative process to which you are going to be introduced will take approximately one hour with the client. It will include all of the necessary and traditional components of a consultation: skin analysis, **photographs**, and product and service recommendations, plus differentiation.

It is important for you to understand your clients and their motivation before you can make any substantive recommendations in consultation. To achieve this end you should use several tactics, including a traditional **client information sheet**, a **skin history sheet**, and a **health history sheet**. The client fills out all these documents in the waiting area before seeing the aesthetician. Attach all of the documents to a clipboard, from top to bottom: the *client information sheet*, the *skin history sheet*, and, finally, the *health history sheet*. If you are working in a larger spa, it will be important for you to ask the client to arrive 15 minutes early to complete the required paperwork. This documentation will help guide you through a successful consultation.

The *client information sheet* is the document that captures all of the social, demographic, and contact information: e-mail addresses, telephone numbers, referral sources, and the like. The purpose of this form is to learn about the client and how to reach him or her. It should also capture information about the client's interest in the office, including procedures in which he or she is interested.

A first impression is a lasting impression. Use your knowledge, personality, and skills to make it a good one.

photographs
Necessary component of skin-care treatment program that accurately documents the original skin condition to prove or disclaim treatment results.

client information sheet
Document used to gather social, personal and demographic information.

skin history sheet
Document used to gather information on a client's past and present skin health; includes past treatment, sunburns, and conditions that are necessary for treatment.

health history sheet
Document used by medical professionals to gather information on past and present health conditions, as well as likelihood for future conditions; includes allergies, medical conditions, and prescription information.

The *skin history sheet* is a detailed questionnaire about the client's past and present skin condition. Some of the specific items you will want to know are past and current tanning habits, including sunburns (as a child and as an adult), skin cancer diagnosis, and locations of skin cancers. In addition, ask about moles or lesions that concern the client. Information regarding past and current acne concerns, including the medications used (both oral and topical), is vital. It is important that you are also aware of previous skin treatments, x-ray treatments for acne, ultraviolet light (PUVA) treatments for psoriasis, as well as the usual spa treatments such as facials and body treatments, and any problems associated with those treatments. Furthermore, you will want to ask about any scarring, makeup use, and daily skin care regimens, including products used. You may want to consider using the Fitzpatrick Skin Typing questionnaires (see Chapter 4) to make this information inclusive and complete. Finally, you will want to ask about basics such as skin condition (oily, dry, normal, sensitive, combination) and skin type. This document will help you to really understand the client's overall skin health. It will also give you a clearer history, not just what he or she chooses to tell you verbally.

The *health history sheet* asks for detailed health status. This questionnaire delves into the past and current health of your client. Included on this document are questions regarding allergies, current and past illness, smoking status, pregnancy status, past and present daily medications, and past surgical events. The objective of the health history is to obtain a detailed "snapshot" of the client's health without spending a lot of time. This form should be set up in a check-box format. Although the client may think that some of the health items are irrelevant, the questions may be important in delivering care, and all boxes should be checked *yes* or *no*.

Greeting the Client

The paperwork is finished, and the client is anxious to meet you. This is your opportunity to make a positive lasting impression (Figure 6–1). Respect for the client should be your first objective, though it would not hurt to take a quick peek in the mirror before you meet a new client; make sure your hair is neat, your face is clean, and your makeup (if you wear it) is evenly applied. Greet the client with a smile, and introduce yourself. Be sure to ask the client how he or she prefers to be addressed. For example, the conversation could begin with, "Hello, Mrs. Smith. My name is Susan. It's a pleasure to meet you. Do you prefer Mrs. Smith or Lorraine?" Her preference should be documented in the chart. Remember that coming to the spa as a new client may be intimidating and it can

---

The client information sheet is loaded with information that will help you to promote your business. By entering this information into your computer database, you will have ready access to information you can use for marketing purposes, such as promotions or direct mail. Because it is the source of your referral information, this document is also useful when you are thanking or rewarding referral sources.

The skin history sheet can also help you to understand the segments of your practice. For example, how many clients do you see who have had a skin cancer? How many clients do you see with acne? How many clients do you see who tan? Some of this information would be valuable to your marketing department and possible future promotions.

The first time you "meet" a client may be on the telephone. Clients often want to know the answers to a variety of questions. Most of the answers will require a face-to-face consultation. Setting an appointment should be the objective of the telephone interview.

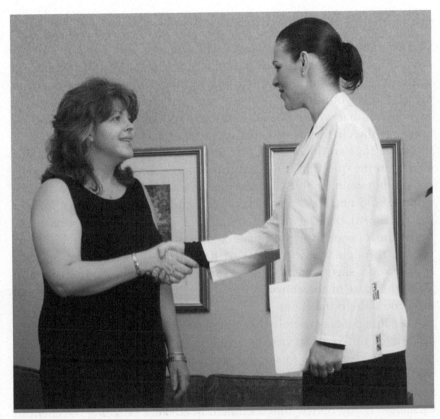

Figure 6–1 The patient greeting is your best opportunity to make a positive, lasting impression.

be a frightening place for many people, even if they are coming for exciting procedures. Take care to explain the physical layout of the facility: restroom location, which treatment or consultation room you will be using that day, and how to exit the facility. A simple tour always helps people to feel more at ease and more confident that they have found the right place.

Reviewing the Client Information Sheet

The *client information sheet* that the client fills out provides a wealth of important data. It tells you where he or she lives, where he or she works (or does not work), if he or she is married or has a partner, and what his or her interests are in your business. Look carefully at the client information sheet; it will give you sales clues and may help you to see the client's motivation—for example, a big birthday, wedding, or recent divorce. All of this information is important and valuable in developing a relationship with the client.

Reviewing the Health and Skin History

Make sure that the client completely fills out the *health and skin history sheet*. This is a great place to start the conversation. For example, you could say, "Mrs. Smith, I am going to take a moment and acquaint myself with your history. Please bear with me a moment while I become familiar with it." Take a moment to look through the information that the client has provided, and ask relevant questions to fill in the areas that are incomplete. An incomplete area usually means the answer to the question is *no*, but sometimes it could mean that the client did not want to give the information or that it was unintentionally skipped. Do not leave any blanks. Ask the client to finish filling out the document if an area is incomplete. Be sure you review both the health history and the skin history sheets. Add anything relevant as you go through the documents with the client. Make notes on your consultation sheet, not on the documents that the client filled out. Take this part of the consultation seriously, and make notes that will help you to help the client.

Because people generally like to talk about themselves (and this situation is no different), reviewing this form is a good place to build rapport with a client. Use this opportunity as an icebreaker to get to know the client. If your client is shy or embarrassed, using this technique will help the client to get comfortable with you and the informational exchange. If you review this document in advance of seeing the client in the treatment room, you lose this momentum.

Health History Updates

At follow-up appointments, or following gaps in treatment, inquire about any changes in the client's health, and update the written documentation. At the very least, this document ought to be completed yearly. Relevant changes to the client's health include medication changes, new diseases and illnesses, or surgeries and treatments. Updates can be extraordinarily important. Take the example of a client recently diagnosed with cancer or diabetes. Health status changes should cause the aesthetician to take pause in the skin care setting. Does this new information require an updated consultation, evaluation, and examination? The answer should be yes. Does the new health status demand a new home program and reevaluation of the microdermabrasion plan? Health changes do not mean the client must forego a skin care program; in fact, treatments and at-home care may be an important part of the client's emotional healing as he or she copes with the disease. However, for his or her safety, the plan needs to be reviewed.

Evaluating the Client's Requests

Once you review the health history and make any additions or clarifications, it is time to identify what the client wants to improve and what the best approach might involve. This process is best accomplished by providing the client a hand mirror and asking him or her to evaluate his or her face. Some clients may find this somewhat intimidating, but it is a useful process if you can encourage your client to talk through his or her concerns and identify any perceived problems. It is helpful to ask clients to start at the forehead, work their way down the face, and include the chest. You may also want to ask them to address their hands. One of the most overlooked areas of treatment is the hands, so you will want their opinion of what they see. This process will give you insight into the client's perceived body image, what is important to the client, and what he or she is willing to do to accomplish the desired result. As you listen to the client's analysis of the problems, try to evaluate if he or she is realistic in the analysis. For example, does the client tell you that he or she is ugly and has big pores and uneven skin, when in reality the pores are of average size and the skin is of normal texture, tone, and pigment for a person of his or her age? Watch for signs of **body dysmorphic disorder (BDD)** (see Chapter 7).

Take notes while the client is speaking to ensure you get all of the information recorded. This will help you to create a useful and complete care plan. Once the client has completed the analysis, ask permission to do the same. Asking permission is an important step in building the relationship. In asking for the client to authorize you to analyze his or her skin, you build on the key concepts of trust and respect. When possible, avoid commenting on just the negative. You don't want the client to leave feeling self-conscious or bad. This is not the impression you want him or her to have of your spa or your person.

When making observations, it is helpful to begin at the forehead and work down to the chest. As you make your way down the face, comments should include what the client said (because you do not want to disregard any of his or her concerns); adding both observations and client comments will make a positive difference in the care plan. Sometimes you will agree with the client's assessment, and sometimes you will not. If you disagree with the client, explain why. It is important to be honest—but in a gentle way.

Many times, clients do not know exactly what they see. They just know that they do not like the way they look. It is your job to identify and elaborate on these issues. Once this process is complete and you have agreed on the specific areas of concern, it is time to do a true skin evaluation.

body dysmorphic disorder (BDD) Psychosocial disease that causes individuals to be inappropriately concerned with their appearance; those affected with BDD are contraindicated for most aesthetic procedures.

Skin Analysis

A skin analysis is performed to evaluate the skin condition and determine the skin type (see Chapter 4). Both of these indicators are important in helping determine which treatment program will be best for the client. Before beginning, have the client change into a wrap or gown, which will allow you a better chance to evaluate the chest and cleanse the face without fear of soiling the client's clothing. With the client changed into a wrap, you will also be able to observe, analyze, and photograph the chest. This skin analysis is a standardized process, but a review is always helpful (Figure 6–2).

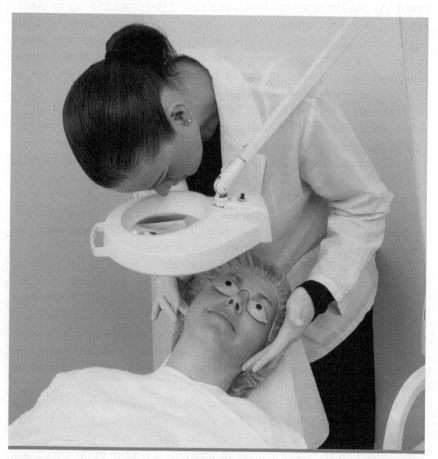

Figure 6–2 A skin analysis is performed to evaluate skin condition and determine skin type.

Cleansing the Client's Skin

Once the client has changed and is made comfortable on the bed, cover the hair with a surgical bonnet or a headband. Using soft gauze or disposable sponge, gently cleanse the face using a mild cleanser and pat dry. Be sure to *gently* cleanse the skin. Your objective is to take off the makeup but not to stimulate the skin. If the skin is overstimulated it will be difficult to observe skin irregularities such as telangiectasias.

Analyzing and Evaluating the Client's Skin

Use a loupe or magnification light to observe the skin. You are looking for hyperpigmentation, telangiectasias, clogged pores, and scarring. On a more subjective level, you are evaluating the skin texture and tone (in other words, aging). Take note of the skin's sensitivity. For example, did it turn pink during cleansing? Discuss now any potential areas of concern that were missed in the initial discussion. Hand the client a mirror and point out your concerns. Ask his or her opinion.

A **Wood's lamp** should be used to evaluate the depth of the hyperpigmentation at this time. Using a Wood's lamp is simple and will only take a couple of extra minutes. Cover the client's eyes with cotton pads or plastic goggles. Dim the overhead lights, and turn on the Wood's lamp. Hold the device close to the skin, but avoid touching the skin because it will burn the client. Then evaluate the skin conditions you see. Be sure to make a note on the chart.

Wood's lamp
Ultraviolet (UV) rays used to detect fluorescent material in the skin that is indicative of certain diseases or conditions.

Interpreting the Wood's lamp

Interpreting what you see with the Wood's lamp can be challenging. However, the following simple cues can make it easier:

Blue-White Spots—Normal and healthy skin

White Spots—Horny layer of the skin (dead skin cells)

Purple Fluorescent Areas—Thin dehydrated skin

Light Violet Areas—Dry skin

Bright Fluorescent Areas—Hydrated skin

Orange or Coral Areas—Oily areas of the skin and comedones (seborrhea)

Brown Areas—Areas of pigmentation; dark spots

Computer Imaging

Many spas have gone to computer imaging to evaluate the skin. These computers scan the skin and take pictures that are very helpful to the aesthetician. Typically, the photographs will show surface and subsurface problems such as pore size, wrinkles, spots, photodamage, unevenness, and telangiectasias. These computer systems are becoming more popular because they not only can track the client's problems and progress, but also can analyze the client's skin compared to others in his or her age bracket. It is a powerful tool for client care.

Documenting Your Findings

Now it is time for you to document your findings. Note the specifics of your findings in the spa chart. For example, if scars exist, note where and how large they are. If the client can elaborate on the history of the scar, document that as well. If an area of hyperpigmentation exists, note its location and color. Make notes about the skin's texture and tone by describing its appearance. For example, "The skin appears to have solar damage at the lateral jawline, exhibited by static lines and roughness." Be sure to note the skin type and condition. If your documentation papers allow for a picture of the face, mark your findings on the picture and make text notes as well. Any information that you can put on the form will help you over time as the face improves with treatment. The next step is photographs.

Taking Photographs

Taking photographs is perhaps the most overlooked but most important part of client care. If you do not have a computer imaging system, digital photographs are a must. Photographs record what the client looked like on the first visit. Most of the time, you cannot recall with accuracy or clarity exactly what the client looked like at the beginning of the treatment. After two to four treatments you may find yourself raving about the results, but the photograph tells the real story. Photographs also may protect you from potential litigation. A digital photography system with computer storage and color printout should be used.

To ensure the accuracy and consistency in photography, a *policy and procedure* should be developed. The policy and procedure should include titles such as *Camera Specifics, Care and Maintenance of the Camera, Flash and Lighting Techniques, Focusing and Framing the Shot, Ensuring Accurate Photographs,* and *Troubleshooting the Camera.* For the purposes of this text we will cover *Ensuring Accurate Photographs*, because many cameras have variable instructions, and not all of the specifics can be covered in this text.

Policy and Procedures for Accurate Photographs

The necessity for accurate photographs cannot be overemphasized. Having a policy and procedure document that accurately depicts the process is a good start. This process creates consistency in the photographs (for example, distance, angle of the face, and color). When comparing before and after photographs, this consistency is critical to the analysis.

Client Expectations

Once all of the documents have been reviewed, missing information has been filled in, and the photographs have been taken, a mini-facial can be done. The facial helps the client relax and consider the options that have been discussed. As the facial nears completion, it is time for the aesthetician to review the findings with the client and confirm the possible actions that can be taken to achieve the client's objectives. When the facial is complete, turn on the lights and review the photographs. At this point, it is time to concur on the home plan and spa treatments. By now it is typical that you have made a connection with the client, and he or she is receptive to your recommendations. If he or she is not receptive to the home and spa program, simply write up the program and try to schedule the client for another facial. If you provided a good facial, surely the client will reschedule and you will have another opportunity for the client to decide when to begin a medical program.

If, on the other hand, he or she is ready to begin the program that day, several steps need to occur. First, an agreement between client and aesthetician on the goals and time frame for the program should be discussed. Next, put together the program. This process will depend on your facility and the approach that is used. Usually the client leaves with home-care products and a schedule for spa treatments. As the aesthetician maps out the plan, mini-goals for improvement need to be set. This plan should be documented in the chart and on a duplicate take-home sheet for the client. It is the aesthetician's job to keep the expectations realistic and to use the care plan as a guide to success. One of the most difficult tasks for aestheticians is to evaluate and project the final result of treatment. Even the best aesthetician with years of experience can be surprised by an unexpected positive result in a case he or she thought was going to be very difficult. The optimum course

Standard Policy and Procedure: Facial Aesthetics

Title: Ensuring accurate photographs

Policy: All personnel will follow the procedures described following.

Purpose: To ensure all photographs are properly focused and framed, providing a documented photographic history.

Scope: All staff

Procedure:

1. Hold the camera at the approximate distance from the subject for the selected magnification. This can be accomplished by providing a specific mark on the floor for the camera and for the client at premeasured distances.

2. Look through the camera to ensure the client is in the frame and the desired shot is in place.

3. Take the photograph.

4. Review the photograph.

5. Ensure that the accurate date is in the system.

6. Take multiple shots of the subject, including:

   A. One full face, straight on

   B. One full face, left side

   C. One full face, right side

   D. One perioral, straight on

   E. One of the eyes and glabella

   F. Any photographs to document specific concern (for example, the neck for poikiloderma, the sides of the face for hyperpigmentation, and the forehead for horizontal lines)

7. Print the photographs that have been taken, and make sure the client's name appears on the photographs.

8. File the photographs in the chart.

---

of action is to *underpromise and overachieve.* You must keep in mind that you are not in total control of the situation. The client bears much of the responsibility for success, including home-care applications—particularly sunscreen—and keeping regular appointments. It is easy for the aesthetician to take too much of the emotional burden of unmet expectations while failing to realize that the client is also responsible.

Realistic Expectations

"My face did not get this way overnight. I guess it will take time to get better." This quote is the sign of a client with **realistic expectations** and an understanding of the possibilities. Setting and maintaining realistic expectations with your client is an ongoing and fluid process. It is

realistic expectations
Belief that a certain outcome is within the realm of possibility or is likely based on unbiased examination of evidence presented.

Table 6–1	What a Client with Realistic Expectations Might Sound Like

I am willing to try something new to look better down the road.

I have spent half my life causing damage, and now I want to take the time to do things right.

I do not expect any miracles, but I would like to see an improvement in my skin's coloring and the fine lines.

I would just like to look better and feel better about myself six months from now.

I think I might need some help deciding if microdermabrasion is the right treatment for me.

also one of the most difficult tasks an aesthetician will do with the client. The best approach is to help the client recognize improvement through three tactics: (1) taking photographs, (2) underpromising, and (3) not aiming for "perfect" results (Table 6–1).

Photographs are the best documentation available to set and sustain expectations. The old saying "A picture is worth a thousand words" is so true. The photographic process is an important one and should not be disregarded. Be sure to share photographs of the progress with the client. This will help him or her to see how much (or how little) improvement has been made, allowing for discussion and alterations in treatments.

Next, you should underpromise and overachieve. Never promise more than you can knowingly deliver, and avoid promising too much too soon. Clients are thrilled when the skin looks better than anticipated, and you are the "skin-care genius" when you are able to achieve reasonable results.

Finally, seasoned plastic surgeons say, "Perfect is the enemy of good." Go for good; it is achievable and believable. For example, someone who is 55 years old is never going to be wrinkle-free and look naturally young. After age 40, crow's-feet are simply part of the physical facial attributes. Help the client to understand that, as we age, we must accept certain changes. As he or she begins to understand the aim of *improvement* rather than *perfection*, it will help you keep the client's expectations in line.

Unrealistic Expectations

Working with unrealistic clients can be one of the most difficult situations you will manage in your career. Clients who have **unrealistic expectations** are unhappy and tell friends and family about their unhappiness. To avoid this problem, you should be aware of the common

unrealistic expectations
Belief that a certain outcome is possible, regardless of merit or circumstance.

Table 6–2 What a Client with Unrealistic Expectations Might Sound Like

I want to look 15 years younger, but I do not want to have surgery.
I want perfectly smooth, evenly colored skin.
I really like my products, and I do not want to have to switch to something new.
I would like to get rid of my crow's-feet, frown lines, and my jowl.
I do not want to have any redness or discomfort.
I have a party to go to tomorrow night, and I want to look like a million bucks!

times within the treatment continuum when clients may become unhappy (Table 6–2).

First, in the consultation process you should be able to identify those clients who will not be satisfied. These clients would be identified by statements such as, "I want all of this loose skin to go away. Will that happen with microdermabrasion?" These clients will also argue with you about potential results. For example, "My friend Sandy had microdermabrasion, and her pores got smaller. I want my face to look like hers." These clients should be referred to the physician or to another aesthetician or spa, if you do not believe you can manage their expectations.

Second, once the process has begun and the results are in the initial stages, unhappy clients will become impatient or believe that they have not had any results at all. This is a time for pictures. Use the initial pictures and take pictures on the day of treatment. Show these pictures to the client. Usually, the improvement is obvious. The client will forget what he or she looked like even a few weeks before. If, on the other hand, not enough improvement exists, a consultation with the physician or a "bump" to the program will be in order.

Finally, once the initial problem is solved, other smaller problems will be uncovered. For example, a client with significant hyperpigmentation may have telangiectasias under the pigment. Many times, the client will accuse the aesthetician of creating these telangiectasias. If you have not previously pointed out to the client the telangiectasias, it could be problematic. Nevertheless, the unhappy client will then focus on a secondary problem, forgetting that the primary problem has been solved. This situation requires a second consultation and a conversation about expectations.

In general, several approaches can be used when dealing with these clients: address the problem head-on, do not treat them, or refer them to the physician for more aggressive procedures that will meet their goals. Sometimes, when you confront the situation and discuss the facts, the client will acknowledge the realities or accept a referral to the physician for surgery. If this approach does not work, be direct: "Mrs. Smith, I am afraid that the service and product I have to offer you will not accomplish your goals. I do not want to waste your money and time. Perhaps you will be able to find another specialist who can achieve your objectives." This is a professional and direct way of managing this client. It also allows you to "take the high road."

Setting Up a Care Plan

The care plan is a roadmap that helps both you and the client understand the process to achieve the goal. Two arms to the care plan exist: (1) the home program and (2) the spa program. The home program is for the client to do at home and is as critical to the outcome as the spa treatments. Clients and aestheticians alike often forget that the best results for a microdermabrasion program are achieved when the client is conscientious about the home program. The second arm is, of course, the spa program. How often the treatment is given, at what intensity, and what other treatments are included makes the difference in the result for the client. These facts and the progression of the process should all be included in the care plan.

Home Programs

Home programs are focused on the morning and evening regimens. Sophisticated medical programs include the use of Retin A, alpha hydroxy acid (AHA), vitamin C, and sunscreen, as well as cleansers and moisturizers that are suited to the program (see Chapter 5) (Tables 6–3 and 6–4). The application of these products is very specific, and the order is important to the final outcome. The use of a home program regimen also helps the aesthetician to evaluate the client's compliance with the program (another component of documenting results and managing expectations).

Spa Programs

Spa programs are those treatments or groups of treatments that will be used in the spa. Initially, the care plan should include a weekly visit by the client. Whether these treatments are always microdermabrasion, or microdermabrasion alternated with a facial, having the client in the spa weekly is important for the long-term success (Table 6–5). In the beginning, you are changing the behavior of the client. You are changing the way he or she washes and moisturizes the face and the commitment made to spa treatments. Keeping the client "close to you" helps the

Table 6-3 Suggested Home Program for Microdermabrasion Treatments—Normal to Dry Skin

Regimen Time	Activity	Product Recommendation
Morning	Cleanse:	Cleanser 5.0 pH
	Medicate:	Glycolic acid 12% 3.8 pH gel
		Vitamin C (*l*-ascorbic acid 3.8 pH)
	Moisturize:	Vitamin E, selenium, and zinc
	Sunscreen:	Chemical blend with zinc oxide
	Makeup:	Client's choice
Evening	Cleanse:	Cleanser 5.0 pH
	Medicate:	Retin A 0.05% cream
		Hydroquinone 4%–6% cream
	Moisturize:	Co-Q$_{10}$, multiple vitamins
	Eye treatment:	Vitamin C eye serum

Table 6-4 Suggested Home Program for Microdermabrasion Treatments—Normal to Oily Skin

Regimen Time	Activity	Product Recommendation
Morning	Cleanse:	With salicylic acid
	Medicate or	Glycolic gel 12%–15% 3.5 pH
	Actives:	*or* peptide serums
		Vitamin C *l*-ascorbic acid
	Moisturize:	Multiple vitamins including zinc
	Sunscreen:	Zinc and titanium oxide blend
	Makeup:	Client's choice
Evening	Cleanse:	1.0 pH with salicylic acid
	Medicate:	Retin A 0.025% gel *or* high-powered
		antioxidant such as Prevage MD™
		Hydroquinone 4% gel
	Moisturize:	Multiple vitamin only in the areas
		needed
	Eye treatment:	Vitamin C eye serum

client through the changes he or she will need to make to be successful. You can encourage and support the client. Additionally, it allows an opportunity to monitor the *realistic expectation* component of your new relationship.

Table 6–5 Example of Treatment Care Plan

Sunday	Monday	Tuesday	Wednesday	Thursday	Friday	Saturday
1	2 *Spa consultation & facial*	3 Begin home program	4 Continue home program	5 Continue home program	6 Continue home program	7 Continue home program
8 Continue home program	9 Continue home program	10 Continue home program	11 *Spa appt: microderm-abrasion, add vitamin C to home care*	12 Post-microderm-abrasion home care	13 Begin phase II home program	14 Continue phase II home program
15 Continue phase II home program	16 Continue phase II home program	17 Continue phase II home program	18 Continue phase II home program	19 Continue phase II home program	20 *Spa appt: microderm-abrasion*	21 Post-microderm-abrasion home care
22 Phase III home program	23 Phase III home program	24 Phase III home program	25 Phase III home program	26 Phase III home program	27 Phase III home program	28 Phase III home program
29 Phase III home program	30 *Spa appt: microderm-abrasion*					

CONCLUSION

First impressions are lasting impressions is a motto to live by, especially the spa business. What you do, how you behave, how you dress, and how you talk will be your ultimate success. Clients look to you for your professionalism and knowledge. It is up to you to deliver the goods. In reality, a consultation is nothing more than an educational process. The client has a need and you have the skills to fill the need. How you impart the information will make the difference as to whether the client hears you. The more experienced you become at the consultative process, the easier it will become.

Finally, setting the road map to get from today's average skin to tomorrow's beautiful skin is all in the care plan you develop. Helping your client to understand the importance of the home plan and the spa plan is an education process. Open communication, a quest for knowledge, and the ability to choose the right programs will set you and your client on the right path.

❯ ❯ ❯ Top 10 Tips to Take to the Spa

1. Keep your hair neatly combed and your makeup conservative; appear professional.

2. Your appearance communicates your ability in the public's mind.

3. At the consultation, you should listen to your client and try to fill his or her needs.

4. You are skilled and are important to the client.

5. Do not forget to take photographs; they provide a visual history of your client.

6. Create realistic expectations for the client and yourself.

7. *Perfect* is the enemy of *good*; accept "good" in your results.

8. Discharge clients that are unrealistic.

9. Care plans help you and the client to work together.

10. Communicate, communicate, communicate!

Chapter Review Questions

1. How do impressions play a role in the aesthetics/spa business? How can an aesthetician improve the impressions of a spa business?

2. What is a consultation? How does it benefit your care and the client's outcome?

3. Why are first impressions important to the aesthetician/client relationship?

4. Explain differentiation. Why is it a valuable component to your success as an aesthetician?

5. What are the two main goals of the consultation?

6. Why is documentation so important? What types of documentation can you use to accomplish this goal?

7. Aside from their intended purpose, what are some of the ancillary purposes for which you can use gathered information?

8. True or False: Clients should only divulge their current sun habits to you.

9. True or False: A telephone consultation is just as good as a face-to-face interview.

10. Match the following documents with their intended purpose:

    a. Client Information Sheet

    b. Photographs

    c. Skin History Sheet

    d. Health History Sheet

    ___ Document used by skin-care professionals to gather information on a client's past and present skin health; includes past treatment, sunburns, and conditions that are necessary for treatment.

    ___ Document used by skin-care professionals to gather information on past and present health conditions, as well as likelihood for future conditions; includes allergies, medical conditions, and prescription information.

    ___ Document used by skin-care professionals to gather social, personal, and demographic information about the individuals who use their services.

    ___ Necessary component of skin-care treatment program that accurately documents the original undisputable, physical skin condition to prove or disclaim treatment results.

11. When greeting a client, what considerations ought to be considered? Why might this be important?

12. Taking the time to ensure that the paperwork is important for what reasons? How can you use this opportunity to advance your relationship with the client?

13. True or False: Client information ought to be updated annually.

14. How should you, as an aesthetician, gauge your client's expectations?

15. A client comes in for a microdermabrasion treatment with unrealistic expectations. How might you handle this client?

16. What is BDD? What are the signs you ought to consider prior to performing a microdermabrasion treatment on a client?

17. True or False: Once you have evaluated client expectations, and determined potential for attainment, then it is appropriate to perform a microdermabrasion treatment.

18. What steps ought to be taken prior to and during the skin analysis?

19. What is a Wood's lamp? How will it help you service your clients?

20. What is a care plan? How will it vary from one client to the next?

Chapter Reference

1. *Random House Dictionary*. (1992). New York: Random House.

Indications and Contraindications for Microdermabrasion

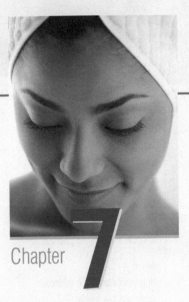

Chapter 7

Key Terms

acne

body dysmorphic disorder (BDD)

Botox® (*Clostridium botulinum*)

burns

cellulitis

clinical indications

comedones

contraindications

crow's-feet

dynamic rhytids

folliculitis

fungal infections

glabella

herpes zoster

hyaluronic acid

impetigo

indications

Juvéderm® and Restylane®

lesions

malignant

pseudofolliculitis barbae

Radiesse®

rashes

Restylane®

ringworm

rosacea

seborrheic keratosis

shingles

static rhytids

tinea corporis

universal precautions

warts

yeast infections

Learning Objectives

After completing this chapter you should be able to:

1. Understand the clinical indications for microdermabrasion.
2. Define the different types of rhytids.
3. Understand the clinical contraindications for microdermabrasion.
4. Understand when physician intervention is required.

167

INTRODUCTION

All one has to do is look around to see that everyone's skin is different. The color, texture, and condition vary from one person to the next, even between people who are closely related. Therefore, not all skin types or skin problems are appropriate for microdermabrasion. It is the aesthetician's responsibility to carefully select the candidates, ensuring that the particular skin condition can be improved or solved by the treatment. The consultation is the obvious time to begin this process. The most common place to begin evaluating a client's potential for treatment success lies with the indications and contraindications for treatment. Indications are the complaints and conditions which warrant treatment. Conversely, contraindications are the situations and conditions in which treatment is unwarranted and can even be detrimental to the well-being of your client.

Indications and contraindications can sometimes overlap, causing a challenging dilemma for the aesthetician. To overcome this, the aesthetician must take the consultation process seriously, listening to the client carefully to identify the primary cause for his or her skin concerns. The problem can then be evaluated based on predetermined indications and contraindications. Using conservative judgment is always the best approach, but sometimes your enthusiasm to help a client's skin can cloud your judgment. Strict adherence to the indications and contraindications as tools in the evaluation process for microdermabrasion treatment will help to avoid poor judgment and, later, poor outcomes.

As you know, microdermabrasion is frequently used to treat a variety of problems and conditions. The broader question which needs to be asked, and which we will be addressing in this chapter, is whether all the conditions treated with microdermabrasion are appropriate for the treatment and, more importantly, why the condition warrants treatment or why the extraneous factors might preclude a client from a microdermabrasion treatment.

The *best* candidates for microdermabrasion are individuals with fine lines, solar damage, hyperpigmentation, rough texture, acne scarring, and variety of skin lesions. Contraindications include active acne, multiple telangiectasias, or immediately after facial plastic surgery (up to one month).

CLINICAL INDICATIONS FOR MICRODERMABRASION

Clinical indications are those conditions suited for a particular treatment or procedure based on specific indicators. In the case of

indications
Any sign or circumstance that a particular treatment is appropriate or warranted.

contraindications
Any sign or symptom that a particular treatment that would otherwise be advisable would be inappropriate.

acne
An inflammation of the sebaceous glands and hair follicles.

clinical indications
Conditions suited for a particular treatment or procedure based on specific indicators.

microdermabrasion, clinical indications cross the boundaries of skin type and include a sophisticated analysis of skin condition beyond the standard normal, dry, oily, combination, and sensitive skin.

In the previous chapters you have analyzed the skin for aging, evaluated the skin for extrinsic and intrinsic aging factors, discussed the consultative processes, and come to understand product use and how it affects the skin. In this section, you will add to your previous understanding, and learn how to analyze the diseases and conditions that affect the skin and may suggest that microdermabrasion is the proper treatment for these problems (or is not). Among the topics in our discussion will be rhytids, solar damage, acne scarring, keratosis, and scars.

> Knowing the indications and contraindications for microdermabrasion will allow safe treatment for all clients.

Rhytids

As we age, wrinkles are the most obvious change we see in our skin (Figure 7–1). For some, these changes in the texture of their skin can be bad news. The good news is that these lines, also called *rhytids*, will

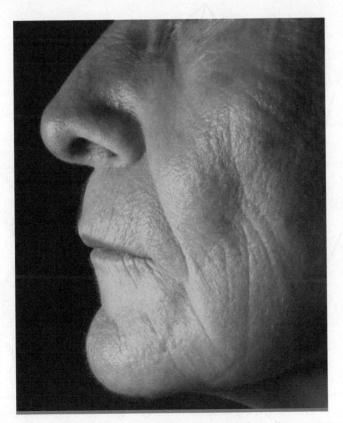

Figure 7–1 As we age, wrinkles (or rhytids) are the most obvious change we see in our skin.

respond to regular microdermabrasion treatments depending on the depth of the wrinkle itself. Rhytid depth can be divided into three classes: (1) fine, (2) medium, and (3) coarse. The rhytids themselves are classified as **static rhytids** (those that occur independent of facial movements) and **dynamic rhytids** (those related to facial movements).

Because rhytids are the main complaint of clients and the first sign of aging, you should look at the different types of rhytids, how they occur, and whether microdermabrasion will resolve or minimize their appearance.

Static Rhytids

Static rhytids are caused by both intrinsic and extrinsic aging. Static rhytids are those found in the morning after sleep, from sun exposure (usually on the sides of the face), or from the effects of gravity (Figures 7–2 and 7–3). Static rhytids are present in the passive face and are not a result of facial movement. These lines respond nicely to microdermabrasion as

static rhytids
Wrinkling that occurs without reference to facial movement.

dynamic rhytids
Wrinkling that occurs because of facial movement.

Clients with deeper rhytids, static or dynamic, are less likely to be satisfied with the end results; therefore, it is important to adjust their expectations before treatment.

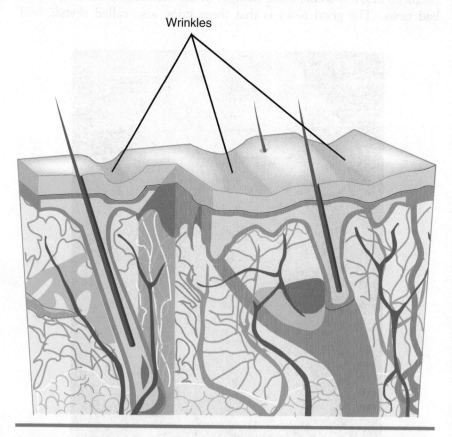

Wrinkles

Figure 7–2 Wrinkling is the result of prolonged exposure to gravity and the sun's harmful rays.

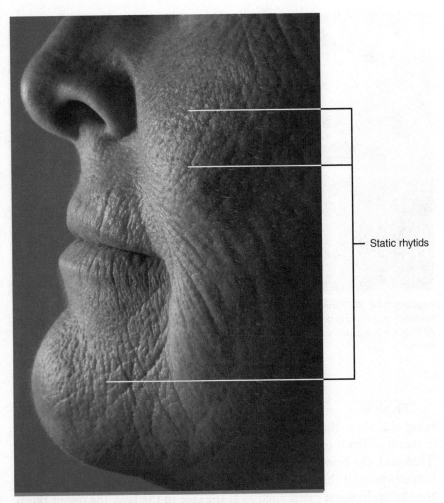

Static rhytids

Figure 7–3 Both intrinsic and extrinsic aging factors cause static rhytids.

long as they are not too deep. Deeper rhytids in this category are a result of skin laxity. Clients whose lines are too deep may not benefit from microdermabrasion to their satisfaction, and may require an adjustment of their expectations or a referral to a surgeon.

Dynamic Rhytids

Dynamic rhytids are lines that are created by muscle movement over a period of time. Those with expressive faces and animated features have far more lines than those with stoic faces. These rhytids usually appear in the forehead (for example, frown lines in the glabella), the sides of the face from robust smiles, and on the upper and lower lip from pursing (Figure 7–4, *A*, and 7–4, *B*).

glabella
Area between the eyebrows with underlying muscle groups that cause creasing (frown lines) as a result of repeated squinting or frowning over time.

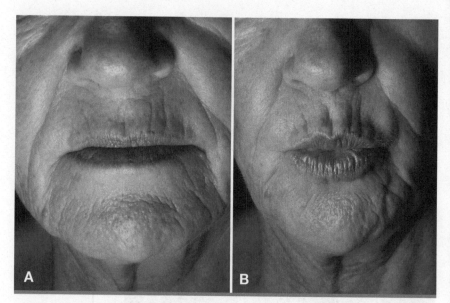

Figure 7–4 *A*, Dynamic rhytids are lines that are created by muscle movement over a period of time. Evaluate this woman in the resting position. *B*, Now, evaluate the lines in motion. Repetitive motion can predict life's later lines.

These lines are deeper and correspond to the muscle groups underlying the skin, dimpling the area. The continued muscle movement makes it difficult to effectively treat these lines with microdermabrasion. That said, the lines can still be treated and will respond better to microdermabrasion if the muscle movement is eliminated with a **Botox**® pretreatment. In some cases, such as at the side of the face, the use of Botox is not indicated; therefore, a therapeutic home program that includes Retin A is required. Microdermabrasion will still improve the lines and the skin, but proper expectations are required in this case.

Fine Rhytids

Fine rhytids are the first to appear in the aging face. These lines are usually found at the eye area and are referred to as **crow's-feet** (Figure 7–5). Crow's-feet can be seen on individuals as young as 18 or 19 years old. Fine rhytids can also be seen along the sides of the face, are either static or dynamic in nature, and may be the result of solar damage or smiling. Obviously, greater success will be found with the static lines and microdermabrasion treatment. Dynamic lines with a mild degree of severity are still indicated, and the treatment program can still yield moderate success.

Botox® (*Clostridium botulinum*)
Trade name for small doses of the botulism toxin that are injected into the wrinkle-causing muscles; toxin blocks the release of the chemicals that would otherwise signal the muscle to contract, thus paralyzing the injected muscle.

crow's-feet
Dynamic rhytids next to the eyes, caused by repeated muscle movement from expression over time.

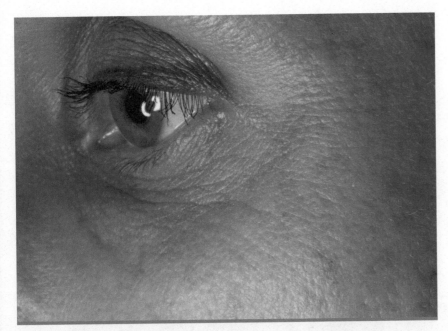

Figure 7–5 Fine rhytids are the first to appear in the aging face, sometimes as early as the late teen years. Fine rhytids most commonly seen in crow's-feet.

Solar Damage

Bronzed skin has long been synonymous with health and leisure. Unfortunately, the consequence of such thinking is the expanding problem of solar damage for the general population. Many of us sat for hours in the sun with baby oil using aluminum foil reflectors to enhance our tans. Now it is time to pay the price. Solar damage can be as simple as fine lines associated with the deterioration of dermal health, or it can be much more severe, resulting in hyperpigmentation, actinic keratosis, and superficial and invasive skin cancers (including melanoma).

Solar damage does not occur just in people in their 50s and 60s, but increasingly in men and women in their 20s and 30s. Sun exposure and the subsequent damage that occurs before the age of 18 is the leading cause of skin cancer and accelerates the aging process (Figure 7–6). As a result, many young men and women will appear significantly older than their chronologic age. The skin types at greatest risk are Fitzpatrick I, II, and III.

Microdermabrasion is an excellent choice for these clients. A full program would include not only the treatment but also an educational program to implement behavior modification. This will be the most difficult part of the program if your client is a "sun worshipper." The client should be encouraged to use sunscreens, hats, and umbrellas.

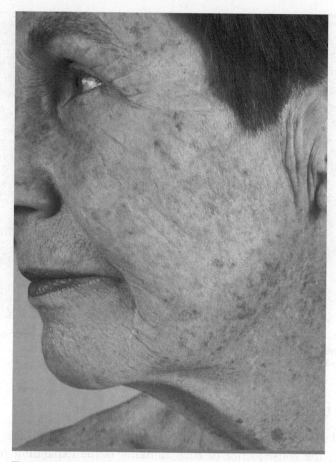

Figure 7–6 Sun exposure and the subsequent damage that occurs before the age of 18 years is the leading cause of skin cancer and accelerates the aging process.

Without behavior modification, the associated microdermabrasion treatments, and home care, these clients will not have the desired long-term results. When your clients are truly committed to making a change in their skin, it can be done; however, it requires effort, expense, and hard work both inside and outside of the spa.

Hyperpigmentation and Telangiectasia

Hyperpigmentation occurs when the enzyme tyrosine triggers the overproduction of melanin (Figure 7–7). Hyperpigmentation is due to a variety of causes, specifically, prolonged unprotected sun exposure, birth control pills, hormone replacement therapy, pregnancy, some antibiotics, and even skin irritation in certain individuals. Hyperpigmentation is often

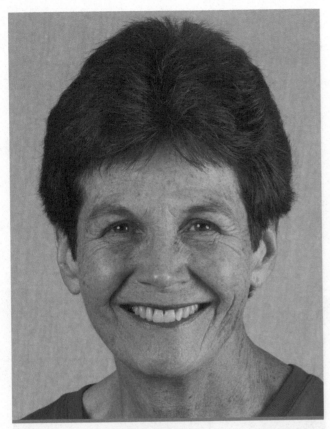

Figure 7–7 Hyperpigmentation occurs as a result of the overproduction of melanin.

difficult to treat, because the source of the problem may remain a constant, such as birth control pills. Microdermabrasion can be an effective tool for the treatment of hyperpigmentation. For a compliant client, a microdermabrasion program with the proper adjunct therapy can usually solve the problem, depending on the depth of the pigment.

Telangiectasias are tiny blood vessels on the face that can become more apparent after microdermabrasion (Figure 7–8). Sometimes referred to as "broken capillaries," telangiectasias are dilated capillaries in the papillary dermis. Because the telangiectasias often become more obvious as the hyperpigmentation is lifted, clients may draw the conclusion that the microdermabrasion has caused the problem. Significant preexisting telangiectasias may be a contraindication to microdermabrasion (see Contraindications to Microdermabrasion). Be sure to look for these little vessels and point them out to the client before treatment to avoid future disappointment on the part of the client.

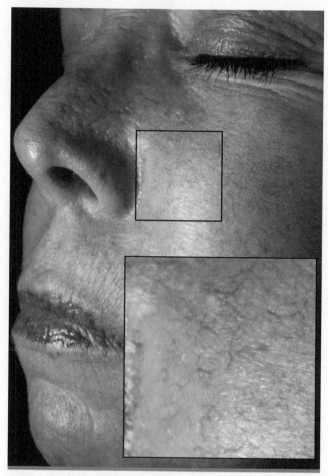

Figure 7–8 Telangiectasias are tiny blood vessels on the face that can become more apparent after microdermabrasion.

Evaluating hyperpigmented skin requires close analysis for telangiectasias. You may be asking yourself, "How do I decide if the treatment should be for the pigmentation or telangiectasias?" That is a good question! The best course of action is to treat the hyperpigmentation first and the telangiectasias second. This course of action allows for clearer skin and the ability to evaluate the telangiectasias clearly (because the pigment covers some of the telangiectasias, their treatment may be partially missed if they are treated first).

Rough Texture

Rough texture is usually the result of unprotected sun exposure but also may be inherited. This phenomenon can be described as the "orange-peel look" or a "pebbly" appearance.[1] Rough texture is many times accompanied by congested pores and usually found on older individuals, sometimes described as "golfer skin." Rough texture responds very well to microdermabrasion treatment.

After Facial Surgery

If an individual has invested in an expensive facial surgery, maintaining that beautiful result is important, and microdermabrasion will help. The results of facial surgery can be dramatic. Taking away a "gobble neck" or wrinkles makes clients look and feel better, but facial surgery cannot improve the color, tone, and texture of the skin (Figure 7–9). These problems are inherent in the skin and require skin treatments. Depending on the skin type and other skin problems, microdermabrasion (not beginning

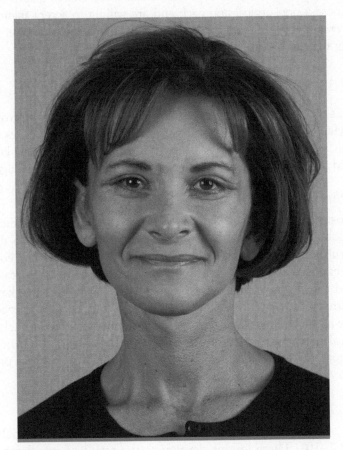

Figure 7–9 Postsurgical presentation of a woman who has had a facelift and eyelid lift three weeks earlier. She still requires skin treatment to improve tone and texture.

until at least one month after facial surgery) is the treatment that will improve the skin and maintain the youthful appearance for this client.

Acne Scarring

Chronic acne is a condition which affects millions of men and women of all ages. Typically associated with teenagers, adult acne is also very common. In fact, acne or acne scarring is one of the most common complaints in the spa setting. In the past, the best treatment for acne scarring was traditional dermabrasion. Dermabrasion is a surgical procedure that takes weeks to heal, months to decolorize, and leaves a potential for hypopigmentation (loss of pigment). Today, microdermabrasion can improve acne scarring, albeit not in one treatment. The best acne scars to treat are the "rolling hill" type of scars versus the "ice pick" kind. Many treatments are required, and completely smooth skin is not a reasonable goal. For those who choose a nonsurgical approach and are willing to accept *improvement* versus *eradication*, microdermabrasion is a good choice. Hence, understanding the client's expectation is of the utmost importance.

Keratosis

Keratosis is described as horny growths (an abnormal overgrowth of cells). Many different types of keratosis exist, but for our purposes we will focus on **seborrheic keratosis** and actinic keratosis. Seborrheic keratosis is related to aging, whereas actinic keratosis is related to sun damage.

Seborrheic Keratosis

The most common type of keratosis is seborrheic keratosis, which does not become **malignant**.[2] Seborrheic keratoses are thought to develop from prolific epidermal cells.[3] They vary in color and are more common on sun-exposed areas of the body.[4] These **lesions** seem to increase with age, and can be problematic to the client. In fact, seborrheic keratoses are so unsightly that clients and aestheticians can become preoccupied with the lesion and overlook a more serious actinic keratosis or melanoma. A clinical program of monthly microdermabrasion can reduce or eliminate seborrheic keratosis, especially when combined with a home program of Retin A and alpha hydroxy acids (AHAs).

Actinic Keratosis

Actinic keratoses are lesions that have become premalignant (Figure 7–10). These lesions develop as the result of sun damage and are sometimes referred to as *solar keratosis*. Actinic keratoses may come and go on the face, ears, neck, shoulders, arms, and, most commonly,

seborrheic keratosis
Benign skin tumor common in the elderly; thought to develop from prolific epidermal cells.

malignant
Resisting treatment, cancerous, or harmful to one's health.

lesions
An area of injured tissue.

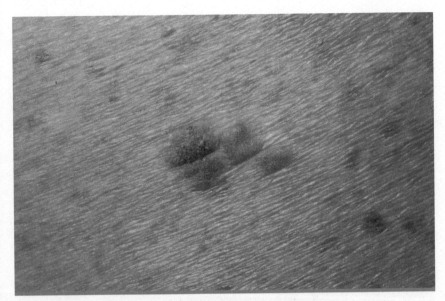

Figure 7–10 An actinic keratosis is a premalignant lesion.

hands. They are pink in color and sometimes peel. Actinic keratoses may evolve into squamous cell carcinomas (SCCs) or basal cell carcinomas (BCCs). If you suspect your client has actinic keratosis, have your physician evaluate this client prior to performing a microdermabrasion treatment on him or her.

Stretch Marks

As any woman who has carried a baby or anyone who has experienced significant weight gain or loss can attest, stretch marks are unsightly and can often be a cause of duress. In the truest sense of the word, a stretch mark is a scar. The skin has been damaged at the dermal layer. Stretch marks have been treated with microdermabrasion for many years. Individual protocols across the country have been somewhat aggressive to address these dermal scars. Some treatment programs have been successful and some have not. Treating stretch marks remains controversial and should be at the direction of your overseeing physician.

Scars

Scars, as you know, are an injury to the dermal tissue and will never go away, but they can be made less noticeable. Scar tissue is never the same as the original tissue and as such will not heal in the same way or at the same rate as the surrounding uninjured tissue.

Treating scars with microdermabrasion has been a common practice for many years, but several caveats hold when treating scars. The *improvement* of the scar will depend on the depth of the scar, the cause (a scar caused from a peel versus a surgical scar), and the location. Scars that are extraordinarily deep (into the reticular dermis and below) will be the most difficult to improve. When you begin therapy on a scar of this depth, have realistic expectations about the potential for improvement. A hypertrophic surgical scar is going to be more difficult to make improvements on than a chemical peel scar, for example. In addition, the location is important to consider. Scars in thinner tissue areas, such as the face, *may* be easier to improve than those on the abdomen. Most scars should respond to *repeated* microdermabrasion treatments by smoothing and minimizing, but use caution to prevent further injury.

CONTRAINDICATIONS FOR MICRODERMABRASION

As you learned in the beginning of this chapter, contraindications are those conditions for which microdermabrasion is not appropriate. In other words, the treatment should not be done when these conditions or diseases are present. A number of skin conditions and diseases are contraindicated for microdermabrasion; they include extensive telangiectasia, rosacea, skin infections, fungal infections, burns, rashes, and viral infections.

Extensive Telangiectasia

Although debated within the aesthetic community, telangiectasias in small patches are not necessarily a contraindication for microdermabrasion; however, skin with large patches of these small blood vessels should not be treated because microdermabrasion may make them worse or more visible. Clients who fall into this category are usually Fitzpatrick I or II. They are the classic ivory-skinned redheads.

Telangiectasias are treatable and should be treated with laser or injection therapy before microdermabrasion. Once they are treated, the microdermabrasion protocol can be implemented. However, do use care because these clients are predisposed to these vessels and can have a reoccurrence. Clients should be made aware of this fact.

Rosacea

Rosacea is an adult form of acne that produces redness, swelling, and obvious telangiectasias with small pustules (Figure 7–11). Over 14 million Americans have some degree of this disease.[5] The disease may start on the cheeks but will gradually spread to the chin and forehead. This condition,

rosacea
Adult form of acne that produces redness, swelling, and obvious telangiectasias.

fungal infections
Any infection caused by the kingdom of organisms that includes yeasts and molds.

burns
Skin injury that occurs as a result of intense thermal, electrical, or acidic agents.

rashes
General term for any topical eruption of the skin.

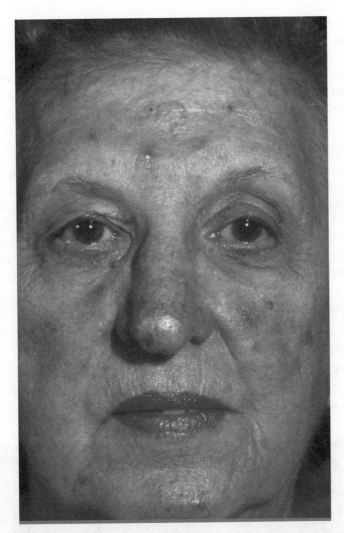

Figure 7–11 Rosacea is most common in women ages 30 to 50 years.

like other forms of acne, is controllable but not curable. Although it is not life-threatening, it is emotionally and socially debilitating. Rosacea is most common in women ages 30 years to 50 years and usually in Fitzpatrick skin types I and II. Since this condition involves telangiectasias, it is important to avoid microdermabrasion with affected clients.

Bacterial Infections of the Skin

Bacterial skin infections occur when a break in the skin occurs and bacteria from the skin's surface or from the environment enter the opening.

Most skin infections are warm to the touch, red, inflamed, and tender. Bacterial skin infections are contraindications for microdermabrasion. Examples of skin infections that the aesthetician might see include cellulitis, impetigo, and folliculitis. All infections require medical attention and antibiotics. If the aesthetician should suspect any skin infection, he or she should refer the client to the physician.

Impetigo

Impetigo is an infection commonly thought to be a childhood affliction, but it can also be seen in adults and occasionally after spa treatments, especially microdermabrasion and peels (Figure 7–12). Impetigo is Group A *Streptococcus* or *Staphylococcus*. The most commonly affected area for impetigo is around the nose and mouth. Impetigo presents itself as blisters of varied appearance, depending on the bacteria. Impetigo itches and is contagious. If the aesthetician suspects impetigo, microdermabrasion should not be done, and the client should be referred to a physician for antibiotics and care.

Cellulitis

Cellulitis is a potentially serious infection of the skin (Figure 7–13). Cellulitis initially appears as a small red area surrounding a skin injury, such as a cut or bite. The skin is red and warm to the touch, and red

cellulitis
Potentially serious infection of the skin that presents as a small red area surrounding a skin injury; those at risk include the elderly and those with compromised immune systems.

impetigo
Skin infection from staphylococcal or streptococcal bacteria.

folliculitis
Infection of the hair follicle, such as ingrown hairs.

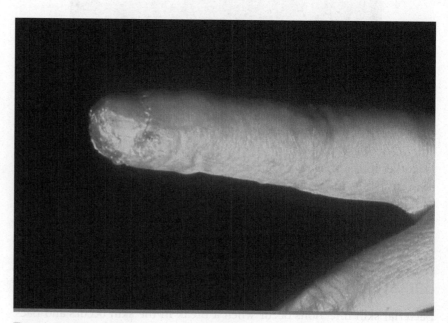

Figure 7-12 Impetigo.

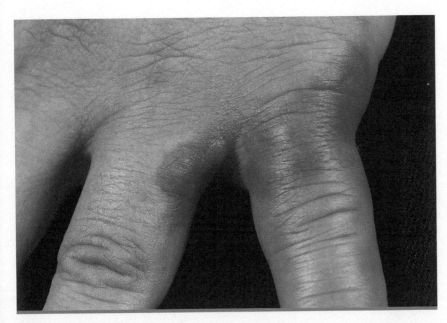

Figure 7–13 Cellulitis.

streaks may appear. The infection can quickly involve the underlying tissues, creating an emergency situation called necrotizing fasciitis or "flesh-eating strep." Clients at risk include the elderly and those with a compromised immune system (human immunodeficiency virus [HIV] or chemotherapy clients), diabetes, chickenpox, or herpes. Microdermabrasion must not be done and the client should be referred to a physician for care.

Folliculitis

Folliculitis is an infection of the hair follicle (Figure 7–14). The hair follicle is irritated and erythemic with pus found in the center. Each infected follicle will have a pimple at the base. Several types of folliculitis exist; the most commonly seen by aesthetician is **pseudofolliculitis barbae**, which is found after shaving or waxing in certain individuals. Refer the client to the physician for treatment with either topical or oral antibiotics before any microdermabrasion treatments.

Fungal Infections of the Skin

Fungal infections of the skin are usually found in the moist, dark areas of the body, such as between the toes. Less frequently fungal infections can also be found on more exposed areas of the body such as the face. Examples of fungal infections include **ringworm** and **yeast infections**.

pseudofolliculitis barbae
Form of folliculitis commonly seen as a result of shaving or waxing.

ringworm
Popular term for dermatomycosis caused by species of fungi from the *Microsporum* family

yeast infections
Viral infection caused by several unicellular organisms that reproduce by budding; oral yeast infections are common in those with compromised immune systems.

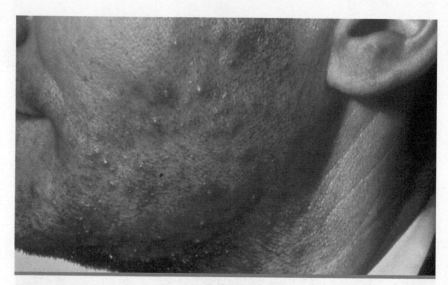

Figure 7–14 Folliculitis.

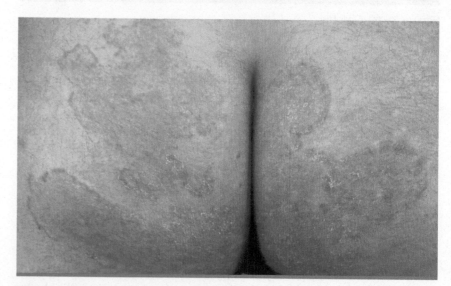

Figure 7–15 Ringworm.

Clients with fungal skin infections should not be treated with microderm-abrasion until their fungal infections are remedied. Refer the client to the physician for treatment.

Ringworm

Several different types of ringworm exist (Figure 7–15). The type of ring-worm most concerning to the aesthetician in the medical spa environment is tinea corporis, or body ringworm. The fungus presents itself as a rash and can appear on the body or the face. Ringworm is circular and has raised edges. The center becomes less red as the lesion grows. The aesthetician should be alert for ringworm in geographic areas of high humidity and high temperatures. Exposure to ringworm is increased when a family has pets that may carry the disease. The physician must treat ringworm before the client undergoes microdermabrasion.

Yeast Infections

When you think of yeast infections, generally you do not think of the face, yet small yeast infections can occur at the corners of the mouth. Yeast is normally not a detrimental component of the skin; however, a yeast infection can appear in clients with depressed immune systems. The aesthetician should be alert to cracks or tiny cuts in the corners of the mouth. To diagnose this problem, a scraping of the skin must be taken and examined under the microscope. The physician may recommend medicated ointments to cure this problem. If a yeast infection is suspected, the client should be referred to a physician before microdermabrasion treatments.

Viral Infections of the Skin

Viruses are parasitic organisms that invade and attach to living cells to survive and reproduce. Viruses cannot be treated with antibiotics. Rather, antiviral medications are the only successful treatments. The most common viral infections of the skin are herpes simplex, **shingles**, and flat facial **warts**.

Active Herpes Simplex

Active herpes simplex, also called (HSV-1), is the virus that causes cold sores (Figure 7–16). These viral infections appear as small clear blisters on the face, most commonly around the mouth.

After the lesion has healed, the virus will be dormant in the body, periodically reactivating. Herpes is contagious and persons with open sores should avoid contact by kissing or other means of person-to-person contact. Microdermabrasion should not be done when a client has active herpes simplex (cold sores).

Shingles

Chickenpox and shingles are both caused by **herpes zoster**. After a person has chickenpox, the virus lays dormant in the nerve endings. It may reappear, usually after the person is past the age of 50 or when the client has a reduced immunity, resulting in shingles. Shingles usually follows

tinea corporis
Body ringworm.

shingles
Sudden, acute inflammation, linked to herpes zoster.

warts
Flat, cutaneous, and flesh-colored lesions caused by papillomavirus.

herpes zoster
Virus responsible for both shingles and chickenpox.

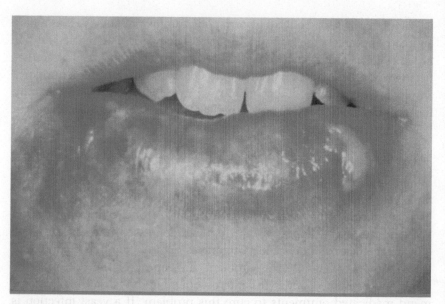

Figure 7–16 Herpes simplex.

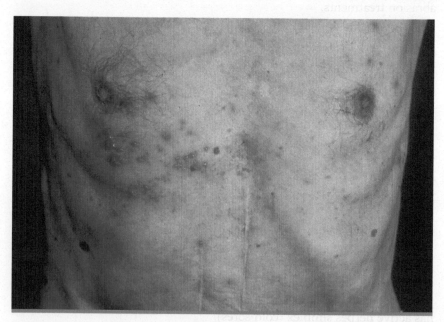

Figure 7–17 Shingles.

a nerve pathway, called a *dermatome*. Shingles can and do occur on the face (Figure 7–17).

Microdermabrasion should never be done when herpes zoster is active. In addition, because the skin is sensitive after a shingles episode, take care to evaluate the appropriateness of microdermabrasion for many weeks after the episode has healed.

Facial Warts

Facial warts appear as flat circular lesions. They are often the same color as the skin of the face and are difficult to see. Most of the time, warts will unexpectedly disappear, other times they require treatment such as cauterization, liquid nitrogen, or salicylic acid treatments. Using micro-dermabrasion on facial warts will cause them to spread and is not advised. Facial warts are easily treated and should be taken care of before microdermabrasion treatments.

Open Lesions, Rashes, and Burns

Open lesions, rashes, and burns are obviously not appropriate for microdermabrasion. Open lesions include areas of surgical treatment such as a keratosis treated with liquid nitrogen. Rashes are generalized skin eruptions that are erythemic and raised (for example, poison ivy, allergic reactions, or sun rashes). Burns include sunburns and other types of burns. Skin that is compromised in any way should be healed through appropriate pathways before microdermabrasion is considered. Once the skin is healed it is important to have clear guidance from the physician before beginning treatments.

Sunburns

No matter how minor, a sunburn is still a skin injury and should not be treated with microdermabrasion. Clients will often be resistant to your refusal to treat them, but this is in their best interest. Healing a simple sunburn, as you know, is just a matter of time and care. Instruct the client to avoid therapeutic products for the next 2 to 3 days and moisturize aggressively. If the sunburn is serious, the client should see the physician for further care.

Atopic Dermatitis

Atopic dermatitis is a rash of unknown cause and can be a very frustrating problem. Many times these problems will appear as acne, with small pustules but without comedones. Dermatitis usually comes from contact with soaps, cleanser, fabrics, or other products such as toothpaste. If your client has a facial rash, it is important to do some investigative work. Ask, "When did the rash start?" "Does it itch?" "Does it hurt?" "Did you change laundry detergents?" Prompting the client with different scenarios will help both of you to understand the potential cause. Has the client been using topical steroids, new facial products, or a new sunscreen? Did the client change toothpaste? Does the client let the

comedones
Typical small lesions associated with acne breakouts; usually raised and red in color.

toothpaste ooze out of the mouth onto the skin when brushing the teeth? These are all important investigative questions. If this problem is significant and does not respond to discontinuation of products, then refer the client to a physician who can implement further treatment. Do not perform microdermabrasion on a client with atopic dermatitis.

Active Acne

Grade II to IV acne is characterized by papules, pustules, and nodules, depending on the severity. A debate is underway concerning the use of microdermabrasion in the treatment of active acne grades II or higher. In published studies, acne clients were evaluated and treated while they continued their oral and topical acne therapy. A 2001 study concerning microdermabrasion and acne indicated that approximately 50 percent of the clients treated with microdermabrasion got better and 50 percent got worse.[6] Carefully consider whether microdermabrasion is the treatment of choice for each individual, generally with your physician's assistance.

Accutane®

Isotretinoin, or Accutane, is prescribed for severe unresponsive acne. Accutane is isotretinoin and is related chemically to retinoid and retinol (forms of vitamin A). It decreases the sebaceous activity in the skin by shrinking the oil glands. The decrease in the sebaceous activity is related to the dose of Accutane and the duration of treatment. Accutane can have minor side effects such as dry and chapped lips, dry skin, and dry hair, but it can also have significant side effects including birth defects, depression, intracranial hypertension, and acute pancreatitis. Therefore, Accutane treatment should be reserved for the most recalcitrant cases of nodular acne. Clients taking Accutane should always be under the care of a physician. The standard of care for those clients that have taken Accutane is to *wait one year to be treated with microdermabrasion*, because the decreased sebaceous activity slows skin healing.[7]

Immediate Postoperative Facelift, Blepharoplasty, or Neck Lift

Clients who have had facial surgery are always excited to get back to their skin-care program. Those who have not been involved in a program are often energized to begin one after surgery. However, care must be taken by the aesthetician and client to avoid potential complications by starting the program too early. Bruising will be present for up to ten days, and hematomas can develop even two weeks after surgery. Numbness can last up to one year in certain areas, so the aesthetician must be careful because the client will not feel the microdermabrasion. The time for beginning a skin-care program for the plastic surgery client is at the sole discretion of the plastic surgeon.

Combining Microdermabrasion with Injectable Treatments

Microdermabrasion can be combined with other treatments to create a more complete result (Figures 7–18 and 7–19). Among the treatments with which microdermabrasion is combined are the cascade of injectables: **Juvéderm®, Restylane®**, Botox, and **Radiesse®**. Careful scheduling of these treatments is required to ensure that the treatments occur in the proper sequence and will suit the aftercare of each treatment. For example, it is generally unadvisable to lay the client flat after Botox therapy. Therefore, the microdermabrasion treatment should be done before the Botox treatment. It is recommended that Juvéderm, Restylane, or Radiesse treatments be done at separate appointments. The skin is somewhat sensitive and perhaps a bit swollen after the microdermabrasion. This slight bit of swelling could cause the misplacement of the dermal filler. It is best to simply wait 1 or 2 days to provide the best result for the client. The preferred course is to do

Juvéderm® and Restylane®
Trade names for hyaluronic acid dermal filler.

Radiesse®
Trade name for dermal filler used to improve laugh lines around the mouth.

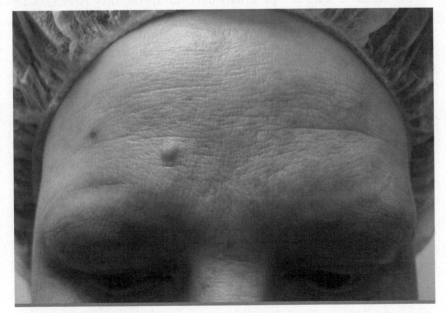

Figure 7–18 Areas of animation, such as the forehead, are difficult to treat with microdermabrasion alone.

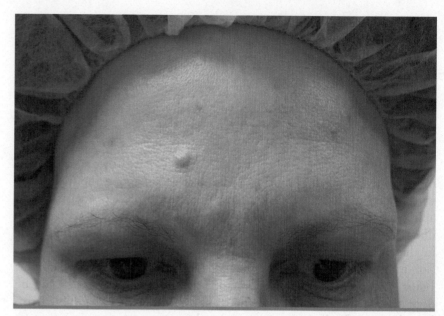

Figure 7–19 The combination of microdermabrasion and Botox therapy provides an excellent outcome.

the microdermabrasion treatment first and injection therapy a few days later.

As aesthetic skin-care programs have advanced, they have become multipronged, using many options to achieve the end result. The aesthetician should be aware of the possibilities in his or her menu of services, including using injectables to achieve a superior result for the client.

Botox

Botox (Allergan, in Irvine, CA), *Clostridium botulinum* toxin type A, is used to paralyze muscle groups by inhibiting the release of acetylcholine at the neuromuscular junction.[8] Once the active muscles are treated and begin to become relaxed or paralyzed, the microdermabrasion will be much more effective in these areas. The areas treated will result in smoother skin and a reduction in lines, specifically in the glabella, crow's-feet, and forehead (the areas most commonly treated with Botox). These areas of animation are difficult to treat with microdermabrasion alone; therefore, the combination of the two treatments provides an excellent outcome. Botox is very safe and there have not been any reported nervous system effects.[9] Botox is a *temporary* solution, and clients should be aware that the treatment needs to be repeated every 3 to 6 months.

Botox and microdermabrasion are good partner procedures. Botox will minimize the muscle movement and improve the appearance of dynamic lines, whereas microdermabrasion will smooth the skin and encourage collagen remodeling in the dermis.

Juvéderm and Restylane

Restylane is a hyaluronic acid dermal filler. It is used to inject wrinkles and fine lines, as well as to augment the lips for a fuller lip line (Figures 7–20 and 7–21). Manufactured as a biodegradable, nonanimal, stabilized hyaluronic acid (NASHA) gel, Restylane is **hyaluronic acid**. This dermal filler does not require a skin test and is very durable. Restylane is versatile and provides many options to the injector. Juvéderm is also a hyaluronic acid filler, used to fill lines and wrinkles as well as lips. The cross linking process is different for Juvéderm than Restylane changing the materials consistency to a smoother and potentially less lumpy product. Both Juvéderm and Restylane are hyaluronic acid and used extensively to inject lines and wrinkles especially in concert with microdermabrasion.

Using a small fine-gauge needle, the product is injected into the areas of defect. The process takes about 30 minutes to 1 hour. The client may exhibit some bruising and swelling that evening and into the next day, generally resolving within one week. On a rare occasion, lumps and bumps can form, but these usually resolve within one week. The treatment will need to be repeated every 8 to 10 months. Combine Restylane or Juvéderm with Botox and microdermabrasion for an outstanding result.

hyaluronic acid
Acid that occurs in intercellular ground substance of connecting tissue; plays an important role in controlling tissue permeation, bacterial invasiveness, and intracellular transport.

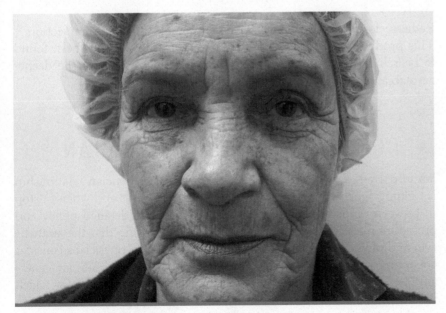

Figure 7–20 Photograph of a woman before receiving a combined treatment of microdermabrasion and Restylane.

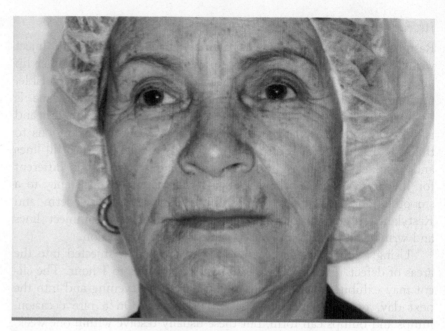

Figure 7–21 Post-treatment photograph visualizing the results of a microdermabrasion treatment with Restylane. Note the improvement around the chin and corners of the mouth.

Radiesse®

Radiesse is calcium hydroxylapatite suspended in a gel or injection.[10] This product has had many uses over the years, and it has been found to be reliable and durable. Radiesse is effective for use in the deeper nasolabial folds (smile lines).[11]

CONSULTING YOUR PHYSICIAN

An important and delicate part of a physician/aesthetician relationship is to know when to consult about the client's progress and when to stop or proceed. This is in large part a function of the detailed policy and procedure manual. However, it is also the relationship that the aesthetician and physician create. In the medical spa setting, physicians consider you a professional and expert. In addition, although physicians are generally performing procedures and caring for clients at the level for which they were trained, they should always be available to you. An aesthetician should never feel uncomfortable or embarrassed to ask for the assistance of his or her physician (Table 7–1).

Table 7–1 When Is It Time to Talk with the Physician?

Concern	Discuss with Physician	Do Not Discuss with Physician
Truthfulness of a client	X	
Ability to achieve desired results	X	
Indications for a possible surgical procedure	X	
Concerns about body dysmorphic disorder (BDD)	X	
Efficacy of the care plan	X	
Client has need for prescription medications	X	
Clarification of medical conditions	X	
Indications of a microdermabrasion treatment	X	
Possibility of an ongoing disease process	X	
Need for advance acne treatment	X	
Suspicious lesions	X	

Microdermabrasion is such a safe treatment that you rarely think about precautions. However, all procedures, including microdermabrasion, have precautions. When treating clients with microdermabrasion, the aesthetician should have a heightened awareness when he or she runs into the following issues: body dysmorphic disorder (BDD), sensitive skin, frequent sun exposure, hepatitis, acquired immunodeficiency syndrome (AIDS) and HIV, pregnancy or lactation, and suspicious lesions or lupus.

body dysmorphic disorder (BDD)
Psychosocial disease that causes individuals to be inappropriately concerned with their appearance; those affected with BDD are contraindicated for most aesthetic procedures.

Body Dysmorphic Disorder

BDD is an emotional disease that causes individuals to be inappropriately concerned with their appearance. People with BDD are focused on the appearance of their skin, hair, nose, or ears, in particular. They may have minor defects of the nose or small scars that they believe are overwhelmingly obvious. Individuals with BDD also are concerned about their eyes and may feel their eyes are too small or otherwise unattractive.

Those with BDD spend at least one hour a day thinking negative thoughts about their appearance.

Unsurprisingly, clients with BDD have difficulty in their social and work lives. While the degree or severity can be highly variable, they can often have difficulty meeting new people or making and keeping friends because they are so self-conscious about their appearance. In the most extreme of instances, they will spend time alone in their home, alienating family or those who care about them.

In the world of cosmetic surgery and medical skin care, some clients are obviously afflicted and others walk in a gray zone between the well-adjusted and the afflicted.[12] Recognizing these clients will become a challenge for the skin-care professional. It will be important for you to be on the lookout for clients who seem overly critical of their skin and appearance. Assuming a psychiatrist is treating the client, one of the easiest methods is to look at the medications that the client is taking. For those under treatment, you will find a medication that is treating mood disorders. However, this can be easily misleading, and not all clients who are on medication for mood disorders have BDD. If BDD is suspected, then the aesthetician should simply ask the client whether he or she is afflicted with the disorder.

Red flags for BDD include depression, anxiety, acute stress, obsessiveness, and compulsiveness.[13] Sometimes individuals with BDD will appear very efficient and organized; however, when the client is under stress, the previously subtle symptoms of BDD will become apparent.

Clients with BDD have a high incidence of dissatisfaction with results, and any small complication can cause undue stress for the aesthetician and client.[14] The most important question the aesthetician should be asking in situations where BDD is suspected is, "Can I satisfy this client?" If the aesthetician has a concern about his or her ability to satisfy the client, the client should be turned away or referred to the physician for further consultation.

BDD (body dysmorphic disorder) can be subtle and difficult to detect. If you are unsure if your client falls into this category, the client should be referred to a physician.

Sensitive Skin

In some spas, sensitive skin is a contraindication for microdermabrasion; however, varying degrees of *sensitivity* exist. At least half of the people who say their skin is sensitive do not have sensitive skin at all. In addition, some clients have environmental sensitivities (such as those to cold and sun), whereas others are sensitive to products and treatments. Investigate what your client means by *sensitive skin,* and use the appropriate precaution.

Sun Exposure

Even with the ongoing media blitz about the hazards of sun exposure, the general population still cannot get enough. A philosophic contradiction exists when the aesthetician tries to improve the skin while the client continues sun exposure without sunscreen. You probably see these clients on a regular basis, counseling them to be careful and wear sunscreen. However, like an addictive drug, clients will return to you time after time with a tan or, worse yet, a sunburn.

Exposure to the sun after a microdermabrasion treatment is a concern. The skin is more sensitive because of the mechanical exfoliation of the microdermabrasion treatment and the home-care products. However, the reality is that everyone has sun exposure. Although you will soon begin to feel that you can recite the dangers of the sun in your sleep, do not give up. Clients need to hear the information at least 5 to 7 times before they embrace it and then, of course, you can begin the behavior modification.

Educate your clients about the effects of direct sun exposure. If they are going to the beach, then they should wear sunscreen, sit under an umbrella, and face away from the sun. Any and all of these tactics will help. You do not have to give up the sun to have nice skin, but you do have to change how you behave *when you are in the sun*.

Finally, the issue of daily sunscreen application is important. If your client is unwilling to wear sunscreen every day, you have a problem. The application of sunscreen is the difference between winning and losing the war, not just the battle. Make sure these clients get a sunscreen in their moisturizer, or microdermabrasion will not be a valid or appropriate treatment.

> Sensitive skin can be frustrating for the client and aesthetician alike. Begin products one at a time and start slowly with microdermabrasion treatments to avoid a potential reaction.

> Hepatitis C is on the rise and is the most likely such infection to affect the aesthetician. Use **universal precautions** to ensure your safety at all times.

universal precautions
Actions taken to prevent the transmission of infectious diseases; involves the use of protective procedures and equipment, such as gloves and masks.

> Individuals with HIV and AIDS are at greater risk for infection.

> Because no one knows the results of certain drugs or topical creams on a fetus all active products should be removed from the program until the pregnancy and breastfeeding are complete.

Hepatitis C

Hepatitis is an inflammation of the liver caused by a number of viruses, including hepatitis A, B, and C. Hepatitis C is of greatest concern because of the chronic nature of the disease. Hepatitis C is transmitted through blood transfusion, unprotected sexual contact, shared needle use, and the mother and infant relationship. Health care workers are at great risk for hepatitis C.

For those of you doing microdermabrasion, coming in contact with blood should be rare. This can happen, however, if the client has small pustules that open during the microdermabrasion process or if the treatment is at the papillary dermis. The greater concern is the next client. Be sure to use disposable tips, if possible. If this is not possible, then ensure the tip is adequately cleaned and sterilized before it is used again. Reusing crystals is an unsafe practice and should never be done.

Human Immunodeficiency Virus and Acquired Immunodeficiency Syndrome

HIV (and AIDS) is contracted through unprotected sexual contact, blood and blood product transfusions, shared needle use, and the mother and infant relationship. As with hepatitis C, the greatest concerns when treating clients with HIV and AIDS is to be sure to use disposable tips and not to reuse crystals. If the tip used does come in contact with blood, it should be disposed of in the sharps container.

Pregnancy and Lactation

Care must always be taken when treating pregnant or lactating women. For these women, microdermabrasion cannot be used with chemical adjunct therapy (peels). Most physicians feel that Retin A, hydroquinone, and AHAs should not be used by pregnant and lactating women. Check your spa protocol for guidance.

Suspicious Lesions

The physician should see any lesion that worries you or looks unusual (Figure 7–22). It may not be a skin cancer, but it could be a lesion of a different type that still requires attention before or concurrent with the microdermabrasion treatment. In addition, your concern for lesions should not stop at the face, neck, and chest. Hands and arms are also at risk for suspicious lesions. Clients depend on you to look at lesions with and for them. When it comes to having lesions examined by the physician, your motto should be: "Better safe than sorry."

Lupus

Lupus is a chronic disease with no known cure. It is also a familiar autoimmune disease for the aesthetician, because it is commonly associated with skin symptoms. Two types of lupus exist: (1) systemic lupus erythematosus (SLE) and (2) discoid lupus erythematosus (DLE). SLE presents on the skin as a red rash on the face in the shape of a butterfly. DLE, on the other hand, exhibits as round red lesions over the skin. Lupus is much more prevalent in women than in men, making it a disease you will tend to hear about frequently. Lifestyle changes are necessary for the lupus client, including reduction of sun exposure, regular exercise, avoidance of stress, and immunizations to avoid disease. If the lesions of lupus (whether SLE or DLE) are active on the face, neck, or chest, the client is not a candidate for microdermabrasion treatment.

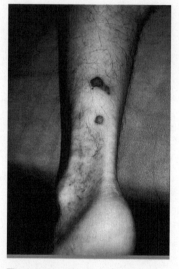

Figure 7–22 Kaposi's sarcoma.

Clients with suspicious lesions should be referred to a physician. Do not be intimidated by the referral process to a proper physician, because such lesions may signal a potential illness. The best interests of your client should be your primary consideration.

Women with lupus may sometimes be treated with oral corticosteroids, making treatment with microdermabrasion slightly more risky because of the potential delayed healing response of the skin.

> Lupus is a common autoimmune disease in women, with markings on the face, hands, neck, and chest.

■ CONCLUSION

The aesthetician will guide the ultimate success of a microdermabrasion program. Proper client selection and education about microdermabrasion is the key to avoiding disappointment for both the aesthetician and the client. The aesthetician's ability to understand when microdermabrasion is indicated, and when it is not, will make the difference between success and failure for the aesthetician and the client. Using proper skills of analysis and communication, the aesthetician can select the right clients and have great success with microdermabrasion. This task is accomplished when all the steps we have covered in this chapter become routine and part of the daily processes of the medical spa.

>>> Top 10 Tips to Take to the Spa

1. Choosing skin problems that are indicated for treatment make your job easier and the outcome more successful.

2. Rhytids are divided into three categories; know these categories.

3. Over 50 percent of daily sun exposure comes through windows; always wear sunscreen.

4. It is better to send a client to consult with a physician about a suspicious lesion than be sorry later. Do not be afraid to "waste" the doctor's time.

5. Sensitive skin falls into two categories: product-sensitive and environment-sensitive.

6. Pregnant and lactating women should not have active products at home or in the spa. They can have basic microdermabrasion with a hydrating mask.

7. If you suspect BDD, take it seriously.

8. Listen and learn from your physician. Follow the physician on rounds and in the spa if possible.

9. Everyone wants to improve the skin of an acne client, but use conservative judgment. Sometimes you can make the situation worse.

10. Combining injections (Botox, Restylane) can provide a great result.

Chapter Review Questions

1. What are rhytids?
2. What is the difference between static rhytids and dynamic rhytids?
3. What is solar damage?
4. What are telangiectasias?
5. What are the different types of acne scarring?
6. Which types of acne scarring respond to microdermabrasion?
7. What is keratosis?
8. What are the types of keratosis?
9. Are stretch marks indicated for microdermabrasion?
10. Name the skin afflictions that contraindicate microdermabrasion.
11. Why is rosacea contraindicated for microdermabrasion?
12. What is BDD?
13. What is Botox?
14. What is Restylane?
15. What is Radiesse?

Chapter References

1. Rubin, M. (1995). *Manual of chemical peels: Superficial and medium depth*. Philadelphia: Lippincott, Williams & Wilkins.
2. Blitzner, A., Binder, W. J., Boyd, J. B., & Carruthers, A. (Eds.). (2000). *Management of facial lines and wrinkles*. Philadelphia: Lippincott, Williams & Wilkins.
3. Balin, A. K. (2002, February 27). *Seborrheic keratosis* [Online]. Available: http://www.emedicine.com
4. Balin, A. K. (2002, February 27). *Seborrheic keratosis* [Online]. Available: http://www.emedicine.com
5. Del Rosso, J. Q., (2003, October). Shining new light on rosacea. *Skin & Aging*, (supp.), 3–6.
6. Lloyd, J. R. (2002, August). The use of microdermabrasion for acne: A pilot study. *Journal of Dermatologic Surgery, 27*(4), 329–331.
7. Bernard, R. W., Beran, S. J., & Rusin, L. (2000). Microdermabrasion in clinical practice. *Spas in Plastic Surgery, 27*(4), 571–577.

8. Fagien, S. & Brandt, F. S. (2001). Primary and adjunctive use of botulinum toxin type A (Botox) in facial aesthetic surgery: Beyond the glabella. *Spas in Plastic Surgery, 28*(1), 127–161.

9. Fagien, S., & Brandt, F. S. (2001). Primary and adjunctive use of botulinum toxin type A (Botox) in facial aesthetic surgery: Beyond the glabella. *Spas in Plastic Surgery, 28*(1), 127–161.

10. Bioform Medical. (2004, April 11). *Product characteristics: Radiance.* [Online]. Available: http://www.bioforminc.com

11. Nassif, P. S. (2004, April). *Radiance, an injectable calcium hydroxylapatite.* [Online]. Available: http://www.plasticsurgery.com

12. Leonardo, J. (2003, August). Negotiating the gray area of BDD, and the bottom line. *Plastic Surgery News, 14*(8), 24–25.

13. Leonardo, J. (2003, August). Negotiating the gray area of BDD, and the bottom line. *Plastic Surgery News, 14*(8), 24–25.

14. The Body Dysmorphic Spa & Research Unit. (2004, January 14). [Online]. Available: http://www.mgh.harvard.edu

Pretreatment for Microdermabrasion

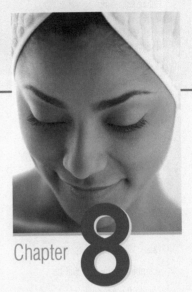

Key Terms

cocamidopropyl betaine

corneocytes

dimethicone

glycerin

hyperkeratinization

octyl methoxycinnamathe

papain

petrolatum

phenylbenzimidazole sulfonic acid

pretreatment

therapeutic program

Chapter 8

Learning Objectives

After completing this chapter you should be able to:

1. Learn the components of a complete therapeutic program.
2. Learn how to educate clients on their pretreatment programs.
3. Evaluate pretreatment conclusions.
4. Evaluate case studies as examples of pretreatment.

INTRODUCTION

pretreatment
Any process that will aid or facilitate a future procedure.

therapeutic program
Program for home use complete with the necessary prescriptions, topical vitamins, and sunscreens.

Prescriptions will improve the condition of the cells; vitamins will attach the free radicals; and sunscreens will protect the skin. When these elements are combined, the skin will be ready for the rigors of microdermabrasion.

In this chapter we will discuss the necessity of pretreatment for microdermabrasion and the products that are required to achieve the desired result. In addition, you will meet our real-life treatment clients for the first time and get to know their current skin-care habits. We will change their home-care programs and introduce them to new ways of caring for their skin, just as you will in the clinical setting (Tables 8–1 and 8–2).

Medical skin care has always ascribed to the notion that pretreatment is the foundation to a good end result. Even in the "old days," Retin A and hydroquinone were considered an important step before a phenol or trichloroacetic peel. The complexity of pretreatment and the understanding of its necessity are now quite advanced. Pretreatment before surgical or nonsurgical procedures with an advanced regimented home-care routine is now considered the standard of care.

Each product in the program should have a specific use. Programs should be very basic, allowing for easy implementation, with recommended adjustments for skin type. A complete therapeutic program, that is, one with prescriptions, vitamins, and sunscreens, will yield the best results (Table 8–3).

Table 8–1 Case Study Home Program—Normal-to-Dry Skin

Time of Day	Activity	Product Recommendation
Morning	Cleanse:	Basic cleanser
	Medicate:	12% alpha hydroxy acid
		Vitamin C
	Moisturize:	Basic moisturizer
	Sunscreen:	20 SPF
	Makeup:	Client's choice
Evening	Cleanse:	Basic cleanser
	Medicate:	Retin A 0.05%
		Hydroquinone 4% cream
	Moisturize:	Heavier moisturizer
	Eye treatment:	Eye cream or serum

Table 8–2 Case Study Home Program—Normal-to-Oily Skin

Time of Day	Activity	Product Recommendation
Morning	Cleanse:	Pamela Hill Papaya Cleanser®
	Medicate:	12% Pamela Hill Alpha Hydroxy Acid®
		La Roche Vitamin C®
	Moisturize:	BioMedic HydroActive Emulsion®
		BioMedic Extra Mild Protection®
	Sunscreen:	BioMedic Facial Shield 20 SPF®
	Makeup:	Client's choice
Evening	Cleanse:	Hymed Liquid Soap®
	Medicate:	Retin A 0.05%
		Hydroquinone 4% Cream
	Moisturize:	Pamela Hill Extra Rich Moisturizer®
	Eye treatment:	Pamela Hill Vitamin C Eye Cream®

Table 8–3 Products and the Effects on the Skin

Product	Changes pH	Affects Dermal Cells	Affects Epidermal Cells	Protects	Hydrates	Exfoliates	Contains Antioxidants
Cleansers	X				X		
Masks	X				X	X	
Moisturizers	X			X			
Alpha hydroxy acids (AHAs)			X		X	X	
Vitamin C							X
Sunscreens				X	X		
Co-Q₁₀							X
Retin A		X					
Hydroquinone		X	X				

COMPLETE THERAPEUTIC PROGRAM

Many clients who will come to your office will be skeptical of medical skin programs. Their body language and attitude say, "Prove it." These clients may be devotees of a particular brand of product, or they may be determined to stick with plain "soap and water." The basis of their skepticism is the result of years of product purchases with limited or no results. Regardless of their product dedication, they still have hopes for improvement. A thorough explanation of the regimen and its importance is necessary to convince the client that the changes and expense are justified.

Retin A and Alpha Hydroxy Acids

Retin A is the gold standard against which all other products are judged. The indicators of efficacy previously included redness, peeling, and irritation, but this is no longer true. In the last few years, improvement in delivery vehicles has made Retin A easy to use, opening the door for use on almost all skin types. Retin A efficacy is now measured by the science, based on years of advanced research. You will remember that as we grow older, cellular movement through the epidermis slows. This process creates a situation called **hyperkeratinization**, or a thick epidermis. One of the effects Retin A has on the skin is to reduce hyperkeratinization and compact the stratum corneum.

The compaction of the stratum corneum allows a superior microdermabrasion result. The results after treatment are quite noticeable compared with those treated without the benefit of Retin A. The use of Retin A will also allow other products in the home program, as well as those used in the spa, to penetrate more effectively. Therapeutic results with Retin A begin at two weeks, and long-term results begin at around seven weeks. We also now know that the results of Retin A therapy will be sustained for several months after the discontinuation of the product. Retin A should be started two weeks in advance of the first microdermabrasion treatment and continued indefinitely.

The scientific research available regarding alpha hydroxy acids (AHAs) is not as extensive as that regarding Retin A. We do know that AHAs loosen the **corneocytes**, which act like cellular glue holding the cells together in the epidermis. The use of AHA improves the cellular movement in the epidermis. In the clinical setting, we observe that AHAs make the skin smoother, softer, and plumper. In addition, we can see that oily areas calm down and become less oily, whereas dry areas are hydrated. It is believed that these results are a function of an increase in hyaluronic acid. Although volumes of general information exist concerning AHAs and their ability to "unglue" or exfoliate, little is known about the science of AHAs or, in other words, *how* this phenomenon occurs. Specifically, no information is available concerning the time it takes for AHAs to begin working on the cells or how long it takes for AHAs to fully integrate into the skin. Anecdotally, from our clinical experience, we know

hyperkeratinization
Thickening of the horny layers of skin, particularly the palmar and plantar areas.

corneocytes
Act as cellular glue in the epidermis, holding cells together.

Pretreatment with Retin A and AHAs will improve the skin's ability to speed cellular movement through the epidermis, increasing hyaluronic acid in the ground substance and enhancing the skin's ability to heal.

that the effects of AHAs will be seen within several days. It is assumed that the cellular effects begin within 1 to 2 weeks.

Because AHAs have the ability to loosen corneocytes, the products work in coordination with Retin A to smooth and compact all the layers of the epidermis. The increase in ground substance is also vital to the improvement in the skin's appearance.

AHA should be started with Retin A two weeks in advance of the first microdermabrasion treatment. This allows both products to work on the epidermis and create an environment for a superior microdermabrasion result.

Hydroquinone

There has been much controversy surrounding the use of hydroquinone. The FDA has investigated this drug and as of this writing is continuing to allow hydroquinone to be available. However, one should know that caution should be exercised recommending especially to Fitzpatrick IV and V skin types. These skin types may have a reaction to the medication and should be carefully monitored. Other skin types fare well with hydroquinone but should be removed from the product once a result is achieved, sustaining the result with sunscreen. Prescription-strength hydroquinone is often overlooked unless the client has hyperpigmentation. But hydroquinone will brighten the skin and improve the glow of the skin in coordination with Retin A and AHAs. Hydroquinone also protects the skin against a potential post-inflammatory hyperpigmentation response to microdermabrasion if the client is predisposed to this problem. When Retin A and hydroquinone are used together, the hydroquinone penetrates more efficiently. Once again, not much data is available to tell us exactly how long it takes hydroquinone to affect the melanocytes and begin to inhibit the production of melanin. Most of the literature simply points to the fact that hydroquinone can cause irritation within 24 hours. However, the actual effect on melanin is gradual, varying from person to person. It may take up to six weeks for the results to become apparent. Hydroquinone pretreatment should begin with Retin A and AHA home therapy.

Vitamins and Enzymes

The superheroes of any skin-care program are the free radical fighters. They generally go unnoticed in favor of products that seem to do the heavy lifting. Although Retin A and AHAs work to improve the cellular health of the skin and hydroquinone works on the discoloration of the skin, vitamins (C and E) and enzymes such as ubiquinone (Co-Q_{10})

or idebenone scavenge free radicals as antioxidants. You will remember that antioxidants hook up with the free radical's unpaired electron to neutralize it and prevent further damage (aging) to the skin. We know the best way to *sustain* the improvement of the skin is through antioxidants. Antioxidants do not directly improve the surface of the skin in preparation for microdermabrasion but rather *sustain* the result.

Vitamin C absorbs into the skin almost immediately; when using *l*-ascorbic acid, it will have a four-day half-life.[1] The pH and the percentage seem to be critical for the absorption, especially when using *l*-ascorbic acid. To ensure proper absorption, the vitamin C should be at a concentration of 15 to 20 percent *l*-ascorbic acid and have a pH of 3.5.[2] Ascorbyl palmitate, like magnesium ascorbyl phosphate, must use enzymes within the skin to convert to *l*-ascorbic acid; however, once converted, the product will remain in the skin up to two days.[3] Daily application is required to sustain optimal levels. Because these products are precursors to *l*-ascorbic acid, a discussion of percentages is not applicable.

Vitamin E (*d*-alpha-tocopherol) is normally found in moisturizers to protect the cellular membranes, but another important function of vitamin E is as an antioxidant. The enzyme ubiquinone (Co-Q_{10}) is particularly effective as an antioxidant. Little is known about the absorption into the skin. Anecdotally, we know that the skin simply looks better when using this product after microdermabrasion.

All vitamins and enzymes play a vital role in sustaining the result of microdermabrasion. The research is conflicting, and the necessary length of pretreatment time is controversial. In our case studies, the clients were put on vitamin C after the first microdermabrasion. Vitamin E and Co-Q_{10} were used immediately as part of the pretreatment program.

Sunscreen

Sunscreen is the component of the program that works to sustain the result and prevent further extrinsic damage (solar damage). A good sunscreen is one that protects against both UVA and UVB rays. UVB is your main consideration because of the decrease in atmospheric ozone; it is responsible for the solar aging familiar to the skin. Sunscreens must be applied daily whether the client is in the sun or not. Retin A, AHA, and hydroquinone make the skin photosensitive. Sunscreen requires 30 to 45 minutes to adhere to the skin and gain efficacy. Reapplication (based on the SPF) of sunscreen is imperative for clients who are playing or working in the sun. The preferred sunscreen for the microdermabrasion client includes both chemical and physical blocking agents. The active ingredients and percentages should closely resemble the following: dimethicone 1.0 percent, octyl methoxycinnamathe 5.5 percent, zinc

dimethicone
Silicone oil consisting of dimethylsiloxane viscous polymers.

octyl methoxycinnamathe
Chemical agent found in sunscreens.

oxide 6.8 percent, phenylbenzimidazole sulfonic acid 2.0 percent, and titanium dioxide 1.9 percent.

Because many clients you meet will not be wearing daily sunscreen, this product should be started at the beginning with Retin A, AHAs, and hydroquinone. At least an SPF 20 should be used and preferably an SPF 30. Remember, it takes a thick layer of sunscreen to achieve the advertised SPF; therefore, if the client is using a very thin layer, a higher SPF is recommended (SPF 20 was used in the case studies in this chapter).

Cleansers and Moisturizers

At first glance, cleansers and moisturizers do not seem to be that important to the overall home program or clinical treatment. We often think of these products as basic and think that any "good" product will do. However, the thought is flawed and requires closer examination: What is a *good* cleanser? What is a *good* moisturizer?

Stabilizing the skin pH begins with proper cleansing and moisturizing. We now know that the proper pH protects us from infection and encourages the penetration of prescription products. The standardized cleansers you choose for a therapeutic program should be slightly acidic with enough sodium lauryl sulfate and cocamidopropyl betaine to dissolve oils, dirt, and makeup.[4] Moisturizers also need to have a lower pH to provide the best penetration. Moisturizers that contain petrolatum or glycerin in large amounts become "heavy moisturizers" and more of a *lubricant* than a *moisturizer*. Although not wrong, this changes the purpose of the product.

Using the proper cleansers and moisturizers can begin to stabilize the skin pH within 36 hours. Establishing a consistent pH before medicinal product application and microdermabrasion creates the best canvas on which to work. (The case studies in this chapter used a cleanser with a pH of 4.51 and a moisturizer with a pH of 5.8.)

Exfoliating Masks

As the Retin A and AHAs begin to exfoliate and compact the stratum corneum, some peeling skin will become noticeable on the face, especially around the mouth. This shedding or peeling, although normal, needs to be cleaned from the face in a gentle manner. The best approach for this exfoliation is an enzyme mask, preferably a papain enzyme mask that is slightly acidic (4.0) and gentle. Papain enzyme masks are usually applied to a wet face in the shower and removed either with the fingertips or with very fine grains. When using the grains the client should be instructed to be gentle; too much rubbing can create raw skin and

phenylbenzimidazole sulfonic acid
Chemical agent found in sunscreens.

cocamidopropyl betaine
Foaming agent used in shampoos and cleansers.

petrolatum
Semisolid mixture of hydrocarbons obtained from petroleum; used in medicinal ointments and for lubrication.

glycerin
Humectant that is a natural by-product of the soap-making process.

papain
Protein-cleaving enzyme derived from papaya and certain other plants.

potentially a deeper-than-intended microdermabrasion if the treatment occurs the next day. If possible, exfoliating *should not* be done the day before the microdermabrasion treatment. The case study clients used a papain mask 2 to 3 times per week during the study.

▪ HOME PRODUCT SELECTION

The home products selected for microdermabrasion clients should be simple so that clients will follow their plans and benefit from the microdermabrasion treatments. The products should be Retin A (or retinol), AHAs (glycolic or lactic acid), hydroquinone 4 to 8 percent (kojic acid, bearberry, or licorice [or a combination of these ingredients]), sunscreen, and the proper cleansers and moisturizers. These products should be in place two weeks before a microdermabrasion treatment and should continue indefinitely.

▪ CASE STUDIES FOR MICRODERMABRASION

The clients for the clinical study group have been divided based on skin conditions: normal, dry, oily, combination, and sensitive. In addition to the basic skin condition, each client has a skin problem (aging, solar damage, hyperpigmentation, or acne) that we will be treating with microdermabrasion through the remainder of this text. You will have the benefit of following each client and evaluating the treatment program, progress, and finally the results of an eight-week program. The individuals are diverse, and each has different concerns and desires. Two pretreatment programs are used: (1) normal-to-dry skin (see Table 8–1) and (2) normal-to-oily skin (see Table 8–2). The basics of the programs are the same as those that have been discussed throughout this chapter. Now it is time to meet our clients.

Group One Pretreatment: Normal Skin with Aging Complaints

Patti is a 45-year-old woman categorized as a Fitzpatrick II and a Rubin two (Figures 8–1 and 8–2). As a young child, Patti never wore SPF while playing outside or during the family's yearly vacation at the shore. She became aware of the importance of sunscreen in high school and began wearing SPF in her twenties. Other than wearing SPF, she has never

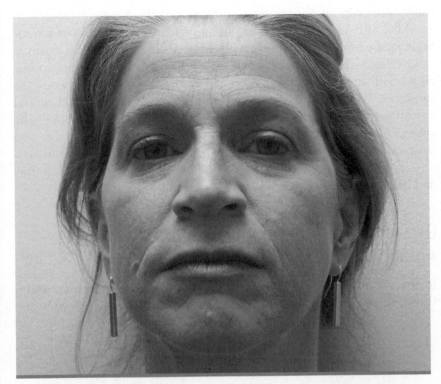

Figure 8–1 Pretreatment–Normal skin with aging complaints.

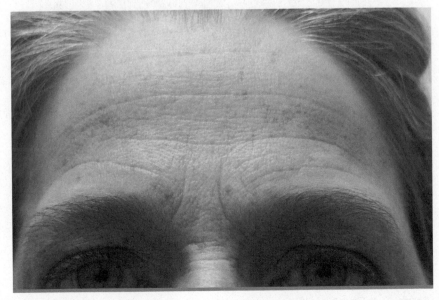

Figure 8–2 Special attention to be given to the forehead area.

really taken care of her skin at a medical spa. She has used Dove with an OTC SPF 15 on a daily basis and a higher SPF if she is outside for prolonged periods. Although as a physician Patti recognizes the extrinsic aging caused by the sun, she is focused on the potential skin cancers associated with sun exposure. It is for this reason alone that Patti wears the sunscreen. Patti is mainly concerned with the appearance of her chest and has little awareness of the hyperpigmentation and lines on her face. She enters this program thinking she looks "pretty good" for her age and believes that fine lines are just part of the aging process. Once again, as a physician, she recognizes that the process of changing the skin takes time and believes that it will take at least two months to see results.

Group Two Pretreatment: Dry Skin with Aging Complaint

Rachael is a 75-year-old woman categorized as a Fitzpatrick IV and a Rubin three (Figures 8–3 and 8–4). As a young child she played in the

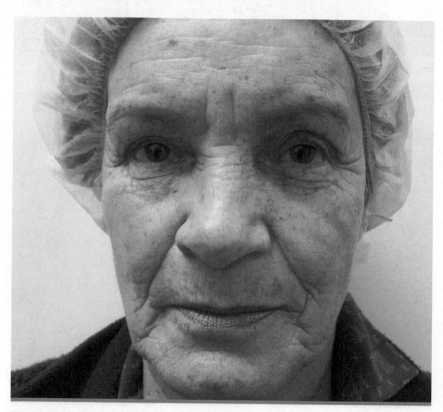

Figure 8–3 Dry skin with aging complaints.

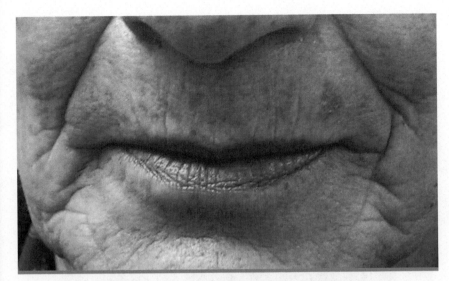

Figure 8–4 Special attention will be given to the upper-lip area.

sun most days and went to the beach every summer. There was not SPF during this time, so her skin was unprotected during her youth and the greater part of her adult life. She still randomly wears an SPF when she is outside or at the beach. She has never been involved in a medical skin-care program, although she has had a lower blepharoplasty. Currently, she washes her face in the shower each morning using an aloe vera cleanser. In the evening she simply washes her face at the sink with the cleanser or soap. Rachael hopes to improve the tone and texture of her skin, including the reduction of freckles and sunspots. She was placed on the normal-to-dry home program (see Table 8–1). Rachael has realistic expectations, hoping to achieve improvement in the color and texture of her skin.

Group Three Pretreatment: Sensitive Skin with Aging Complaints

Kathryn is a 54-year-old woman categorized as a Fitzpatrick I and a Rubin three (Figure 8–5). She spent her childhood on the farm, never using an SPF. Even now, when she is in the sun, she does not use an SPF. Her skin is dry and appears sensitive, although she does not report any incidents of sensitivity to the environment or to products. She currently washes her face with soap from the shower. She applies the remainder of her program, which consists of an OTC moisturizer, in the car on the way to work. She does not wear any makeup. Kathryn has never taken care of her skin and is extraordinarily excited about the

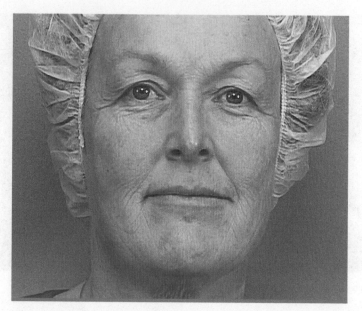

Figure 8–5 Pretreatment—Sensitive skin with aging. This is our only picture of Kathryn. Her skin became too sensitive to continue the program.

program. She has reasonable expectations for a woman with her skin condition. She hopes to have a softer, smoother texture and believes this can be done in about three months. She is placed on the normal-to-dry home program (see Table 8–1).

Group Four Pretreatment: Normal Skin with Hyperpigmentation Complaints

Maria is a 47-year-old woman categorized as a Fitzpatrick IV and a Rubin two (Figures 8–6 and 8–7). As a child and in her teen years, Maria sunbathed with cocoa butter applied to her face and body. Maria vacationed at the beach every year; she never wore an SPF. She was involved with a medical skin-care program about two years ago when she had a previous microdermabrasion treatment resulting in post-inflammatory hyperpigmentation. Her current program includes washing her face in the shower using body soap on the face. She uses an oil-free moisturizer without SPF. She has been reluctant to use an SPF for fear it would cause her to break out. In the evening she uses a cleanser and vitamin E cream or oil only on the eyelids, never on the face. She would like to see the pigment even out and her skin have a peaches-and-cream complexion. She believes this should happen in three months. She was placed on the normal-to-oily home program (see Table 8–2).

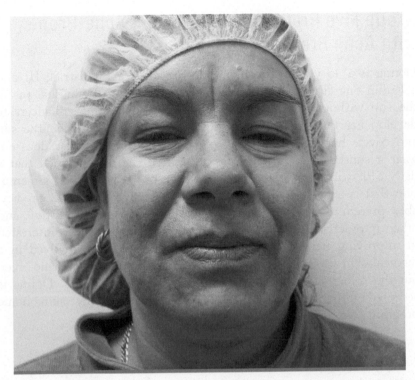

Figure 8–6 Pretreatment—Normal skin with hyperpigmentation.

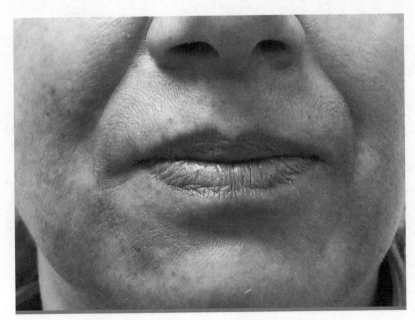

Figure 8–7 Special attention will be given to the perioral region.

Group Five Pretreatment: Oily and Acne-Prone with Acne Breakout Complaints

Donna is a 43-year-old woman categorized as a Fitzpatrick III and a Rubin one (Figures 8–8 and 8–9). As a young person she was in the sun without SPF, using coconut oils and tanning enhancers to develop her tan. As an adult she applies SPF 15 when in the sun and covers her face with a hat or umbrella. She otherwise does not wear a sunscreen on a daily basis, because she is concerned that a daily SPF will cause her skin to break out. She has hyperpigmentation that is acne-related. Donna feels her acne is hormonal, predictably present during her menstrual cycle. She uses ProActiv® and other infomercial products inconsistently. Donna is very interested in improving her skin, although she has never been involved in a medical skin-care program. She would like to control the acne, even out the color, and smooth the fine lines around the eyes. Donna is accepted into the program and placed on the oily skin home program (see Table 8–2).

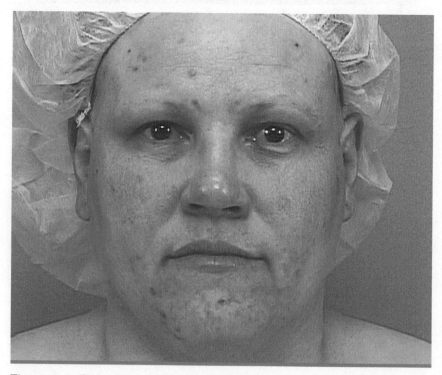

Figure 8–8 Pretreatment—Oily and acne-prone skin with acne breakout.

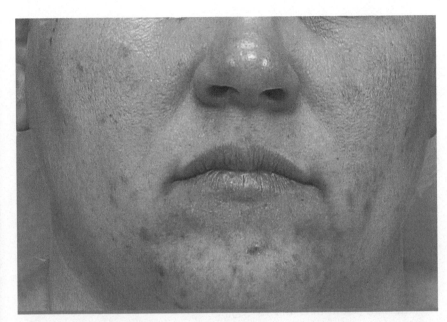

Figure 8–9 Special attention will be given to the perioral region.

■ CONCLUSION

Medical skin care has always ascribed to the notion that pretreatment is the first step to achieve a good end result. In this chapter we discussed the need for pretreatment before conducting a microdermabrasion treatment, as well as using products that are required to achieve the desired result. A complete therapeutic program, with prescriptions, vitamins, and sunscreens, is needed to reach this goal. Because of the complexity of the products used, the aesthetician must know the products, their ingredients, and what results are expected for using as much. Furthermore, the aesthetician needs to act as a coach for his or her client in the weeks leading up to the actual treatment. Being available to answer questions, motivate, and adjust the pretreatment program will have as much of a bearing on the end result as will the microdermabrasion treatment itself.

To this effect, each product in the program should have a specific use. Programs should be basic, allowing for easy implementation with recommended adjustments for skin type. The aesthetician must necessarily tailor the pretreatment regimen to the individual client's needs. Normal, dry, oily, and sensitive skin types will require adjustments, as well as other special nuances or irregularities specific to the individual client.

If administered properly, the pretreatment program will have spectacular effects on the end product. These effects help ensure client satisfaction and aesthetician success.

▶ ▷ ▷ Top 10 Tips to Take to the Spa

1. Pretreatment is critical to the success of a microdermabrasion program.
2. Finding the client's motivation will help you to provide the proper home program.
3. Each individual product has a place in a program.
4. Exfoliating masks should be chemical (papain) in nature versus physical (grains).
5. Vitamin C is the most important antioxidant for the skin.
6. A moisturizer should also provide nutrients and antioxidants to the skin (vitamin E and Co-Q_{10}).
7. Sunscreen will improve the skin and is required in a therapeutic program.
8. Cleansers of the proper acidic pH will sustain the skin's acid mantle.
9. The home program needs to be simple so the client will follow the plan.
10. Simple basic programs work for any age and are adjusted for skin type.

Chapter Review Questions

1. What are the primary skin considerations with regards to sunscreen? Why is it so important?
2. Describe the benefit of using vitamins as a pretreatment for microdermabrasion.
3. What is the skin's normal pH? How do cleansers affect the skin's pH?
4. When does Retin A begin to work on the cells of the skin?
5. What does AHA do for the cells of the skin?
6. Why should you include hydroquinone in every skin-care program?
7. What is the benefit of vitamin C in a skin-care program?

8. Why must every client use a sunscreen?

9. Why are medical cleansers important to a microdermabrasion program?

10. What constitutes a complete therapeutic program?

11. Why is pretreatment important?

12. How do Retin A and AHAs prepare the skin for microdermabrasion?

13. True or False: A skin-care client's microdermabrasion outcome can be dependent upon the client's dedication to the home-care program.

Chapter References

1. DeBuys, H. V., Levine, M., Omar, M., Pinnell, S., Riviere, N. M., Wang, Y., & Yang, H. (2001). Topical *l-ascorbic acid: Percutaneous absorption studies. Dermatologic Surgery, 27*(2), 137.
2. DeBuys, H. V., Levine, M., Omar, M., Pinnell, S., Riviere, N. M., Wang, Y., & Yang, H. (2001). Topical *l-ascorbic acid: Percutaneous absorption studies. Dermatologic Surgery, 27*(2), 137.
3. Blanock, K., Chie, S., Koichiro, K., Kozo, Y., Masato, T., Quigley, J., Shigeo, K., Tomoji, M., & Toshio, M. (1993). Inhibitory effects of magnesium ascorbyl phosphate on melanogenisis. *Nippon Kesho-hin Gijutsusha Kaishi, 27*(3), 409–414.
4. Vermont Soapworks. (2004, March 2). *Sodium laurel sulfate* [Online]. Available: http://www.vermontsoap.com

Microdermabrasion Treatments

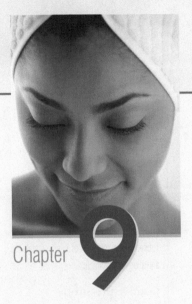

Chapter 9

Key Terms

ablation
APIE
bloodborne
  pathogens
charting formats
contaminated
diamond crystals
diamond-encrusted
  tips
Environmental
  Protection Agency
  (EPA)

LED
medical waste
muscle memory
Occupational Safety
  and Health
  Administration
  (OSHA)
oxidized
PIE
pinpoint bleeding
positive pressure
preauricular

red bagging
Safety Bill of Rights
safety coordinator
safety manual
salt crystals
SOAP
SOAPIER
Soiled
ultrasound
vacuum settings

Learning Objectives

After completing this chapter you should be able to:

1. Identify the protocols for safe microdermabrasion treatments.
2. Identify the acceptable microdermabrasion techniques.
3. Identify the required safe practices used with microdermabrasion.
4. List potentially unique treatments available.

INTRODUCTION

Aconcept that ought to be well-understood by this point in the book is that variations are a constant in the aesthetics industry. When it comes to actually performing the microdermabrasion treatments on the clients, the same will apply. Variations in the techniques used, the machine selected, the aesthetician's level of comfort and experience with the treatment itself, and the condition of the client's skin will all have a noticeable affect on the microdermabrasion result. Because the goal in the spa environment is to have predictable, positive outcomes, each of these variables creates questions in the minds of physicians and/or spa operators. So many decisions need to be made and so many opinions exist, all seemly defensible. The choice of which type of crystal, **vacuum settings**, **positive pressure**, and which clinical and home products to use in tandem with treatment, as well as the perceived risks of aluminum oxide, all create fodder for continued debate. This chapter will attempt to tackle the intricacies of microdermabrasion technology, technique, and result. Due to the possible variables in the results, microdermabrasion has not garnered the respect it deserves among physicians or, for that matter, among some consumers. Opinions become more powerful than facts, especially with your clients and their friends.

With the hopes of quieting the discussion and debate, the focus of your attention should lie with the client and the potential result. Simple as it may sound, doing so will require you to use guidelines that reduce, as much as possible, the variability found in microdermabrasion treatments. Within this chapter we will discuss those subjects that will help to simplify and demystify microdermabrasion and direct the aesthetician to a predictable and repeatable outcome.

MICRODERMABRASION TECHNOLOGY

As with most businesses, the greatest expense which will be incurred is in the technology. Furthermore, the choice in machinery will have a great bearing on the services offered. In the aesthetic arena, the same holds true, particularly with regard to selecting a microdermabrasion device. Which is the best microdermabrasion machine, and why? Who is the best vendor to buy from, and why? As with many of the decisions you make in business, these questions must be answered individually, focusing on the issues that are most important to the individual facility. In the end, the most important consideration when it comes to choosing

vacuum settings
Adjustable setting on microdermabrasion machine that is responsible for the rate at which crystals strike the skin, as well as the subsequent elimination of used crystals and bio-waste particles.

positive pressure
Specific vacuum pressure applied while administering a microdermabrasion treatment.

the best machine becomes what is best for the user and for the particular spa. So many machines are available and so much must be understood, especially about the technology of microdermabrasion. As an aesthetician, you will likely first work in a spa where the device already exists. In order to have a machine preference you will need to have an understanding of their commonalities and their basic operation. Other preferences will naturally follow with experience. The obvious place to start is the advent of the microdermabrasion machine itself.

Microdermabrasion machines began as simple units that used vacuum to exfoliate the skin, aided by pure aluminum oxide crystals. Aluminum oxide, or corundum, was chosen as the exfoliant for several reasons; it is inert, it is hard, it is stable, and it does not cause skin irritation. In the 1990s, many companies saw the manufacturing or sale of microdermabrasion machines as the next great opportunity in the skincare industry and scrambled for market share. The business environment shaped the opportunity for technologic advancements and, as with any situation in which many newcomers are found, the cream always rises to the top. Now, although many microdermabrasion machine companies exist, only a few are recognized and respected.

Technology continues to advance. Improvements in machine precision, reduction of machine size, and increased safety mechanisms have created machines that are easy and safe to use. Now, microdermabrasion is as widely accepted as the routine facial. Technology has also improved the result of the treatment by adding *attachments,* such as **ultrasound** or **LED**. Also, tips that secrete a serum during the treatment have been added to machines, creating a specialized microdermabrasion treatment called the "serum-based exfoliation." In addition, combining treatments, such as enzyme peels, chemical peels, and masks, is common with microdermabrasion. Importantly, manufacturers have made significant strides in developing advanced machines for the medical environment while maintaining the salon version.

The current generation of microdermabrasion machines has improved on the original technology to include options in crystal types (salt versus corundum) or the use of **diamond-encrusted tips**. Safety issues have been addressed by the development of "closed systems" to prevent corundum from spilling or the dust from flying. Machine performance has been improved by addressing filter issues and receptacle canister size. The ergonomics of the handpiece have been given special attention, as manufacturers have recognized that this particular issue makes a significant difference to the daily user.

Before we discuss the methods and techniques that you will use in the treatment of clients, we should talk about the technology differences found in microdermabrasion machines.

ultrasound
Use of high-frequency sound waves to increase the intercellular spaces of the epidermis and dermis, allowing penetration of a topical product during treatment.

LED
In electronic devices, a semiconductor device that emits a light when charged with an electric current. Used in many aesthetic devices including lasers and specialized microdermabrasion devices.

diamond-encrusted tips
Reusable microdermabrasion system that has varying wands for specific regions and coarseness.

> Improvements in machine precision, reduction of machine size, and increased safety mechanisms have created machines that are easy and safe to use.

Aluminum Oxide Machines

The original microdermabrasion process used aluminum oxide machines. These machines were developed using a vacuum which moved crystals via a handpiece that moved over tautly held skin to "polish" and exfoliate the stratum corneum. Much has changed since then: the angle at which the crystals hit the skin, the design of the handpiece, the size of the machine, and the internal system.

While most manufacturers have addressed the ergonomics of the handpiece, there remains a controversy as to the best size and shape, because the handpieces direct the crystals. Opinions differ about the best angle for the crystals to impact the skin. Some manufacturers continue to prefer a 90-degree angle, whereas others have embraced a 45-degree angle (Figure 9–1). It seems that those machines that use the 90-degree angle have a greater propensity for scraping the skin and provide less exfoliation. At the 90-degree angle the crystals simply "bounce" against the skin before returning to the system. This problem is solved when the angle at which the crystals hit the skin is adjusted to about 45 degrees. At this angle, the crystals impact the skin, gently exfoliate it, and then are returned to the system.

The early machines were "open systems," requiring crystals to be poured into the machine and drained out. The potential for spillage and compromise of the corundum was great. The more sophisticated "closed system" machines have overcome these elementary issues, although this open technology still exists today. Open technology created two problems: (1) the temptation to reuse crystals and (2) the controversy regarding the safety of aluminum oxide crystals.

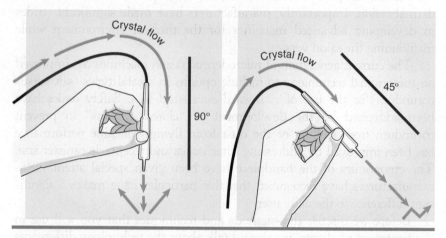

Figure 9–1 Differences between the 90-degree handpiece and 45-degree handpiece.

For obvious reasons, the reuse of crystals is strictly forbidden. This is unsanitary and would create the opportunity to pass contagious diseases onto unknowing clients. Although there is documentation suggesting that there is a reduction in the efficacy of crystals once they have been used, in reality this is a meaningless discussion. The most important point to understand is that diseases can be passed on when crystals are reused; therefore, reuse is absolutely unacceptable. To truly understand the safety issues involved with corundum, you need to know a little about metals, in particular, aluminum. Aluminum is the third-most common element in the Earth's crust;[1] it becomes aluminum oxide when it is oxidized, or exposed to oxygen. The two are, in fact, different substances. Aluminum oxide has been used for years in construction for sandblasting, in dentistry (polishing your teeth after cleaning), and even on emery boards. The FDA has not questioned the safety of aluminum oxide crystals; it considers the crystals inert and a different compound from aluminum metal. Aluminum oxide was once thought to be a cause of Alzheimer's disease, but that theory has since been disproven. Instead, the **Occupational Safety and Health Administration (OSHA)** "… considers aluminum oxide dust a nuisance dust in the workplace."[2] Nuisance dusts are not linked to problems with the health of those using the product and do not cause cancer. The most disconcerting exposure to aluminum oxide may be through inhalation; therefore, it is highly recommended that all aestheticians wear surgical masks during treatment. Based on this information, aluminum oxide is considered quite safe for the purposes of microdermabrasion.

Additional advancements in the aluminum oxide machine include the type of filter and its location within the machine. Originally, "wet" crystals (those that had touched wet skin debris or absorbed air humidity) would clog the filter, requiring a service call or, at the very least, a talented aesthetician to dismantle the machine and clean the filter. While advanced filter technology has solved many of these problems, crystals can still absorb the humidity in the air, and care should be taken to avoid keeping the machine in the same room with traditional facial steamers.

Another improvement in the aluminum oxide microdermabrasion machine is the size. As with your computer or mobile phone, microdermabrasion equipment has slimmed down and become easier to manage, especially if it is on a custom cabinet that has wheels. This is a benefit to everyone, especially the aesthetician.

Overall, aluminum oxide microdermabrasion machines are tried and true. They have a track record many years long and a number of consistent manufacturers with which you can feel comfortable doing business. Aluminum oxide microdermabrasion machines have sustained popularity over the years and remain some of the most popular types of machines.

oxidized
Prolonged and damaging exposure to oxygen; oxidized materials are usually brown in color.

Occupational Safety and Health Administration (OSHA)
Federal agency responsible for defining and regulating safety in the workplace.

Salt Crystal Machines

Salt crystals are an alternative to aluminum oxide crystals for microdermabrasion. Using the same principles as aluminum oxide, salt machines have created a niche based primarily on the different physical characteristics of crystals. The replacement of aluminum oxide with salt gives those with concerns about aluminum oxide an opportunity to use the process without the perceived risks. However, a consideration when evaluating the salt machine is the actual result. Salt particles are softer than aluminum oxide crystals and may result in unsatisfactory outcomes. Additionally, some data suggest that the salt is more uncomfortable than aluminum oxide because of the crystal's irregular shape and the potential for scraping the skin.

The manufacturer of the salt machine suggests that it has many benefits compared with other types of machines. These benefits include the use of a nontoxic, water-soluble material. Salt treatments are said to provide a deeper abrasion, producing results in fewer treatments and the ability to integrate skin-care products during the treatment using ultrasound. Obviously, some of these benefits are available for all machines. The salt machine, however, may still have a place in the microdermabrasion treatment world and is still recommended.

Diamond Crystal Machines

Two types of diamond machines exist: (1) the type that uses **diamond crystals** and (2) the type that uses diamond-encrusted tips. Originally developed in Australia in 1996, diamond-encrusted tip machines reflect the most advanced technology microdermabrasion has to offer. This machine has several varying sizes of reusable wands for specific areas of the face, neck, chest, and body. These wands work together with a vacuum to create the microdermabrasion effect. In addition to the available wand sizes, different textures are available, beginning with coarse (significant enough to cause **ablation**) and moving to fine (gentle enough to treat upper and lower eyelids). This design, of course, eliminates the need for crystals—a positive characteristic that saves on *direct costs* (see Chapter 10) and eliminates the potential for leaving behind crystals in a wound. This machine also requires limited replacement of canisters (because no crystals are used), and it uses a disc filter, which prolongs the life of the machine.

There are two downsides to using diamond machines: First, the technique varies from the traditional technique and has a learning curve. Second, the wand must be sterilized between treatments.

Infusion Microdermabrasion

The infusion, or suffusion, system is the newest technology in microdermabrasion treatments. The systems use specific tips that resurface the skin while introducing topical serums to the skin (Figure 9–2). The benefit of this treatment is the versatility of the treatment. Microdermabrasion is still being done, but the advanced technology allows for the treatment of hyperpigmentation, fine lines, and oily or acne-prone skin with specific serums. Among the serums are growth factors (peptides), acne treatments, bleaching for hyperpigmentation, antioxidants, and hydration. These serums improve the skin beyond traditional

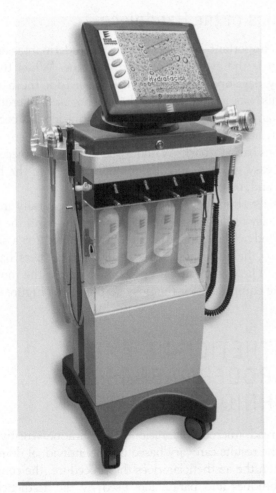

Figure 9–2 The infusion, or suffusion, system is the newest technology in microdermabrasion treatments. (Courtesy of Edge Systems Corporation)

microdermabrasion. Infusion microdermabrasion, while seemingly still in its infancy, will be the next generation of microdermabrasion. It provides the client with an advanced treatment with multiple steps that improve the skin beyond what traditional microdermabrasion can do.

That said, these machines are expensive and require the ongoing purchase of serums to complete the treatment. Good investigative work must be done by the practice manager to ensure that the machine being purchased is the best machine for the practice. Most manufacturers suggest the use of LED light with this treatment along with the use of lymphatic drainage. Both of these treatments add benefits to microdermabrasion treatments.

Ergonomics of the Handpiece

A subtle yet important advancement in microdermabrasion equipment biotechnology is the evolution of the handpiece. When the equipment was originally developed, there was little regard for the handpiece style and size. This was a problem for those who used microdermabrasion equipment many times a day. As microdermabrasion has become increasingly popular, aestheticians find that they are doing many treatments a day, sometimes back-to-back. Without the proper handpiece—one that is comfortable, easy to hold, and fits ergonomically into the hand—hands become tired and, on occasion, disabled.

A handpiece should be lightweight and fit naturally into the hand. It should be easy to hold and easy to maneuver around the face or other areas of the body. Many manufacturers have opted for a slender cylinder, similar to the size and shape of a pencil. Others have chosen a *trigger design*. The design alterations rank as one of the most important changes in the equipment for the busy aesthetician (Figure 9–3).

■ AESTHETICIANS AND MICRODERMABRASION TECHNIQUES

As you have read, microdermabrasion is a technique-sensitive procedure. This means the results can vary based on the individual doing the procedure, how often the aesthetician does the procedure, the condition of the skin, the techniques and parameters used by the aesthetician for each treatment, and the equipment itself, especially the newer technologies. Because of these variables, the aesthetician needs to learn the proper techniques and practice them often. The more treatments the aesthetician

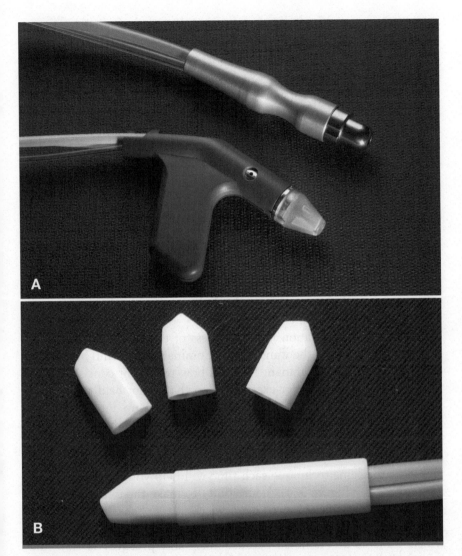

Figure 9–3 Design alterations of the handpiece rank as one of the most important changes in the equipment for the busy aesthetician.

does, the better he or she becomes at performing the treatment. Now, that may sound simple, but if it were that simple, there would not be so many variables in the results clients receive.

Aestheticians should consider several factors before they begin to provide microdermabrasion treatment. Some of these considerations may seem elementary, but when doing microdermabrasion several hours a day, a failure to consider these factors can affect the consistency of the result. We should begin by answering the question of whether to sit or

When an aesthetician is doing several microdermabrasion treatments each day, the hands can become tired. This may cause pain for the aesthetician over time and the inability to properly perform microdermabrasion. This is why the ergonomics of the handpiece are important.

stand during the treatment. Although it may seem silly, the decision to sit or stand is an important first step. The aesthetician must choose the position in which he or she is most comfortable and which allows the aesthetician to sustain his or her energy. The aesthetician should also consider how easy it is to move around the client's head, control and move the machine, and reach the equipment on the back bar. The aesthetician should try both approaches during the training process to decide which is best. Once the decision is made, he or she should be consistent.

The next consideration to be aware of is the power of the dominant hand. Whether you are cleansing the treatment area or using the microdermabrasion wand, always use your dominant hand. For aestheticians, this is a change (because the idea of using both hands has been your training). However, the dominant hand is stronger, and the firmness of the preparation and the handling of the wand make a difference; therefore, the dominant hand is the best choice. The management of the wand is particularly important; the lightness or the firmness of the touch will affect the result.

The next consideration is the tautness of the skin held in the *nondominant hand*. Using the wand (in the dominant hand) and holding the skin taut (in the nondominant hand) is how treatment consistency will ultimately be achieved. For example, skin that is not held taut is more likely to be affected by a high vacuum (sucked up into the wand). A wand that is given pressure and moved slowly over the skin will give a different result than a wand that is held lightly and moved quickly over the skin. Using the same hands for the steps of the procedure and repeating the same technique each time will help you to develop a consistent process (Figure 9–4). Your ability to make the treatment consistent depends on your ability to *teach the muscles* to behave the same way each time. It is the process called **muscle memory**—a process with which athletes are familiar because this (and practice) is how they become better and more consistent in their chosen sports. It is also the way a physician excels in a surgical procedure. The repetitive nature of surgery helps the surgeon's hands to remember the movements and improves his or her ability each time he or she does the same surgery. In a sense, you are similar to the surgeon; repeating a procedure over and over, creating motor skills that are fine and detailed.

An important and often-forgotten step in creating consistency is setting up your environment. Knowing where things are on the back bar, understanding how your machine moves and how flexible the tubing is (you do not want to hit someone in the face with the tubes), and draping the client are all important. It sounds simple, but it takes practice. This process eliminates the variables you can control in the treatment. Create

muscle memory
Ability of muscles to behave the same way after a repeated action.

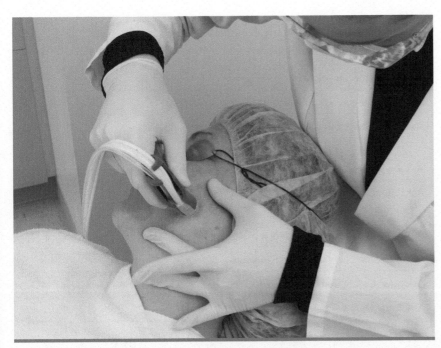

Figure 9–4 To provide a reliable, reproducible treatment, the clinician must create a consistent routine.

a routine for yourself; this will do away with any worries during the procedure (Table 9–1).

Finally, remember to consider client sensitivity issues, such as the inability to see. Because eyes will be covered with goggles and the client will be unable to see, you should touch the client on the shoulder and explain what you are going to do before you do it. Respect his or her privacy, and make sure the chest is well-draped and not exposed. Ask about the comfort level. Is he or she hot or cold; does he or she need a blanket? Is the client's phone ringing? Some of these distractions take away from the enjoyment of the treatment. Sometimes the client may be uncomfortable and not say a word. Be intuitive and sensitive to your client.

In summary, many important steps should be considered when providing microdermabrasion: First, your configuration to the client, whether you sit or stand, and your proximity to the back bar. Remember to use your dominant hand during the treatment; consider the use of the nondominant hand and the importance it plays in a treatment. Set up your environment carefully and do so the same way every time. Last, be respectful of your client. Making these steps a priority and following the same process each time will decrease the variability in the result.

> To provide a reliable, *reproducible* treatment, the aesthetician must create a consistent routine to follow each time the procedure is performed. A clinical treatment should be like a ballet; you should know each step before it comes, anticipate it, and carry it out beautifully.

Table 9–1 Pre-Procedure Checklist		
Did You Do the Following?	**Yes**	**No**
Have consent form signed.		
Ask if any new skin problems exist.		
Ask if any new medications (oral or topical) are being taken.		
Ask if any new medical history updates are available.		
Ask if the client has adhered to the daily home-care program.		
Ask when the last exfoliation took place.		
Ask when the client last used Retin A.		
Ask how the last treatment was.		
Ask if the client will be in the sun.		
Ask about the client's last exposure to the sun or sunburn.		
Ensure the client is draped.		
Provide eye protection.		
Provide a bonnet.		
Provide a gown or towels.		
Check the machine to ensure it is in working order.		

Condition of the Skin and Microdermabrasion Results

Skin condition is an important consideration when trying to develop consistent treatments. Skin that is dry will have a different result than skin that is oily. Combination skin will be more of a challenge than skin that is normal. This is just common sense. However, how do you determine the treatment settings that will work best for the skin condition with which you are presented?

The first question you will want to ask yourself is: What is the condition of the skin? Is it dry, normal, oily, combination, or possibly more sensitive than the last treatment? The next consideration is what you trying to treat. Is it hyperpigmentation, solar damage, or mild acne?

Next, evaluate any changes that may have taken place since that last treatment. Are there areas of the skin that may require more attention today than other areas? For example, is the skin more pigmented in a particular location, or do you have a persistent texture problem in an area? Look at the skin carefully, determine the answers to these questions, and take the necessary steps to provide proper treatment. Those necessary steps might include increasing the crystal flow for oily skin or adding a hydrating mask after the microdermabrasion if the skin is dry. If you are still concerned once you have a plan in mind, use a *test spot* to determine your settings. These tests are best done in front of the ear (**preauricular**) or near the hairline.

Because so many of your clients will be seeking acne treatments, including microdermabrasion, you might think that extraction may be a requisite precursor. In actuality, extractions are generally not recommended with the microdermabrasion treatment, as crystals will enter the open wound. However, if there are one or two stray blackheads or a single pustule that needs to be extracted, try to do this after the treatment. The skin may be more pliable and easier to extract; in addition, you will avoid getting crystals into the open wound. In general, if the client needs to have multiple extractions, consider combining the microdermabrasion with a facial so that the skin can be warmed and softened to allow for easier extraction.

Having determined a treatment for the skin condition, other things (such as the technical parameters, including the settings on the machine as well as the direction and number of passes) must be adjusted to accommodate said considerations.

Technical Parameters (Vacuum and Crystal Settings)

The technical parameters are the settings for the vacuum suction and crystal penetration rates. In other words, they are the dials that control the outcome of the treatment. As an aesthetician in training, less familiar with the processes than you someday will be, you may wonder if the setting affects how you guide the handpiece over the skin. Are there a standardized number and direction of passes for each area of the face? After the aesthetician has established his or her style, attention should be directed toward the next phase of clinical education—understanding technical parameters.

As mentioned above, the *technical parameters* refer to the settings for the vacuum and crystals, which, in part, determine the penetration depth and final outcome of the treatment. A vacuum and crystal setting that is too low will not provide an aggressive treatment. On the other hand, a

Determine the skin condition; *then* determine the settings and any add-on treatments needed to treat the skin condition, such as an exfoliating mask, hydrating mask, peel, or facial.

preauricular
In front of the ear.

setting that is too high may be responsible for **pinpoint bleeding**. As you know, each machine has different settings. Some have dual controls (one for the crystal and one for the vacuum); others have a single control. Unfortunately, it is impossible to standardize this variable for a textbook. Each machine must be evaluated for protocol individually.

Machines with dual controls for vacuum and crystals are more refined than the standard machine with a single dial for both. You will need to work with your microdermabrasion machine vendor to determine the best settings for each skin type and condition (Table 9–2). Finding the correct settings will take time and practice. Do not be afraid to ask a couple of models to come in so that you can practice. This will help you to understand the settings and set up protocols for your particular machine.

Table 9–2 Technical Parameters for Dual-Control Machines

Vacuum Setting	Crystal Flow	Description	Skin Considerations
High	High	Aggressive—*faster* passes with the wand will be necessary to avoid pinpoint bleeding	Oily, thicker skin
High	Medium	Moderate treatment	Normal skin
High	Low	Won't achieve a meaningful result in most skin areas, but recommended for thin skin areas (e.g., around the eyes)	Thin skin
Medium	High	Moderate treatment	Normal skin
Medium	Medium	Moderate treatment	Normal skin
Low	High	(positive pressure) *controlled* passes of the wand will be necessary to avoid pinpoint bleeding	Thicker skin
Low	Medium	Recommended for skin with acne	Acne skin
Low	Low	Won't achieve a meaningful result in most skin areas, but recommended for thin skin areas (e.g., around the eyes)	Thin skin

Several general statements can be made with regard to vacuum and crystal settings. If both the vacuum and crystal settings are high, the treatment will be the most aggressive. If the vacuum is low but the crystals are high (commonly called *positive pressure*), a greater volume of crystals will strike the skin. In this case, the crystals may cause greater exfoliation, but the treatment result also depends on the speed with which the handpiece is moving over the skin. If the vacuum and crystals are both set low, the treatment will be lighter.

The settings should be increased as much as the skin can tolerate. Conservative treatments (low vacuum and low crystals) given without adjusting for skin type will not achieve a meaningful result. Therefore, the settings must be adjusted for skin type and condition, as well as for different areas of the face. For example, the thicker skin of the forehead should be at a higher setting than the delicate skin of the upper cheeks or lower eyelid.

The pressure of the handpiece against the skin will also affect the result. If you push the wand against the skin, you will increase the potential for injury to the skin and also create a more uncomfortable treatment. The wand should be held lightly on the skin, lifting slightly, almost *pulling* the skin into the wand. The approach allows the crystals to hit the skin evenly and for the treatment to be more comfortable.

The end point of the treatment is erythema. Erythema is achieved through the vacuum and crystal flow and the number of passes. The settings should not be so high that it does not allow the required passes; therefore, it is important that the aesthetician is clear on the number of passes that should be made in a traditional treatment.

Number of Passes

One of the greater concerns with regard to unsatisfactory outcomes with microdermabrasion is passing the wand too frequently over the skin. The simplest way to quantify this (barring machine-specific aspects) is that the ideal number of passes is directly related to the thickness of the skin (location). The problems occur at the point at which erythema appears. Generally, three passes is a good place to start on normal or oily skin. Dry skin or skin that has some sensitivity should begin with two passes until you reach a comfort zone with the client and your observations of the skin. Always talk with the client during the treatment. Ask how the treatment is feeling; is it too intense or too scratchy? The clients should always feel something; they should not, however, be extraordinarily uncomfortable. The tauter the skin, the less discomfort the client will have during the treatment.

Some articles recommend up to seven passes when doing microdermabrasion, but this number of passes should not be the initial goal.

> The microdermabrasion result is affected by several variables: the thickness of the skin, the number of passes, the vacuum and crystal settings (whether independent or a single setting), and the speed at which the handpiece is moved over the skin.

Remember also that the settings have much to do with the skin's ability to tolerate multiple passes. Finally, the other variable is your hand. Is the skin taut? Are you using the handpiece lightly or firmly? How was the skin prepped? Which machine are you using? Do you use the same machine each time? Keep all of these issues in mind when you choose the number of passes and remember that erythema is the end point.

Tight Skin Is the Key to Good Treatment

Hold the skin taut between the thumb and middle finger to achieve the tightness you will need to accomplish the treatment. When treating the upper lip, either use the thumb or first finger horizontally across the lip or have the client bite the lip to achieve tightness of the skin. Use the same technique on the chin or lower lip area. When treating the neck, have the client lift the chin to the ceiling and turn the head away from you to achieve tightness.

Direction of Passes

The direction of the pass should be the next item with which an aesthetician ought to concerned. On the first pass, a horizontal pattern should be used. The second pass should be a vertical pattern, and the third pass should be a diagonal pattern (Figure 9–5). This will help to achieve a complete treatment in all areas (treating areas that may have been missed in one of the previous passes, if you were careless). Remember, the speed of the passes, the skin thickness, and the technical aspects are also determining factors in the erythema and thus the end result. Do not hold the handpiece in one place for too long or move the handpiece too slowly; otherwise, you will not be able to complete the recommended three passes.

Charting and Documentation

Any skilled professional would agree that success lies in the details. To this effect, charting and documentation are an important step in the treatment process. As with any procedure in the medical spa, the treatment history helps to provide continuity in care and treatment planning for the client. It is often said, "If it is not written down, it did not happen." Therefore, all of the information about the treatment should be included in the record each time the client is seen. Charting and

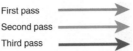

First pass

Second pass

Third pass

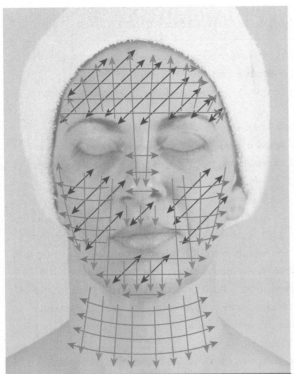

Figure 9–5 The first pass uses a horizontal pattern, the second pass should be a vertical pattern, and the third pass should be a diagonal pattern of the passes.

documentation is one of the hardest tasks an aesthetician must learn when entering into the medical spa. Writing notes in the record and ensuring all of the information has been included can be challenging for anyone, especially someone with little medical experience.

Many different **charting formats** exist, all of which include the same basic information (Tables 9–3 and 9–4). The preferred approach today is *problem-oriented charting*. Several approaches to problem-oriented charting exist; the most common and easiest to use is **SOAP** (subjective data, objective data, assessment, plan). This format has been expanded to include is **SOAPIE** (subjective data, objective data, assessment, plan, implementation, evaluation) and **SOAPIER** (subjective data, objective data, assessment, plan, implementation, evaluation, revision). Some of these categories become too complex for the simple charting necessary in the medical spa. Two other problem-oriented charting formats exist: (1) **APIE** (assessment, plan, implementation, evaluation) and (2) **PIE** (problem, intervention, evaluation).

charting formats
Any method meant to document or record the events, consequences, or abnormalities associated with a microdermabrasion procedure.

SOAP
Problem-oriented charting aid that emphasizes subjective data, objective data, assessment, and planning.

SOAPIER
Problem-oriented charting aid that emphasizes subjective data, objective data, assessment, planning, implementation, evaluation, and revision.

APIE
Problem-oriented charting aid that emphasizes assessment, planning, implementation, and evaluation.

PIE
Problem-oriented charting aid that emphasizes planning, implementation, and evaluation.

Simple Steps for Microdermabrasion

Step One: After making the client comfortable and draping, wash the client's face with a mild cleanser.

Step Two: Using regular gauze, de-oil the skin with 70 percent isopropyl alcohol.

Step Three: Apply the eye shields.

Step Four (optional): Apply the peel solution, and allow it to sit for the amount of time recommended by protocol (use a hand-made fan to keep the client comfortable).

Step Five: Remove the peel solution and dry the skin.

Step Six: Begin the microdermabrasion process. Remember: If the skin is not dry, the handpiece will drag over the skin, increasing the potential for untoward results. Hold the skin taut between the thumb and third finger; lightly move the wand over the skin. Begin on the forehead, working around the face, first to the right and then to the left. If you wish to stand, you can move from side to side. If you sit, turn the client's head from side to side. When doing the neck, have the client lift the chin to the ceiling.

Step Seven: After the first pass, remove the crystals as necessary. Evaluate the skin's response and adjust the machine to provide the result you want to achieve.

Step Eight (optional): Apply a cooling mask to comfort and hydrate the skin.

Step Nine: Cleanse the skin.

Step Ten: Remove the eye pads.

Step Eleven: Apply moisturizer.

Step Twelve: Apply sunscreen.

Step Thirteen: Answer any questions the client might have, review the discharge instructions, and set up the next appointment.

The SOAP approach is easy for two reasons: (1) it is simple and inclusive, and (2) it specifically asks for subjective data or information that the client specifically states. The best way to use a formal charting format is to create a form. This way, aestheticians and other team members know the specific information that is being collected and documented. However, the specific charting method is specific to the aesthetician. While one might say that less is more with regard to treatment, the opposite is true for documentation. Room should be provided for all documentation types.

Table 9–3 Types of Documentation	
Documentation type	**Description**
SOAP	**S**ubjective data
	Objective data
	Assessment
	Plan
SOAPIE	**S**ubjective data
	Objective data
	Assessment
	Plan
	Implementation
	Evaluation
SOAPIER	**S**ubjective data
	Objective data
	Assessment
	Plan
	Implementation
	Evaluation
	Revision
APIE	**A**ssessment
	Plan
	Implementation
	Evaluation
PIE	**P**roblem
	Intervention
	Evaluation

Forms for Microdermabrasion

With that in mind, the documentation forms ought to be clear, easy and simple to use, and include as many checkboxes as possible, while leaving room for written notes. Subtle information, such as any recent minor illness (flu, colds, headaches), medications the client is taking (including OTC medications such as Advil® or Motrin®), the consistency of the home program, and sun exposure should be included on each treatment record. Because any of the aforementioned conditions could easily affect the outcome of the treatment, failure to document will cause a "hole" in the client care history. Additionally, any changes in the settings of the

Table 9–4	Documentation Acronym Definitions
Subjective data	Reviewing and documenting complaints and physical evidence, including photographs
Objective data	What you as the aesthetician see
Assessment	Your professional opinion of the complaints, the client's observations, and the treatment options available
Plan	The agreed-upon course of action for treatment, including dates, expectations, and home treatment
Implementation	Applying the plan
Evaluation	Determining if the plan is working to achieve the goals of the assessment
Revision	What might be done differently at the next treatment

machine and the reasons why those settings were changed should be documented. Each microdermabrasion treatment should have a separate treatment form, because it is a new visit and new problems or concerns may exist.

Starting at the top, we will discuss what should appear on a microdermabrasion treatment form. First, of course, are the client's name, the date, and the results of the last treatment. Next should appear a list of checkboxes that reflect the focus of the current day's treatment. These checkboxes would include acne scarring, scars, rhytids, texture, and hyperpigmentation. Next is a list of checkboxes that answer questions about the compliancy of the client to the home-care program. The next section of the document reflects the actual treatment, in other words, what is being done that day—the settings used on the machine, the preparation of the skin, and the additional treatments provided. Finally, the last section of the document will have a series of checkboxes that reflect discussions of post-treatment, when the client should return to the spa, and which treatment will be given.

> SOAP charting collects four types of relevant information: (1) subjective data (what the client says), (2) objective data (what you see), (3) assessment (your evaluation), and (4) plan (what you are going to do).

Progress Tracking

Because microdermabrasion, or even infusion microdermabrasion, is a progressive treatment (that is, it takes many appointments to achieve the result), the form that is used should reflect the progression. The signals for improvement (changes in hyperpigmentation, texture, rhytids, or scars) should be included. Both written documentation and a scale of improvement should be reflected in this assessment.

Treatment Form for Microdermabrasion

Client name: _____   Date: _____

Aesthetician: _____   Photos today?   ☐ yes   ☐ no

Consent date: _____

Skin Type and Aging Classification:

☐ Fitzpatrick I   ☐ Fitzpatrick IV   ☐ Rubin one

☐ Fitzpatrick II   ☐ Fitzpatrick V   ☐ Rubin two

☐ Fitzpatrick III   ☐ Fitzpatrick VI   ☐ Rubin three

Skin Conditions:

☐ Telangiectasias; improvement since last treatment: ☐ yes   ☐ no

☐ Wrinkles; improvement since last treatment: ☐ yes   ☐ no

☐ Scarring; improvement since last treatment: ☐ yes   ☐ no

☐ Rough texture/solar damage; improvement since last treatment: ☐ yes   ☐ no

☐ Hyperpigmentation; improvement since last treatment: ☐ yes   ☐ no

☐ Acne; improvement since last treatment: ☐ yes   ☐ no

☐ Other:

   ☐ Regular home-care program use   ☐ yes   ☐ no

   ☐ Recent illness   ☐ yes   ☐ no

   ☐ Medication changes since last visit (oral or topical) ☐ yes   ☐ no

   ☐ Home product change since last visit   ☐ yes   ☐ no

   ☐ Sun exposure since last treatment   ☐ yes   ☐ no

   ☐ Results of last treatment: ☐ Minimal   ☐ Moderate   ☐ Extensive

Comments about last treatment: _____

Number of days since last treatment: _____

Treatment Specifics

Prep Solution: ☐ 70% alcohol   ☐ Acetone   ☐ Beta wipes   ☐ pH cleanser

Microdermabrasion Settings:

☐ Face_____cm/mm Hg   ☐ Eyes_____cm/mm Hg   ☐ Hands_____cm/mm Hg

☐ Neck_____cm/mm Hg   ☐ Back_____cm/mm Hg   ☐ Other_____cm/mm Hg

☐ Chest_____cm/mm Hg   ☐ Arms_____cm/mm Hg

Comments: _____

Continued

Treatment Form for Microdermabrasion—cont'd

Peel Solutions Used:

Number of Coats	**Minutes**	**Neutralized with**
_____ 20% glycolic	_____	☐ Water
_____ 30% glycolic	_____	☐ Alpha lotion
_____ 50% glycolic	_____	☐ Anti-inflammatory gel
_____ Jessner's solution	_____	☐ Spring water mist

Other Applications:

☐ Enzyme mask   ☐ Sunscreen SPF

☐ Hydrating mask   ☐ Moisturizer

☐ Soothing mask

☐ Facial added to the treatment?   ☐ yes (see facial sheet)   ☐ no

Aesthetician signature: _____

Return for next treatment (date): _____

Single treatment?   ☐ yes   ☐ no

Package: _____ of _____ treatments

Within the facility there should be a **safety coordinator** who is responsible for maintenance of the OSHA or safety manual. The manual is the guideline for communicating the safety practices for the business, maintains all the required documents, and houses the safety training protocol for the facility.

safety coordinator
Specially designated person in a business who is responsible for updating the OSHA safety manual as warranted.

Health Insurance Portability and Accountability Act and Record Keeping

Every aesthetician working in the medical spa recognizes the importance of confidentiality. HIPAA (Health Insurance Portability and Accountability Act) requires that every employee working in the medical field (hospital, doctor's office, medical spa) follow the rules of HIPAA. For the working medical spa aesthetician, this means care in the daily management of charts. Several *dos* and *do nots* should be memorized and implemented into daily behavior (Table 9–5).

▪ SAFE PRACTICES AND SANITATION

It is hard to separate the concepts of safe practices and sanitation. Although they seem like separate concepts, they are quite intertwined. For example, leaving dirty implements on the counter (including used lancets) is unsanitary, but it can also be dangerous to the client and the aesthetician. Having electrical cords strung across a room collecting dust is unsanitary, but walking across in the room and tripping over the cord is dangerous. Keeping the environment clean and safe is the priority of everyone in the facility. Sometimes these issues are points of contention between employers and aestheticians. This is always surprising because the idea is really to protect employees. Nevertheless, spas, regardless of

Table 9–5 Dos and Do Nots of the Spa

Do	Do Not
Ask the client for permission when an accompanying friend or family member wants to enter the treatment room with the client.	Leave charts lying on counters where other clients can read or take them.
Keep your charts/records for the day in a locked drawer or safely filed at the front desk before use.	Leave or post your daily schedule where clients can see it.
Make phone calls to clients or pharmacies and do confirmations in a closed area where the clients in the waiting area cannot overhear the conversation.	Mention one client's name in front of another client.
Chart immediately and file charts by the end of the day.	Assume that client's family members are authorized to have information.
Lock your files at the end of the day.	Allow the scheduling book or screen to be seen by a client.
	Have a sign-in "guest book."

their individuality, are universally required to observe OSHA rules to protect their employees and clients.

OSHA has many rules and regulations—far too many for us to cover in this small section. However, it is necessary for us to discuss the rules of OSHA that generally apply to microdermabrasion, of most significance, protecting the aesthetician and client from **bloodborne pathogens**. The use of universal precautions and crystal management fall into the category of disposal of hazardous waste. The protocol you will be concerning yourself with should be outlined specifically in your spa's **safety manual**.

Universal Precautions

The subject of bloodborne pathogens is in itself an extensive subject that includes a variety of issues, mostly related to needle sticks, recapping needles, and exposure to body fluids (usually blood). Because it is possible to become exposed to blood or other bodily fluids during microdermabrasion, it is important for the aesthetician to use universal precautions. By assuming that all body fluids you come into contact

OSHA was originally known as the **Safety Bill of Rights** It was developed by the federal government to protect workers, initially those in hazardous work environments.

bloodborne pathogens
Infectious substances present in the blood that can cause infection or disease; human immunodeficiency virus (HIV) is a bloodborne pathogen.

safety manual
OSHA document that outlines the hazardous materials and equipment specific to each location, as well as the safety protocols for each.

Safety Bill of Rights
Original name of OSHA manual.

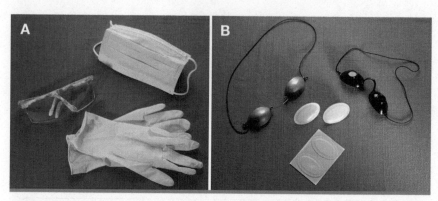

Figure 9–6 *A,* For protection during a microdermabrasion procedure, you must always wear a mask, protective eye goggles, a lab coat or scrubs, and gloves. *B,* The patient's eyes should also be protected during the procedure.

contaminated
Act of making an item or compound nonsterile or impure.

with are **contaminated**, you will be protecting yourself as well as your clients. For secure protection during a microdermabrasion procedure, you must always wear a mask, protective eye goggles for you and your client, a lab coat, and gloves (Figure 9–6, *A*). This may all seem like much ado about nothing; however, these rules are for your safety and protection. You must be prepared by always using universal precautions. For example, what if your machine malfunctions and sprays crystals toward your eyes or the eyes of your client? During the procedure, your client's eyes should also be protected. Remember, you can never be too safe (Figure 9–6, *B*)!

Gloves

Gloves are probably the single most important component of self-protection for an aesthetician performing microdermabrasion or any other aesthetic treatments (Table 9–6). Two types of gloves are available: (1) latex and (2) non-latex. Latex allergies have become more common and can be significant. If your client states that he or she might have a latex allergy, be sure to use a non-latex glove to prevent the allergic reaction from occurring. The allergic reaction presents as erythema, and a rash or even systemic symptoms can occur. Needless to say, this reaction will be aggravated by the microdermabrasion treatment. Latex allergies are also common in aestheticians who wear gloves every day. Obviously, those with latex sensitivities or allergies should wear gloves without latex.

Masks

Masks are one of the aggravating yet necessary additions to an aesthetician's protective wear. They will prove to be inconvenient because they can steam up the eyewear. Therefore, the mask should be one that

Table 9–6 Protective Glove Materials[3]

Material Type	Tensile Strength	Softness	Elasticity	Tear Strength	Cost
Natural rubber	Good	Very good	Very good	Good	Low
Polyisoprene	Good	Very good	Very good	Moderate	High
Nitrile	Good	Good	Good	Poor	Moderate
Neoprene	Good	Good/ very good	Good/ very good	Poor	Moderate/ high
Block copolymers	Good	Good	Very good	Fair	Moderate/ high
Polyvinyl-chloride (PVC)	Fair	Good	Poor	Poor	Low
Polyurethane	Very good	Good	Good	Good	High

is designed to avoid that problem. Because the long-term effects of inhaling aluminum oxide dust are unknown, it is important for aestheticians to protect themselves and use masks whenever they are doing microdermabrasion.

Eyewear

Using protective eyewear is simple and will protect the aesthetician from spraying crystal or body fluids. They do not need to be laser-safe (you are not operating a laser), and they do not need to be construction-grade (you are not hammering nails); they just need to protect the eyes from sprays. As mentioned earlier, the client's eyes also need to be protected (Figure 9–6, *B*). Some spas prefer to use the metal goggles that are meant for laser treatments; other spas use the plastic goggles used for tanning salons. Another type of eye protection available for microdermabrasion is adhesive protection. If the choice of eye protection is goggles, be sure they do not just sit on the face; they need to be attached to an elastic band and secured to the client's head. Some aestheticians like to place a gauze pad under these goggles to make them more comfortable. If you choose adhesive ovals, be sure you get them to stick. They can sometimes pull at the corners, allowing crystals to blow inside to the eye.

Microdermabrasion Tips

Since the microdermabrasion tip is the point of contact with the skin, it requires the same degree of caution, if not higher, as other areas of concern. The microdermabrasion tip should be able to easily disconnect from the handpiece for cleaning. The tip can be either disposable or reusable. Disposables have become a way of life in the medical world and have made their way into the spa world, specifically for microdermabrasion. Although the risk of communicable diseases is low, it cannot be disregarded; disposables are a safe way for the aesthetician and the client to feel comfortable that the treatment is free from contamination. Some spas have begun to use the disposable tip as a reusable tip. They clean them and soak them in a medical-grade sterilizing solution. Although this practice may seem acceptable, the reality is the tips were meant to be disposable for a variety of reasons (not the least of which is to allow the aesthetician to skip the step of cleansing and soaking, or doing so ineffectively). Additionally it is reported that the plastic tips can become sharp and cause scratching or possibly small cuts.

Reusable tips are usually metal and bring with them not only the cleansing dilemma but also a residue that is left on the skin. This will appear as blue or gray streaks on the client's skin. Those reusable tips that are not metal are glass. Glass tips bring a whole host of problems such as breaking, chipping, and potential injury (cuts) to the aesthetician and client. Try to avoid glass tips.

In the end, the best choice is disposable tips that are treated as disposable. Use them once and throw them away.

Crystal Management

Disposal of crystals, like other subjects within microdermabrasion, is a controversial issue. Many of the machine vendors tell you to throw them in the trash, but no doubt many of you are red bagging the crystals. According to the **Environmental Protection Agency (EPA)**, **medical waste** (red bag) is defined as "… **soiled** bandages, culture dishes, surgical gloves, and instruments (including needles), as well as human tissue."[4] *Soiled* is the operative word.

Because you do not know what has been vacuumed from the skin, and because caution should be your first course, the crystals should be red bagged and considered contaminated trash. Your gloves are not soiled with blood or human fluids, they are simply used. Yes, they may have some occasional specks of blood (not unlike a used bandaid), but they are not soiled. Obviously, gloves should never be reused regardless of the

---

When doing microdermabrasion, the aesthetician must use four protective components: (1) a surgical mask to protect from dust inhalation, (2) gloves to protect from body fluids, (3) eyewear to protect from sprays, and (4) a lab coat to protect street clothes from crystals and body fluids. Additionally, using disposable tips will act as an important extra measure to protect the client as well.

red bagging
Slang term that means placement of a medical waste material into an appropriately marked and sealed biohazard receptacle.

Environmental Protection Agency (EPA)
Federal agency responsible for monitoring the environment and regulating waste disposal.

medical waste
Waste resulting from medical activity that includes human blood and blood products, and used or unused sharps (syringes, needles, and blades).

soiled
Any item that is contaminated or formerly in contact with medical waste.

level of debris on the surface of the glove. Soiled items include sponges and gloves in the operating room, or used wound dressings.

Finally, if your machine is not closed and requires that you pour crystals into the machine receptacle, you must wear a mask and protective eyewear when performing this task. This is also true if your machine requires the crystals to be drained out of the machine for disposal. If you spill crystals on the floor, immediately clean them up. The crystals will grind into the tile and cause damage to the flooring. In addition, they will attach to your shoes and track throughout the spa.

▪ PREDICTABLE OUTCOMES

For aestheticians and their clients alike, one of the best things about microdermabrasion is that outcomes are predictable and complications rarely occur. Once you become familiar with your machine, its limits and capabilities are more easily appreciated. With regard to predictable outcomes, you must return to the subjects of skin typing (see Chapter 4), home treatment (see Chapter 5), consultations (see Chapter 6), and indications (see Chapter 7). The knowledge you have gained in these subjects will allow you to control your outcome. Specifically, four simple rules will ensure you will control the outcome and have a positive result: (1) choosing the proper skin types and aging categories, (2) setting up and monitoring the home program, (3) setting client expectations, and (4) staying within the boundaries for proper indications.

If, for whatever reason, you stray outside the guidelines, your result will not be as predictable and may actually cause a complication. When you are strict about the categories, the treatment will go well and the client's skin will improve.

For the beginning aesthetician, learning this information can be stressful; even for those who are more experienced, applying this information can be overwhelming. Although the process does become easier with time, it is made simpler by putting together a questionnaire and creating an easy selection process. This questionnaire will allow you to take a quick glance, once you have gathered the data, to ensure your client is in a qualified category. That said, what about the exceptions to the rule? Exceptions do exist, and they usually come in the form of client demands. People who do not fit into other treatment modalities may include those with health concerns (too sick to undergo surgery), financial issues (unable to manage the surgical fees), or simply those who have their hearts set on microdermabrasion. Of course, the answer in these situations is to ensure that reasonable expectations are set for the client.

Once a client selection has been made, the next concern is the actual treatment. Ensure that you have chosen the right treatment, for the right reason, and at the right time. Once again, using a questionnaire will help you to ensure that the right treatment plan is selected.

Finally, the last step of ensuring a predictable outcome is getting the client to make an appointment for the next treatment. It may sound silly to focus on the next appointment at this step, but microdermabrasion is a progressive treatment. Without a plan for continued care, the result and the client's perception of the end result will be flawed.

Proper Client Selection

When choosing the clients who will be best suited for microdermabrasion, first, consider the indications. You need to be sure that what you are trying to solve falls into the categories of *indications*. If not, the outcome you are predicting will be difficult to achieve.

Skin typing is the second category for the aesthetician to evaluate. As you will remember, the best candidates for microdermabrasion are those who are Fitzpatrick skin type I, II, or III. Although of course you should not disqualify skin types IV, V, and VI, you should prefer lighter-skinned individuals. Next is the aging category on the Rubin scale. You should prefer those in Rubin levels one and two.

Reasonable expectations are next on the evaluation list. Be certain that your client clearly understands what can be accomplished. Those who believe microdermabrasion is going to lift the loose skin of the neck should be educated on the benefits and limitations of the treatment. However, those people probably should have been disqualified when evaluating the aging analysis.

Finally, the outcomes will have much to do with the pretreatment and post-treatment home programs. Home programs require cosmeceuticals, balanced cleansers, moisturizers, sometimes prescription products (if available), and most certainly sunscreen. Remembering that microdermabrasion can dry the skin is an important component for recommending a balanced home-care product program. Part of the home-care program is motivating your client to adhere to his or her assigned regimen. The degree to which you choose to do this will depend on your customer service skills and your personal relationship with your clients.

Assuming you have correctly identified your client, the outcome should be very predictable. The changes to the skin that you should be able to expect include even texture, even pigment, minimization of fine rhytids, improvement in solar damage, and improvement in the appearance of scars.

Aftercare

Caring for the skin after the microdermabrasion treatment is important but certainly not tricky. Only a few basic considerations are necessary in the aftercare phase of treatment. First, did another procedure accompany the microdermabrasion, such as a peel, that may cause additional considerations, such as peeling skin? If so, the care of the skin from this perspective needs to be a priority. However, the main issues to be concerned about should be dry skin, streaking (from excessive suction), and sensitivity. Because the skin is often a little sensitive after a treatment, the products the client uses for the first 24 to 48 hours after treatment may be different. Make the aftercare instructions clear by providing written instructions that are basic and applicable for most of your clients. A handful of clients will not need special instructions after the treatment, because their skin is hardy and they can return to their home-care programs the next day. Nevertheless, the instructions should be written down for the client so that no misunderstandings occur.

Aftercare Kits

Aftercare kits are a terrific idea. The kit should contain only the products you would like the client to use for 24 to 48 hours after the treatment, such as a mild cleanser, a heavier moisturizer, a sunscreen, and an exfoliating product. The aftercare kit should also contain the instructions for the care of the skin after the treatment, when they should return to their normal routine, and any additional information the client should know or be aware of, such as sensitivity to the sun, dryness, or anticipated results.

Kits are usually available from the machine manufacturer but can also be put together by a product company. The use of prepackaged aftercare kits also limits the number of phone calls you will have to return, especially if the post-treatment information in the kit is well-worded and well-thought-out.

Cleansers

Remember, cleansers can cause the skin to be dry by changing the acid mantle pH. It is important that the client is using a cleanser with a slightly more acid pH after this treatment. A mild cleanser without active ingredients (glycolic or salicylic acids) is the best choice. Just be gentle to the skin for a day or so; then go back to the cleansers with active ingredients.

Client Skin Typing Evaluation Form

1. Does the client exhibit any of the following?
   - Rhytids
   - Solar damage
   - Hyperpigmentation
   - Acne scarring
   - Keratosis
   - Scars
   - Rough Texture
   - General wish to improve the skin

   ☐ yes   ☐ no

   If *yes*, move on to question 2; if *no*, STOP. This client is not a good candidate for microdermabrasion.

2. Does the client present with any of the following ailments?
   - Excessive telangiectasia
   - Rosacea
   - Bacterial skin infections
   - Fungal infections
   - Viral infections
   - Open lesions and rashes
   - Active acne

   ☐ yes   ☐ no

   If *no*, move on to question 3. If *yes*, STOP. This client is not a good candidate for microdermabrasion.

3. Is this client using Accutane?

   ☐ yes   ☐ no

   If *no*, move on to question 4. If *yes*, STOP. This client is not a good candidate for microdermabrasion.

4. Does this client have realistic expectations for treatment?

   ☐ yes   ☐ no

   If *yes*, move on to question 5. If *no*, STOP. This client is not a good candidate for microdermabrasion.

5. Does the client have Fitzpatrick skin type I, II, or III?

   ☐ yes   ☐ no

   If *yes*, move on to question 6. If *no* (the client is Fitzpatrick IV, V, or VI), STOP. This client is not the best candidate for microdermabrasion.

6. Does the client have Rubin skin aging level one or two?

   ☐ yes   ☐ no

   If *yes*, move on to 7. If *no* (the client is Rubin level three), STOP. This client is not a good candidate for microdermabrasion.

7. This client is the best candidate for microdermabrasion!

Caring for the Skin after Microdermabrasion

Aftercare is where some clients get into trouble with home remedies and listening to friends. Make sure you are the authority.

WHAT CLIENTS CAN EXPECT FOLLOWING MICRODERMABRASION:

After microdermabrasion you will need to provide your clients with an *aftercare kit* as well as emotional and physical guidance. Emphasize how important it is that they follow the instructions carefully. Immediately following the procedure, clients may be slightly dry and may even peel slightly. This is normal. If any blisters, sores, or other types of concerning problems arise, advise clients to call your office immediately. They should not try to care for these problems without the assistance of the aesthetician, or possibly a physician. Your instructions and those in the aftercare kit *are not recommendations; they are vital to the outcome*. This must be stressed to the client in the best manner possible. Clients will often be tempted to use home-care remedies as a shortcut or cost-cutting effort. Advise them not to use home remedies which haven't already been specified in the aftercare kit. The only products they ought to use, as a general rule, are those supplied to them by you prior to leaving your facility. Finally, if they have questions, advise them to call your office. This ought to be documented clearly and discussed with the client both prior to and following a microdermabrasion treatment.

SAMPLE OF INSTRUCTIONS FOR CLIENTS IN AFTERCARE KITS:

Evening After Your Treatment:

Use the gentle cleanser found in your aftercare kit. After cleansing, use the night moisturizer found in the kit.

Day One:

Use the gentle cleanser found in your aftercare kit. Apply moisturizer and sunscreen as directed in the kit. Do not use any active ingredients such as glycolic or lactic acids, Retin A, Renova, or hydroquinone unless instructed by your aesthetician. In the evening, use the gentle cleanser again and follow with the nighttime moisturizer.

Day Two:

Use the gentle cleanser found in your aftercare kit. Apply moisturizer and sunscreen as directed in the kit. Do not use any active ingredients such as glycolic or lactic acids, Retin A, Renova, or hydroquinone unless instructed by your aesthetician. In the evening, use the gentle cleanser again and follow with the nighttime moisturizer.

Day Three:

In the shower, exfoliate your face with the mask provided in the aftercare kit. Begin your usual therapeutic home program.

Moisturizers

Moisturizers are important because the skin can become dryer after microdermabrasion (aluminum oxide is an absorbent). Even if you are using a different type of machine (salt or diamond tip), you are still taking down the stratum corneum and increasing the TEWL. Clients should use moisturizers with vitamins and antioxidants to heal the skin and promote skin health. Although the everyday moisturizer you recommend for the client should be robust and full of vitamins and antioxidants, after a treatment these ingredients should be increased.

Sunscreens

Obviously, sunscreen is required after a microdermabrasion. In fact, it is simply something that should be used every day.

Hydroquinone

If you are permitted to dispense prescription in a medi-spa, and your client has pigment problems, you will probably want to implement hydroquinone into the immediate post-treatment skin program. If the client is inclined toward hyperpigmentation, some physicians like a higher dose of hydroquinone and little bit of topical steroid after a treatment. Check with your overseeing physician on the protocol if you work in a medical environment. Meanwhile, if you are just attempting to reduce pigment, you can add hydroquinone into the post-treatment program for greater impact and improvement. This would be a special instruction that would need to be written down for this particular client.

Complications

Complications with microdermabrasion are rare. Properly trained aestheticians who understand their machines and who have directed care plans for clients rarely run into problems. However, an unforeseen event will occasionally arise. Among those complications of which the aesthetician should be aware are infections, abrasions, sunburns that occur after treatment, and the use of an unapproved topical. If a problem occurs, handle it professionally. Complications can happen to everyone, no matter how experienced you are.

The protocol for complication care is very straightforward. The client must always be seen in the office. Clear and concise documentation is required, creating a "story" in the chart (to leave a good paper trail). Next—and this step is often forgotten—take a photograph. You need a *visual history* of the injury. Finally, the client must always see the physician. If you are in a situation where no physician is available in the facility (luxury or day spa), refer the client to the physician with which your facility has a relationship, or one whom you trust.

Once a treatment plan is put in place to solve the problem, make sure the client has a follow-up appointment. Sometimes aestheticians have an out-of-sight-out-of-mind attitude. Avoiding the client will not make the problem go away and will often make it worse. If the physician takes over the care of the client through the complication period, make a point of accompanying the physician when the client comes in for follow-up appointments. This keeps you in the loop and shows concern for the client. In addition, you will learn from the physician about the process of solving a problem. Do not be afraid; problems happen. Luckily, in microdermabrasion, they do not happen often.

Infections

Infections are rare but do occur, especially when the implements (micro-dermabrasion tips, in particular) are not properly cleaned. Follow the protocol for cleaning and sterilizing your tips if they are reusable. If they are disposable, then throw them away (Table 9–7). Be sure that all of your instruments are properly sterilized.

Infections can happen if an unexpected break occurs in the skin of which the aesthetician is unaware at the time of treatment or just after treatment. Clients who touch their faces with dirty hands or allow other people to touch their faces immediately following treatment will be at a greater risk. Remember, the skin has *Staphylococcus* and *Streptococcus* that normally live on the surface. When you abrade the skin, you are creating the opportunity for a small scratch and a subsequent infection. This is unusual and should not concern you; however, do not disregard a client who calls to tell you he or she has a "sore" after microdermabrasion. These clients should be seen, a photograph taken of the area, and the case referred to the physician. Remember, if the wound is deep (in the midpapillary dermis), then it will leave a scar. Once again, do not worry, because this rarely happens; however, you need to be aware that it could happen, especially if the problem is disregarded. Infections, on the rare instances in which they occur, usually heal nicely without scarring.

Corneal Abrasions

The cornea is a thin transparent coating over the inner workings of the eye. A scratch in the cornea is called a *corneal abrasion*. A corneal abrasion can occur when the eyes are not protected throughout the micro-dermabrasion treatment. This means that the eyes need to be covered during the *entire* treatment. Clients are especially vulnerable at the end of the treatment when the face is being wiped clean of crystals. Some aestheticians have found it helpful to put eye pads (oval cotton gauze pads) under the goggles to ensure that the eyes are fully protected.

Table 9–7 Commonly Used Disinfectants, Sterilizers, and Antiseptics

Disinfectants and Sterilizers

Name	Form	Strength	Use (Per Manufacturer's Instructions)
Quaternary ammonium compounds (quats)	Liquid or tablet	1:1000	Immerse implements in solutions for 20 minutes or longer.
Formalin	Liquid	25% solution	Immerse implements in solutions for 10 minutes or longer.
Formalin	Liquid	10% solution	Immerse implements in solutions for 20 minutes or longer.
Alcohol (ethyl or isopropyl)	Liquid	70% or 90% solution	Immerse implements or sanitize electrodes and sharp-cutting edges for 10 minutes or longer.
Autoclave	Heat sterilizer may be used as steam or dry heat.	–	Sterilize for 30 minutes.

Antiseptics

Name	Form	Strength	Use (Per Manufacturer's Instructions)
Boric acid	White crystals	2%–5% solution	Cleanse the eye.
Tincture of iodine	Liquid	2% solution	Cleanse cuts and wounds.
Hydrogen peroxide	Liquid	3%–5% solution	Cleanse skin and minor cuts.
Ethyl or grain alcohol	Liquid	60% solution	Cleanse hands, skin, and tiny cuts. Do not use if irritation is present.
Formalin	Liquid	5% solution	Cleanse sinks and cabinets.
Chloramine-T (Chlorazene; Chlorozol)	White crystals	0.5% solution	Cleanse skin and hands, and for general use.
Sodium hypochlorite (Javelle water; Zonite)	Liquid	0.5% solution	Rinse the hands.

Leave the eye protection in place until the treatment is complete. If the client complains of *something in the eye,* then use an eyewash to irrigate the eye. Pain, tearing, and redness also accompany corneal abrasions. If this does not solve the problem, the client will need to be seen in the emergency department or by an ophthalmologist. The treatment for a corneal abrasion is antibiotic drops or ointment, and a patch.

Skin Abrasions

Abrasions are possible if (1) the microdermabrasion tip is being reused and is sharp or (2) the treatment was aggressive (both the crystals and the vacuum volume setting are high) (Figure 9–7). Sometimes this is intended, and the post-treatment should be adjusted to manage these small skin scrapes to prevent infections and scabs. Remember that scrapes on the skin or exposure of the papillary dermis (where bleeding occurs) places the skin at greater risk for infection. After these areas heal, they may be a little pink for a short time; this is normal.

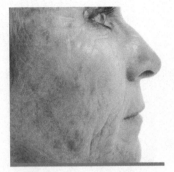

Figure 9–7 When you are too aggressive with the settings, abrasions or even pinpoint bleeding can occur.

Topical Antibiotic Ointments

Topical antibiotic ointments should be avoided. On closed skin they disrupt the bacteria counts, causing rashes and irritation. Even under applicable situations the client can develop allergies to the antibiotics in the ointment, causing a rash, swelling, and client discomfort. To avoid all of these potential problems, simply stay away from antibiotic ointments unless your physician directs you accordingly.

Vitamin E Oil

Many clients are attracted to vitamin E oil because of the positive coverage it has received in the lay press. The most problematic vitamin E comes from the capsules that are broken open and applied directly onto the skin. In reality, vitamin E oil is not beneficial, and in at least 30 percent of the cases atopic dermatitis will result. Once again, the best answer is to keep the client focused on the aftercare kit and away from home remedies and friends' advice.

Sunburn after Treatments

On occasion, a client will be outdoors and develop a sunburn after the microdermabrasion treatment. This is somewhat worrisome, because the stratum corneum has been significantly exfoliated. Alert your clients to the possibility of sun sensitivity, and educate them about the use of sunscreen. Sometimes your best efforts will go unheeded, and a problem will arise. If this happens, always see the client in the office to evaluate the status of the skin. Gentle cleansing, heavy moisturizing, and eventually exfoliating is in order. If the sunburn is significant, the client should see the physician.

Psychosocial Attitudes

Clients have varying emotions about having treatments. As an aesthetician, you will see the entire gamut over time. Some clients are happy to tell anyone who will listen that they are having the treatments. Others will not tell a soul but will be proud of their commitment to themselves and their skin. Some will be excited to have the procedure and eagerly anticipate the change in the way they look and feel, while others will be terrified. The last group is those who want and need the procedure but feel guilty for taking care of themselves. This is the group who needs your support because they may find themselves being ridiculed by friends or family members who find out they are taking the time and making a commitment to do something for themselves. Continued encouragement and support is the right answer. Additionally, this group needs a mild treatment that will not compromise their personal situations or cause conflict in their lives.

▪ GROUP STUDY EXAMPLES

The clients for the clinical study group were divided into groups based on skin conditions: normal, dry, oily, combination, and sensitive skin. Additionally, each client had a complaint of aging, solar damage, hyperpigmentation, or acne. The clients have been in the program for at least eight weeks. Remember, each client was put on a specific home-care program that was simplified into either normal-to-dry skin or normal-to-oily skin. In addition to the study groups, photographs are available of long-term results. These photographs will help you to understand and predict the benefits of microdermabrasion.

All of these microdermabrasion treatments were done with a clinical pretreatment of glycolic acid and the use of a Parisian Peel microdermabrasion machine.

Group One Pretreatment: Normal Skin with Aging Complaints

Patti is a 45-year-old woman categorized as a Fitzpatrick II and a Rubin two (Figure 9–8). She has been in the program for 12 weeks, totaling five visits. Home care was begun two weeks before the first treatment. The microdermabrasion treatments included a 30 percent glycolic acid

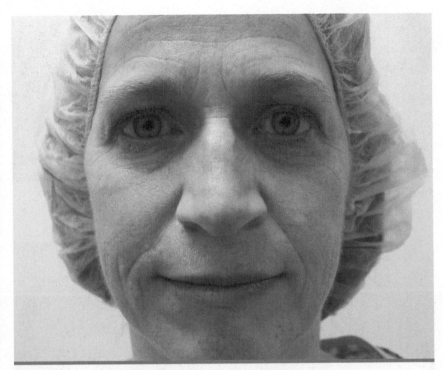

Figure 9–8 Normal skin with aging after treatments.

(2.7 pH) that was applied to clean and prepped skin. The glycolic acid was left to sit for three minutes, watching for areas of redness and potential overexposure to the glycolic acid. At the end of three minutes, the glycolic acid was removed and neutralized. The skin was cleansed with water and dried. The microdermabrasion treatment was then begun. As stated earlier, the Parisian Peel microdermabrasion machine was used. The setting for this treatment plan was −10 mm Hg.

Patti began to notice a difference after the first appointment; after the third appointment she began to see an improvement in the fine lines around her eyes. At the fifth appointment she reported that friends and family were noticing a difference but were unable to identify the change. This is a common response—the client just looks better, but people are unable to identify the source of the change (Figures 9–9 and 9–10).

Patti's after-treatment photographs show improvement in several areas of note. First, the pigment is beginning to diminish. Definite improvement is seen in the crow's-feet, and the forehead lines are much improved. This result is standard for this skin type and the number and type of treatments.

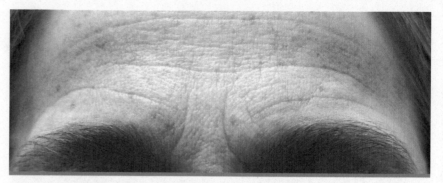

Figure 9–9 The forehead before treatments.

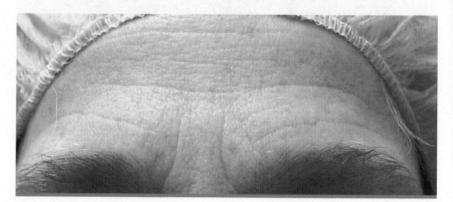

Figure 9–10 The forehead after treatments. Notice the improvement in depth and length of forehead lines.

Group Two Pretreatment: Dry Skin with Aging Complaints

Rachael is a 75-year-old woman categorized as a Fitzpatrick IV and a Rubin three (Figures 9–11 and 9–12). Rachael is, according to our protocol, outside the optimum age bracket to show significant improvements with microdermabrasion. Her lines are actually deep folds, and the pigment in her skin is both freckling and deep solar damage. However, for our benefit we included Rachael to prove just how much improvement can be made with microdermabrasion. Additionally, Rachael had realistic expectations that made our job easier.

Rachael was put on the standard home-care program for dry skin. As with the previous protocol, Rachael was treated with a 30 percent glycolic solution (2.7 pH) before the microdermabrasion. The solution was allowed to sit for four minutes, watching of course for redness and

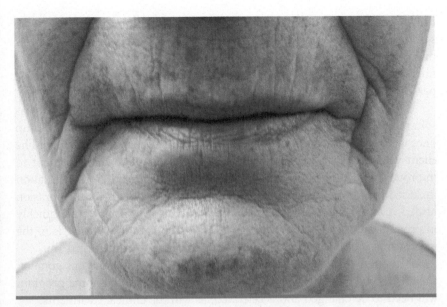

Figure 9–11 Dry skin with aging before treatments.

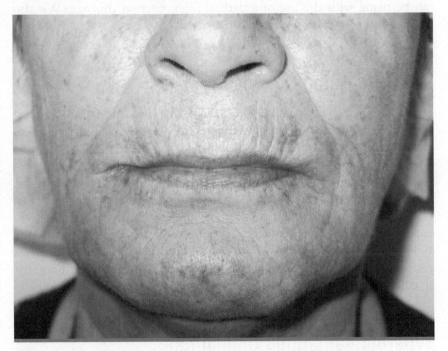

Figure 9–12 Dry skin with aging. This woman, although not a likely candidate for microdermabrasion, had extraordinary results. Note the improvement of the lines of the upper lip. This photograph was taken immediately after Restylane® and Botox® injections, hence the slight redness and bruising.

tissue injury from the peel solution. After four minutes the glycolic solution was neutralized and the skin was cleansed and dried. The microdermabrasion treatment was then begun using the Parisian Peel microdermabrasion machine set at −10 mm Hg. The standard three passes were made at each treatment visit.

After the second appointment, Rachael reported that her skin was softer and smoother to the touch. At the third appointment the upper lip lines were treated aggressively, bringing the skin to pinpoint bleeding. The client was flexible, allowing us to increase the depth of the treatment to improve the quality of the result. Her post-treatment care in this situation included the application of Aquafor® for 48 to 72 hours until the abrasion healed. Once healed, it was apparent that this approach would quickly improve her upper lip lines. However, her most significant result is in the improvement of her hyperpigmentation also notable on the upper lip.

Although Rachael had quick, immediate results, as time has gone on she has reached a plateau. This will often happen, and the home program will need to be changed and accelerated, as will the clinical treatments.

Rachael is our model for the use of Restylane with microdermabrasion. You can see from the photographs that significant improvement can be made with the use of a dermal filler, even at this age. We also added a little Botox to her upper lip areas.

Group Three Pretreatment: Sensitive Skin with Aging Complaints

Kathryn is a 54-year-old woman categorized as a Fitzpatrick I and a Rubin three. We noted in the pretreatment analysis that Kathryn's skin appeared sensitive, even though she denied this observation at the time of the consultation. She was placed on the normal-to-dry home program, and within one week she had a significant response to the home product regimen. Her response included hives, itching, and redness. We attempted to provide a milder program for home use, but she was unable to tolerate the therapeutic products (Retin A, retinol, or alpha hydroxy acid [AHA] of any kind, including a mild lactic acid). She was also intolerant of the microdermabrasion treatment, even without the glycolic acid. Therefore she was removed from the program.

Group Four Pretreatment: Normal Skin with Hyperpigmentation Complaints

Maria is a 47-year-old woman categorized as a Fitzpatrick IV and a Rubin two (Figure 9–13). You may recall from Maria's pretreatment information that she had had a previous microdermabrasion treatment, resulting in

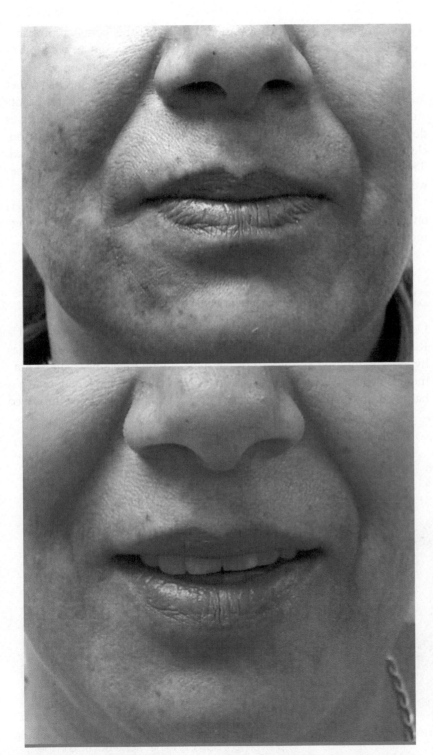

Figure 9–13 Normal skin with hyperpigmentation after treatments.

post-inflammatory hyperpigmentation. Because of this potential problem, we began Maria's clinical treatment slowly, trying to avoid any redness or potential opportunity for post-inflammatory hyperpigmentation.

Maria was put on the home program for normal skin and began her microdermabrasion treatments after two weeks. The clinical treatments still included the application of glycolic acid; however, the time was decreased to two minutes. After the standard process of neutralization, cleansing, and drying, the microdermabrasion treatment was performed. The Parisian Peel machine was set at −10 mm Hg, and three passes were performed.

Maria's hyperpigmentation seemed to be quite resistant; however, on photographs we can make note of improvement not only in the pigment but also in the smile lines (especially on the left side).

Group Five Pretreatment: Oily and Acne-Prone Skin with Acne Breakout Complaints

Donna is a 43-year-old woman categorized as a Fitzpatrick III and a Rubin one (Figures 9–14 and 9–15). You may recall that Donna has hyperpigmentation secondary to her acne. Donna feels her acne is hormonal, predictably occurring during her menstrual cycle. Donna has had over six treatments (one every other week). Her skin has improved

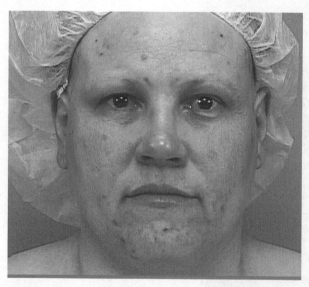

Figure 9–14 Oily and acne-prone skin with acne break out.

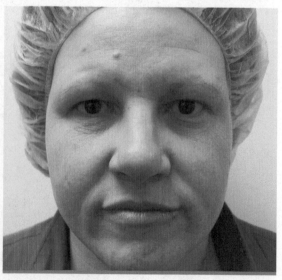

Figure 9–15 Oily and acne-prone skin. Donna had improvement not only in her acne but also in the tone and texture of her skin.

dramatically. As with the other study candidates, Donna's treatments included an application of glycolic acid before the microdermabrasion treatment. The microdermabrasion treatment was done with the Parisian Peel machine at −10 mm Hg.

Donna had improvement not only in the status of her acne but also in the lines and wrinkles around her eyes and in the forehead area. Donna's hyperpigmentation has also improved.

• CONCLUSION

Microdermabrasion treatments have been on the receiving end of factual and fictitious analysis. Some recipients report a healthier, more youthful appearance as a direct result of the treatments. Others say that the treatment was unsuccessful. With such a varying chasm between those who loved it and those who hated it, the need for the aesthetician to exercise thoughtful consideration as to whom he or she selects to be a candidate becomes that much more critical. In addition, the aesthetician needs to be well-practiced in the logistical and procedural components of the treatment (Figures 9–16 through 9–21).

To have this depth of knowledge, the aesthetician should have an understanding of the technological advancements in microdermabrasion machines, crystals, and processes.

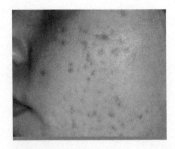

Figure 9–16
Microdermabrasion can be very effective on acne scarring. This photograph shows scarring before treatment.

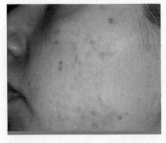

Figure 9–17 The result of microdermabrasion on acne scarring.

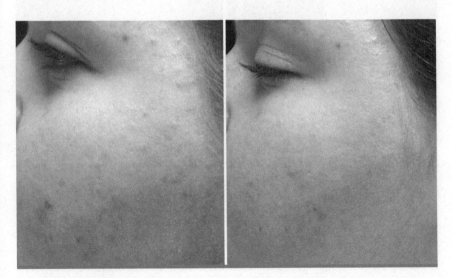

Figure 9–18 Microdermabrasion can be effective for oily skin that is congested. (Photograph courtesy of Aesthetic Technology.)

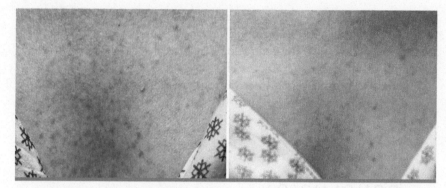

Figure 9–19 Microdermabrasion can be effective on the chest.

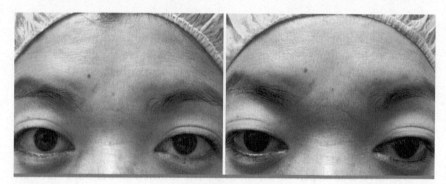

Figure 9–20 Microdermabrasion can improve very fine forehead lines.

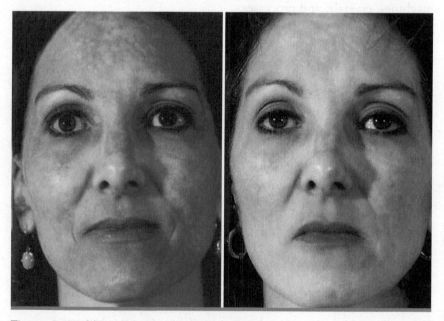

Figure 9–21 Microdermabrasion is excellent treatment for melasma. (Photograph courtesy of Aesthetic Technology.)

However, true optimal outcomes require that the aesthetician know the indications and contraindications to select the candidates who will most likely benefit from the procedure. Doing so will be beneficial to the client, aesthetician, and spa.

⟩ ⟩ ⟩ Top 10 Tips to Take to the Spa

1. Select your clients carefully.
2. Make sure the handpiece you use is comfortable in your hand for hours at a time.
3. To be really good at microdermabrasion treatments, you must get a great deal of practice.
4. *Always* use universal precautions.
5. Use aftercare kits to ensure the client follows your instructions.
6. Use disposable tips.
7. Get to know your machine, and create standardized setting protocols for the skin conditions you see.
8. Dispose of crystals in the hazardous waste containers.
9. Do not avoid clients with complications.
10. Create unique multi-treatment procedures using microdermabrasion.

Chapter Review Questions

1. Variation is a constant in the spa industry. Describe some of these variables and how each ought to be overcome.
2. Microdermabrasion is technique-sensitive. This can be both a benefit and a disadvantage. How so? How can you, as an aesthetician, overcome the negative aspects of this quality?
3. What are the technical components of the microdermabrasion device? How do they affect the outcome of treatment?
4. Identify some of the characteristics all machines share. Identify some differences.
5. True or False: Aluminum oxide machines are far superior to and safer than other types of microdermabrasion machines.
6. True or False: Open system machines are not as safe as closed system machines because it has been proven that aluminum oxide causes cancer and Alzheimer's.

7. What is ergonomics? How does it apply with regard to handpiece and position?

8. Name the proper methods of microdermabrasion?

9. What special considerations should the aesthetician be aware of when using microdermabrasion?

10. Why should the aesthetician wear a mask during the treatment?

11. Why are gloves necessary during the treatment?

12. What are the appropriate recordkeeping measures for microdermabrasion treatments?

13. What is the proper method for disposal of microdermabrasion crystals?

14. How does the aesthetician create unique treatments?

15. What are some of the complications that are seen with microdermabrasion?

16. What is the recommended aftercare program for microdermabrasion clients?

17. What skin improvements can be seen with microdermabrasion?

Chapter References

1. Powerpeel.com. (2004, March 27). *Aluminum oxide: What is aluminum oxide?* [Online]. Available: http://www.powerpeel.com

2. Powerpeel.com. (2004, March 27). *Aluminum oxide: What is aluminum oxide?* [Online]. Available: http://www.powerpeel.com

3. Health and Safety Executive. (2004, April 11). *Nonlatex glove alternatives* [Online]. Available: http://www.hse.gov.uk

4. Environmental Protection Agency. (2004, March 29). *EPA topics: Medical waste* [Online]. Available: http://www.epa.gov

Bibliography

Deitz, S. (2004). *Milady's the clinical esthetician*. Clifton Park, NY: Thomson Delmar Learning.

Dermaster. (2004, March 27). *Dermaster salt macrodermabrasion* [Online]. Available: http://www.spaline.ca

Freedman, B. M., Rueda-Perez, E., & Waddell, S. P. (2001). The epidermal and dermal changes associated with microdermabrasion. *Journal of Dermatologic Surgery, 27*(12), 1033–1034.

Gail, S. (2003, May 1). *Managing your patients' expectations: A fresh approach* [Online]. Available: http://www.cosmeticsurgerytimes.com

Gerson, J. (2004). *Milady's standard: Fundamentals for estheticians* (9th ed.). Clifton Park, NY: Thomson Delmar Learning.

Guttman, C. (2001, August). *Microdermabrasion with diamond dust coated wand has foundation in traditional dermabrasion* [Online]. Available: http://www.cosmeticsurgerytimes.com

NewApeel® aesthetic exfoliation system. (2004, March 27). [Online]. Available: http://www.newapeel.com

Root, L. (2001, January). *Buying power: A guide to purchasing a microdermabrasion machine* [Online]. Available: http://www.skinforlife.com

Shelton, R. M. (2003, October). Prevention of cross-contamination when using microdermabrasion equipment. *Journal of Cutis, 72*(4), 266–268.

Slimtone USA Diamond Medical Aesthetics. (2004, March 27). *Microdermabrasion* [Online]. Available: http://www.slimtoneusa.com

United States Department of Health and Human Services. (2004, March 9). *Fact sheet* [Online]. Available: http://www.hhs.gov

U.S. Department of Labor Occupational Safety & Health Administration. (2004, March 28). *OSHA's mission* [Online]. Available: http://www.osha.gov

U.S. Environmental Protection Agency. (2004, March 29). *EPA topics: Medical waste* [Online]. Available: http://www.epa.gov/ebtpages/wastmedicalwaste.html

Wang, C. M., Huang, C. L., & Chan, H. L. (1997, January). The effect of glycolic acid in the treatment of Asian skin. *Journal of Dermatologic Surgery, 23*(1), 23–29.

Creating Unique Treatments

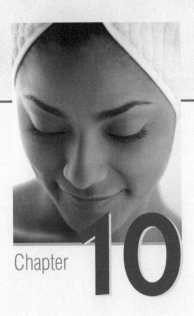

Chapter 10

Key Terms

cavitation   collagenase   photomodulation

Learning Objectives

After completing this chapter you should be able to:

1. Describe the benefits of enhancing microdermabrasion treatments.
2. Discuss the unique treatments currently available.
3. Identify the treatments that work best with microdermabrasion.
4. Identify the risks associated with combination treatments.

267

INTRODUCTION

Creating a unique treatment with your microdermabrasion equipment is one of the most exciting reasons to offer microdermabrasion in your spa. If you are currently offering microdermabrasion as a simple, independent treatment, read carefully—this section will be important to you.

A microdermabrasion treatment that is unique to you and differentiates you from your competition can be created in many ways. Because it seems like everyone is doing microdermabrasion, the ability to develop a treatment that is uniquely yours is important. Aside from the commonly thought of peels, facials, and masks (enzyme, hydrating, or soothing), think *outside the box* to create a treatment that is all about your facility. This is especially true for those who have invested in an infusion machine. For example, add a vitamin C eye treatment with each microdermabrasion; if the upper lip is a problem, add a lip treatment. If you have an ultrasound, be sure to use it with each treatment and let the client know what is special about the ultrasound and microdermabrasion combination. In addition, consider the idea of complementary makeup application after each treatment. These simple ideas will enhance your treatment, make you different, and capture your client's loyalty. Another idea that is gaining popularity is the use of microdermabrasion on body parts other than the face such as the hands, arms, or chest. This is an excellent use of microdermabrasion and should be suggested to the client. One can always tell about the client who takes care of the face but ignores the other areas of the body. The hands, especially, will show the true age unless the client has regular spa and home treatments.

Once you create something special, add in the *tried and true*. It cannot be denied that the use of peels, masks, and facials brings great benefit to the microdermabrasion treatment. Perhaps *your* microdermabrasion treatment includes a peel and an eye treatment as standard; that would be a terrific treatment that covers all the common aging concerns a client might have.

The next issue to address is time and cost. It may take you an hour to do this treatment, so charge fairly for your time, but do not price yourself out of the market. You may want to consider inclusive packages or a menu of "add-ons." Be creative about the unique microdermabrasion treatment you will offer to your clients.

MICRODERMABRASION AND FACIALS

Facials are one of the most requested treatments at spas, if not the single most requested treatment. Aside from being effective and noninvasive, they are beneficial in balancing, restoring, and nourishing the skin, and relaxing the client. Today, there exist a variety of facials that are desired by clients. Among them are microdermabrasion facials, which are combination treatments (Figure 10–1).[1] All basic facial treatments including microdermabrasion facials share several commonalities, including cleansing, toning, exfoliating (microdermabrasion), massaging, and mask treatments. Microdermabrasion facials provide benefits such as general relaxation, deep exfoliation and cleansing, stimulating circulation and lymphatic drainage, and corrective properties. Just because the microdermabrasion is being used as the exfoliation component of the facial doesn't mean that all the other steps should not be followed as they would in a normal facial.

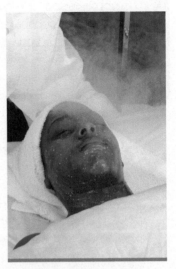

Figure 10–1 Client having a facial with microderm-abrasion.

Pre-Treatment Setup

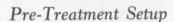

1. Prepare the facial bed in the following manner:
   a. bed warmer
   b. fitted sheet on top of bed warmer
   c. flat sheet draped
   d. light blanket placed over sheet
   e. bath sheet on top of flat sheet, leaving space at top for hand towel
   f. headband positioned on top of towel
   g. cotton towel folded diagonally with points facing out (head wrap)
   h. facial gown folded on top of facial bed
2. Be certain that the room contains every supply that may be needed for the aseptic procedure, such as gloves and EPA-approved, hospital-grade disinfectant. General supplies used during the treatment should be organized for easy use during the procedure.
3. Place products on the shelf of a cart in an organized fashion. Use small dispensing containers or those with pumps to easily dispense the products.
4. The microdermabrasion machine should be close at hand.

Suggested Steps for a European Facial with Microdermabrasion

1. <u>Light cleansing</u> – Remove all makeup and prepare for skin analysis.
2. <u>Analysis and consultation</u> – Establish skin type and conditions to determine treatment.
3. <u>Deep cleansing and exfoliation</u> – Perform deeper cleansing, exfoliate the buildup of dead skin cells, and extract comedones.
   a. Apply deep cleansing solution to the face.
   b. Cleanse with a hand-held manual brush, sponge, or gauze (depending on the client's skin type and sensitivity level) or use a deep cleansing massage with a milky cleanser (clients will prefer the deep cleansing massage if they are seeking a relaxation based facial).
   c. Perform the microdermabrasion (crystal or crystal-free), using 1 to 2 passes in each direction (vertical, horizontal, and diagonal).
   d. If you have an exfoliation mask such as an enzyme that may require processing time, a nice relaxing massage can be performed on the foot and legs. If you want to further pamper the client you may also add heated foot booties after the massage sequence. Reflexology may be substituted at this time. If you use an exfoliation mask, be careful to avoid overtreating the skin. After microdermabrasion, the mask may only require 1 to 2 minutes to be effective. The aesthetician should also be alert to the possibility of stinging. If the mask stings, it should be removed immediately and the facial should be continued without the exfoliating mask.
   e. Remove the mask with sponges or warm towels.
4. <u>Massage and corrective treatment</u> – Delivers specialized ingredients, offers relaxation to the client, and stimulates blood and lymph circulation and cell turnover. (In European facials, the massage also is used to loosen comedones for easy removal during extractions.)
   a. Apply a specialized serum or ampoule and lightly massage into the skin.
   b. Apply a massage cream appropriate to the skin type. Use the massage technique appropriate to skin type. Omit the massage if the client's facial skin is fragile and concentrate the massage on the shoulders and upper arms.
5. <u>Correct</u> – Perform extractions and a corrective treatment for specialized skin conditions.
   a. Use a warm towel to steam the face for one minute, then repeat.
   b. Place moistened eye pads on eyes.
   c. Move magnifying lamp over face.
   d. Perform extraction using light pressure with moist cotton or a comedone extractor tool.
   e. Rinse skin with warm water.
   f. Apply an antiseptic toner or corrective treatment.
6. <u>Mask</u> – Place concentrated nutrients on the skin for an extended period of time to help correct the skin.
   a. Choose a mask that is appropriate for the skin type.
   b. Prepare the mask in a small bowl.
   c. Apply with a clean brush at medium thickness, using upward strokes and avoiding the eyes and nose membranes.

   d. Place eye pads on the eyes and leave the mask on the face for 10 to 15 minutes.

   e. An eye and lip treatment may be integrated at this time by applying specialized eye and lip serums under a specialized eye and lip mask and cover with cotton pads moistened with toner.

   f. At this time, a nice, relaxing massage can be performed on the hands, arms, and shoulders. If you want to further pamper the client, you may also add heated hand mitts after the massage sequence. Reflexology may be substituted at this time.

   g. Rinse thoroughly with sponges or warm moist towels.

7. <u>Completion</u> – Restore and rebalance the skin. Discuss home skin care regimen.

   a. Apply freshener/toner.

   b. Apply eye cream.

   c. Apply light moisturizer.

   d. Apply sunscreen.

   e. Discuss home skin care regimen.

   f. Schedule client's next appointment.

When adding a microdermabrasion treatment to a facial package, it is important to determine what the goals are and what should to be done to achieve them. Some aestheticians improve the results of their facials by replacing standard products, such as exfoliating masks, with microdermabrasion. One example for a client who has a buildup of excess dead skin cells is replacing exfoliating granules with micro-dermabrasion. Lymphatic drainage is another step that may be added into the normal facial and microdermabrasion protocol.

MICRODERMABRASION AND ULTRASOUND

In a physical therapy setting, ultrasound is used to stimulate blood flow, increase metabolic rate, and warm up tissues to promote temporary pain relief. Ultrasound used for cosmetic applications has increasingly gained popularity. Its current applications include its use to penetrate products or provide deep-cleansing action. For the purpose of deep cleansing, a spatula-like handpiece is used in conjunction with water-based cleansers and steam to perform a deep cleansing (Figure 10–2). It is believed that the ultrasound helps to dislodge any surface contaminates or impurities embedded in the follicles. In the case of product penetration, a circular, flat handpiece or the opposite side of the spatula is used in conjunction with serums and ampoules for deeper penetration of products. When using

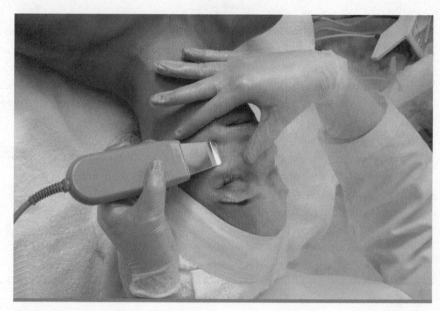

Figure 10–2 Client having ultrasound.

microdermabrasion in combination with ultrasound, the objective is to use the ultrasound first as a cleansing device, followed by microdermabrasion. The microdermabrasion protocol is followed as it normally would be, with three passes: vertically, horizontally, and then diagonally. Finally, the treatment can be ended with the use of ultrasound and product such as moisturizer to intensely moisturize the skin.

When determining the proper application parameters for the cosmetic application of ultrasound, it is first important to understand that the depth of tissue penetration is not intensity-dependent, but frequency-dependent. When using ultrasound with microdermabrasion, the application usually consists of a tissue penetration depth of less than two centimeters, which can be obtained by using a 3 MHz frequency. Most of the ultrasonic energy with a 3 MHz frequency will be absorbed in the superficial tissue. In contrast, the slower, 1 MHz frequency will have less energy absorbed superficially, allowing for deeper penetration and heating tissue up to 3 to 5 centimeters deep.

One important aspect to remember is that if the ultrasound is placed directly on one part of the skin for too long, the excessive heat buildup can cause unstable **cavitation**. During treatments, it is important to remember that the technician should maintain constant movement of the handpiece on moist tissue. Damaged, thin, or fragile skin are contraindications for ultrasound and, therefore, ultrasound should never be performed close to the periocular (around the eye) area. Other

cavitation
The formation of gas bubbles in a liquid.

contraindications include clients with heart conditions, pacemakers, or electrical implants; pregnant women; or clients with diabetes.

▪ MICRODERMABRASION AND MASKS

Masks have long been used in aesthetics, thanks to their ease of use, potential for success, and immediate, noticeable effects. Furthermore, most clients find the mask experience to be a soothing and gentle experience. However, masks can potentially contain active ingredients in high concentrations. They are normally applied as the next-to-last step of a microdermabrasion facial treatment. Masks intensify the treatment and work on the principles of occlusion.

There are three standard types of masks:

- Gel-based masks can be used on all skin types and are very hydrating. Their gel form increases the moisture content of the skin.
- Cream-based masks are nondrying, usually have calming and hydrating properties, and typically contain water-soluble ingredients as the main components.
- Clay masks are drying by nature and draw out impurities. They offer a balancing and tightening result. Manufacturers may design their clay masks to be setting (drying) or "non-setting" or hardening types.

Aestheticians are increasingly recognizing the benefits of adding specialty masks to a microdermabrasion treatment (Figure 10–3). Layered treatment masks are those which involve the use of multiple masks for an improved microdermabrasion result. Aestheticians use freeze-dried collagen sheets to offer surface hydration, especially after microdermabrasion. These masks deliver specialty ingredients incorporated into the sheets targeted for specific skin types and conditions. These sheets are commonly used alone or in conjunction with ampoules for increased results.

▪ MICRODERMABRASION AND LYMPHATIC DRAINAGE

Lymph drainage is also known as *lymphatic drainage* or *lymphatic drainage massage*. It is an excellent adjunctive therapy to microdermabrasion. Since its development in the 1930s, there have been leaps and bounds in research focused on lymphatic drainage and its techniques. More scientific studies have been conducted, and research and advances in technology have given rise to more effective techniques of lymphatic drainage than the original version of the earlier methods. Research has demonstrated that lymphatic drainage accelerates the flow of lymphatic fluid in the

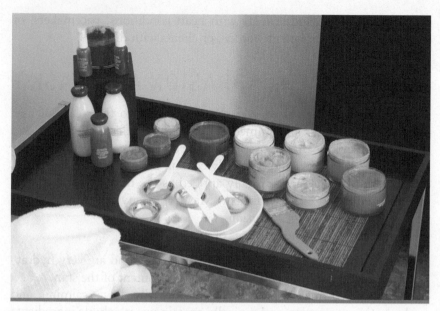

Figure 10–3 Different masks used with microdermabrasion.

lymph ducts to the lymph nodes, where toxins are filtered and eliminated. As a result, the skin is better able to purge the toxins that build up from chemicals as a result of normal cellular metabolism.

Lymphatic drainage can be done manually or with a vacuum/suction lymphatic drainage machine. The machine will have a push/pull action, achieved with a computer-controlled pump or compressor. Some microdermabrasion machines come equipped with a lymphatic drainage system in addition to the microdermabrasion system. The compressor lymphatic system is used after the microdermabrasion treatment and before the mask. The intensity of the vacuum apparatus will need to be set at low for the face and neck areas. The vacuum/suction action will mimic the contractions made within the lymph vessels and assist with the movement of the lymphatic fluid. Many aestheticians find that using these machines will allow them to complete a greater number of clients in a day versus laborious manual methods of lymphatic drainage. Others argue that the machines are not as effective as manual therapies, and there has been much discussion over this debate. Scientific studies tend to support the greater effectiveness of manual therapist but, as with anything, it is dependent on the skill and knowledge of the therapist.

Whichever method is used, the benefits of combining microdermabrasion and lymphatic drainage cannot be underestimated. Each procedure has its benefits and, when combined together, improve the final result for the client.

Suggested Steps for Machine-Assisted Lymphatic Drainage with Vacuum Machines

Begin with light effleurage movements.

Have the client turn his or her face to one side and place the handpiece just on the postauricular area (behind ear, under hairline). Move the handpiece down the neck to clavicle. Repeat the sequence 3 to 5 times.

Have the client straighten their head to supine position.

Separate handpieces so that you have one in each hand. Place the handpieces just below the preauricular area one (in front of the ear) and move downwards to the clavicle. Repeat the sequence 3 to 5 times.

Separate handpieces so that you have one in each hand. Place the handpieces on the submental area (under the jaw) and move downwards to the clavicle. Repeat until you have cleared the front of the neck but exclude the trachea area. Repeat the sequence 3 to 5 times.

Separate handpieces so that you have one in each hand. Place the handpieces so that they are touching side by side on the top of the chin just above the above the submental area (above the jawline) and move downwards to the clavicle. Repeat the sequence 3 to 5 times.

Separate handpieces so that you have one in each hand. Place the handpieces so that they are touching side by side on the top of the lip, just below the nose, and move out to the ear area and continue to move downwards to the clavicle. Repeat the sequence 3 to 5 times.

Separate handpieces so that you have one in each hand. Place the handpieces on both sides of the face so that they are level with the tops of the ears, and move downward to the jawline. Repeat the sequence 3 to 5 times.

Separate handpieces so that you have one in each hand. Place the handpieces on the either side of the nose and move out to the ear area and continue to move downwards to the jawline. Repeat until you have moved progressively up to the area just under the eye. Typically, this can be achieved with three points. Repeat the sequence 3 to 5 times.

Separate handpieces so that you have one in each hand. Place the handpieces just under the eye, gently move out to the ear area, and continue to move out to the corners of the eye and to the lower temple area. Repeat the sequence 3 to 5 times.

Separate handpieces so that you have one in each hand. Place the handpieces on the brow line and move out to the temples. Repeat the sequence 3 to 5 times.

Separate handpieces so that you have one in each hand. Place the handpieces on the forehead just above the brows, move outwards to the hairline, and continue to move downward to the temples. Repeat until you have cleared the middle forehead and upper forehead areas. Repeat the sequence 3 to 5 times.

Separate handpieces so that you have one in each hand. Place the handpieces on the either side of the temple, continue to move downward to the jawline, and proceed to the clavicle. Repeat the sequence 3 to 5 times.

End with light effleurage movements.

▪ MICRODERMABRASION AND LED

Lasers and lights have been used in aesthetics for some time. In fact, one of their first applied uses was on skin. It took much time to advance the technology and refine the technique, and some debate still exists, but lasers have proven most beneficial to many skin conditions, including treatment of mild to moderate rhytids and dyschromias. To accomplish this, most lasers have traditionally used pulses of heat and light that could potentially cause burns and scarring. In contrast to the thermal laser of years past, there is an exciting new technology of a non-thermal, non-ablative cellular stimulator called photomodulation. Unlike other laser/light-based procedures, which rely on heat and thermal injury to improve the skin's appearance, LEDs trigger a photobiochemical response. The process involves using low-level light energy to modulate or activate cellular metabolism. LED devices are designed to include panels of tiny diodes that are pulsed at an exclusive array sequence (Figure 10–4). LED photomodulation can suppress collagenase, a collagen-degrading enzyme that can accelerate our skin's aging process. This process is extraordinarily helpful to the microdermabrasion client. When the microdermabrasion is completed first and the LED is applied after the treatment, it not only activates the cellular metabolism to improve the result of the microdermabrasion, but also can stimulate the energy-producing mitochondria to enhance wound healing and decrease the inflammatory response. LED

photomodulation
To use controlled light therapies to regulate irregularities of the skin.

collagenase
Any enzyme that catalyzes the hydrolysis of collagen.

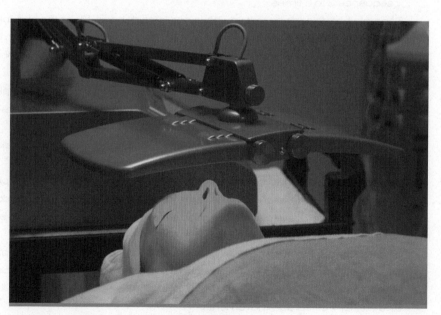

Figure 10–4 Client under the LED light.

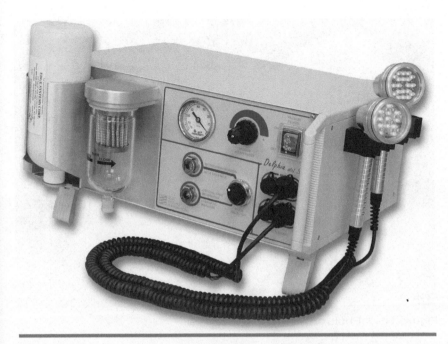

Figure 10–5 LED lights can be separate, or in this case, handheld and part of the microdermabrasion machine. (Photo courtesy of Edge Systems Corporation.)

devices are becoming more accepted as a treatment adjunct for improving the signs of aging and bolstering collagen production. LED is the perfect adjunct to microdermabrasion and is being used on a daily basis by progressive practices (Figure 10–5).

■ MICRODERMABRASION AND FOTOFACIAL

IPL or photorejuvenation treatments use a noncoherent, broadband, pulsed light source to treat vascular and pigmented lesions of the skin. IPL (intense pulsed light) skin treatments use specific wavelengths of light to achieve what is called photorejuvenation and is sometimes referred to as PhotoFacial or FotoFacial. Photorejuvenation is typically used to treat a wide of variety of benign conditions such as vascular lesions, pigmented lesions, and skin laxity. Aging, sun exposure, and other factors can cause the appearance of broken capillaries and blood vessels on the face, also known as telangiectasia or spider veins (Figure 10–7). Rosacea is also a common skin condition noted to respond well to IPL. In the case of lax skin and loss of tonicity, the IPL treats imperfections in

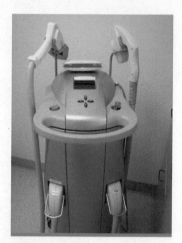

Figure 10–6 Photo of Fotofacial machine.

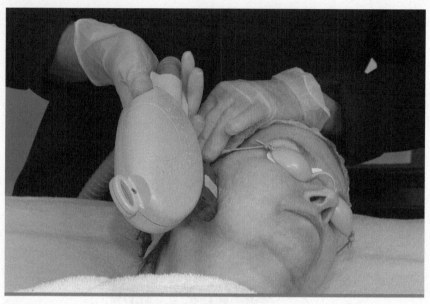

Figure 10–7 Photo of client having Fotofacial.

the superficial layers of the skin while delivering thermal energy to deeper tissues. It is believed this energy has an effect on collagen production and helps to firm and tighten the skin (Figure 10–6).

On average, 4 to 6 treatments are recommended, scheduled at three-week intervals. Each session usually lasts about 20 to 30 minutes. Microdermabrasion is typically combined with FotoFacial for several reasons. First, it will continue to improve and stimulate the skin between FotoFacial treatments. Next, it has the ability to polish the skin and remove any dead cells or dry skin left behind after a FotoFacial treatment. Typically, the microdermabrasion is scheduled about 7 to 10 days following the FotoFacial. During this treatment, a mild peel (20 to 30 percent glycolic acid or lactic acid) can be done with the microdermabrasion to encourage the improvement in the skin's tone and texture, and to help remove the remaining debris from the FotoFacial. In most medical spas, the treatment is always concluded with an LED treatment.

The Use of Levulan®

Levulan prescription therapy is used with FotoFacial to improve the results of extensive solar damage and actinic keratosis. Levulan is unique because it is light-activated and, when applied to the actinic keratoses, will destroy them in combination with FotoFacial or the BLU-U Blue Light Photodynamic Therapy Illuminator (BLU-U®).

It is a two-step treatment procedure:

1. Application of the Levulan Kerastick® Topical Solution to individual actinic keratoses

2. BLU-U treatment or FotoFacial

After the treatment, clients should avoid sun exposure to treated areas for 48 hours. Any sun exposure can intensify the production of the Levulan and overtreat the skin. The overtreatment will present as intense stinging or burning and may cause swelling or redness. A sunscreen will not protect the skin against the potential complication of treatment.

Once the treatment is complete and the skin has had the opportunity to heal, a microdermabrasion is often recommended. This is typically 10 days following the treatment. The microdermabrasion will polish the skin and remove loose actinic keratoses and other skin debris.

▪ MICRODERMABRASION AND PEELS

Combining aggressive peeling and microdermabrasion has always been controversial. Common questions are whether to do the peel before the microdermabrasion or after the microdermabrasion, and how much of a solution to use. Obviously, the questions of results and safety come to mind when doing the combination of peels and microdermabrasion.

Microdermabrasion and glycolic or lactic acid peels are often used together at the same treatment to gather the benefits of both treatments. While some aestheticians use the peel after the treatment, the best results comes when the glycolic or lactic acid peel solution, in low strengths, is used as a keratolic agent prior to the microdermabrasion treatment. Glycolic and lactic acid peels that are used after microdermabrasion risk uneven uptake and possible unintentional deep peeling in the areas where the microdermabrasion abraded the skin aggressively. In order to avoid this phenomenon, it is important to remember that it is a combination treatment. Therefore, depending on skin type, tone, and texture, it may be important to decrease the number of passes with the microdermabrasion treatment before applying the peeling agent. For example, a client with extensive solar damage may be able to take two passes with the microdermabrasion machine (Figure 10–8) and a coat of 30 to 50 percent glycolic or Jessner's, whereas someone with less solar damage or slightly thinner skin might only be able to tolerate one pass with the microdermabrasion before the peel. Combining peeling and microdermabrasion is an advanced technique that requires the ability to properly skin type and access the client's skin before, during, and after the treatment. Common peel solutions used with microdermabrasion

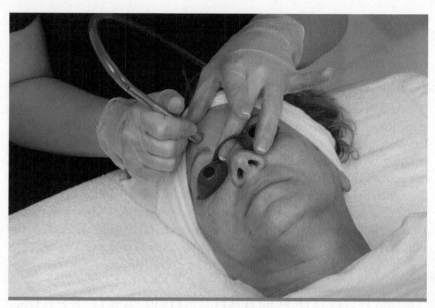

Figure 10–8 Client having microdermabrasion.

include: glycolic and lactic acid 20 percent, glycolic acid 30 percent, 50 percent, and Jessner's. While glycolic and lactic maybe common to the aesthetician, the Jessner's peel has a safer uptake than the glycolic solution since it does not need to be neutralized. As such, Jessner's can be a very useful solution when combined with microdermabrasion.

▪ MICRODERMABRASION AND THE EXTREMITIES

Microdermabrasion of the extremities is becoming more popular as IPL is used on the extremities. Microdermabrasion of the extremities is used to treat all of the problems associated with solar damage and aging skin found on the face. Among the important issues to remember is that, like the face, the extremities must also have a home care program. Many medical spas use a combination of Retin A and bleaching cream called Kligman's cream, while others prefer a prepackaged program such as Décolletage System® by Obagi. Whatever the choice, the extremities or chest must be treated with home care products as well as in the spa to achieve a meaningful result.

Like the face, using a peel solution with the microdermabrasion can be useful when treating the extremities. Often, the solar damage found on the legs and arms can be stubborn and require more aggressive attention. That said, it is easy to overtreat the legs and arms. The extremities heal slower than the face and this should be taken into consideration when a treatment plan is developed.

CONCLUSION

Microdermabrasion is not what it once was. Now, combined with many other treatments, microdermabrasion is often a step in a multi-faceted treatment program. Whether the treatments are high-tech treatments such as FotoFacials, or everyday treatments such as peels, microdermabrasion has found a new niche in clinical skin care.

Top 10 Tips to Take to the Spa

1. Microdermabrasion treatment that is unique to you and differentiates you from your competition.

2. Facials are one of the most requested treatments at spas.

3. Ultrasound is used to penetrate products or provide deep-cleansing action. It can be used to improve the benefits of microdermabrasion.

4. Masks intensify the treatment and work on the principles of occlusion. They can make a significant difference in the microdermabrasion result.

5. Lymph drainage is also known as lymphatic drainage or lymphatic drainage massage. It is an excellent adjunctive therapy to microdermabrasion.

6. Microdermabrasion is used to polish the skin and remove any dead skin following a FotoFacial.

7. Microdermabrasion and glycolic or lactic acid peels are often used together at the same treatment to gather the benefits of both treatments.

8. Microdermabrasion of the extremities is used to treat all of the problems associated with solar damage and aging skin found on the face.

9. The extremities or chest must be treated with home-care products as well as in the spa to achieve a meaningful result.

10. The extremities heal more slowly than the face and this should be taken into consideration when a treatment plan is developed.

Chapter Review Questions

1. Why is the peel solution used before the microdermabrasion treatment?

2. Why is microdermabrasion used with FotoFacial or BLU-U light?

3. What is the LED light used for?

4. What does lymphatic drainage do for the body?

5. Why are facials and microdermabrasion a good combination?

Chapter Reference

1. Hill, P., & Todd, L. (2008). *Advanced Face and Body Treatments for the Spa*. Clifton Park, New York: Delmar Learning.

The Business of Microdermabrasion

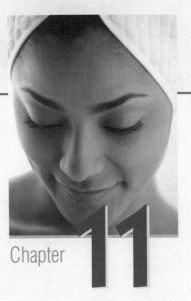

Chapter 11

Learning Objectives

After completing this chapter you should be able to:

1. Understand the business environment for a microdermabrasion.

2. Learn about the components of a business plan.

3. Learn how to establish and evaluate goals and indicators.

4. Understand the components of cost analysis.

5. Define the direct and indirect costs associated with microdermabrasion.

INTRODUCTION

Microdermabrasion is an essential component of many individual aesthetic skin care programs and, from a business perspective, an essential service for all types of spas. Effective, popular, and safe, its intrinsic need for repeat visits is an important aspect of the business of providing skin care. After all, repeat business is the cornerstone of any spa business's success. As reiterated a number of times in the course of this text, microdermabrasion treatments are progressive in nature. The more the client has the treatments done, the greater their chance for success—and the greater the chance for success for your spa business. Microdermabrasion can be the vehicle both to get a potential client in the door, and to keep him or her returning.

Along these lines, the business of providing microdermabrasion includes a mastery of the subjects discussed thus far, including client selection, consultations, and technique. It also demands an understanding of some fundamental business knowledge. In the context of capitalism, a business goes into business for one purpose alone: to make money. This may sound harsh, but it is an important point to understand. Without profit, a spa, or any business, will fail to exist. This would make your employment options fairly scarce. In this context, making a profit seems to be more of a critical matter, doesn't it?

Whether you are the owner, operator, or an aesthetician at a spa, the financial success of the *business* of providing the microdermabrasion service depends on understanding and analyzing several crucial, but basic, business concepts. For the aspiring aesthetician, starting, maintaining, or directing a spa business may seem too distant to envision, but employing these principles and engaging yourself in the spa in which you are employed will make you that much more prepared to own and/or operate a spa business of your own.

Any business idea, regardless of industry, has its origins within the development plan. A development plan is the design by which you will plan, implement, and profit from the implementation of a new product or service.

At the beginning, writing a development plan looks simple, but it will be wrought with details about which you usually do not think. Doing so will help you to anticipate logistical problems. The beauty of a development plan is that it makes its creators *think* and *plan*. In the process of thinking about how you or your spa will develop your microdermabrasion business, a few questions will require foresight to prevent or solve these initial problems. The sections of the development plan are simple: *getting the microdermabrasion business started* and *keeping it moving to the point of profitability*.

GETTING THE MICRODERMABRASION BUSINESS STARTED

Getting a microdermabrasion business started can be both exciting and challenging. Microdermabrasion can provide a spa with the opportunity to take the business to the next level. The startup process involves evaluating microdermabrasion machines, learning how to use them, understanding the cost and price relationship, and creating **marketing strategies** to bring the clients through the door. Adding this service to the menu will require hard work. Without as much, the fruits of labor won't yield as much or as rapidly. To accomplish this, strict and methodical processes ought to be implemented. The development plan for getting started with microdermabrasion should address three issues: (1) equipment, (2) pricing, and (3) marketing (Table 11–1).

In the equipment category, one ought to be looking at microdermabrasion machines and deciding which machine best fits the spa's needs. The best approach for accomplishing this goal is to make a list of the desired **machine features**. This approach will formulate the questions for vendors, assist in deciphering their information, and help you to better choose from the machines available.

Pricing is the next category in the development plan. The plan should begin with market research (both inside and outside your spa). Inside market research is what your clients think is fair price for a microdermabrasion treatment. Outside market research is how much the competitors are charging. In addition to this information, one will want to consider the operational costs associated with performing the service and how to create a margin wide enough for profit to occur.

The last category is usually everyone's favorite—marketing. It is great to watch satisfied clients come through the door. However, without proper planning in the previous two categories, marketing is of no use.

marketing strategies
Planned use of marketing elements and media pathways to create a strategy to introduce new clients or reactivate former clients.

machine features
In relation to microdermabrasion, the specific components of a machine that separate it from its competition; some features include type of filtration system, type of crystal supply system, ergonomic handpieces, and portability.

Table 11–1 The Development Plan	
Equipment	Evaluate different machines, prices, and features to decide which will be best suited for your business.
Pricing	Research demographic information, cost analysis, and competition to set a fair market price for your service while allowing for profit.
Marketing Strategies	Develop a marketing strategy that is both cost-effective and will bring in new clientele.

Buying a Machine

The success of the microdermabrasion business begins with the selection of the equipment and its associated components. Whether it is a new spa business or an expansion of the service menu, buying the right equipment is key to the microdermabrasion service's ultimate success. Given the options and devices available, shopping for a new machine can be difficult. As of 2001, there were 40 different microdermabrasion machines on the market,[1] and the number increases regularly. Although price is obviously important, it is not the primary consideration. To ensure that you get a machine that fits your budget and meets your needs, begin by evaluating the features you are looking for rather than just the price. The cost of microdermabrasion machinery will vary quite a bit, depending on these features. You should know exactly what you are getting for the price. What does it include? Think of the details; for example, does it come with a cart or will you need to purchase this separately? Be sure that you are comparing "apples to apples" when comparison shopping. Remember the old adage, "You get what you pay for." With regards to microdermabrasion devices, this remains true.

A reliable place to start looking is with the machine manufacturers. When considering a manufacturer, find out if the company is well-established. Do they have reliable safety and performance records? Do their existing and former customers believe the manufacturer has a reputation for quality and service? *Will the company be here today and gone tomorrow?* A safe place to look for this information is in trade magazines, trade organizations, and industry peers. Be certain to look in more than one place. For-profit sites may pander to their advertisers, so an informed decision may require a certain amount of legwork. If the company is new to producing microdermabrasion machines, have they been making other medical devices with a solid reputation? Are they the primary manufacturer or reseller? Will they stand behind the machine and provide service and support? What type and duration of warranty comes with the machine? Is the manufacturer registered with the Food and Drug Administration (FDA)? If so, the company will be required by law to continue to provide parts and service for seven years after the discontinuation of the machine's production.[2] In determining the general quality of a machine, you should consider its physical stability, the quality of component parts, the crystal flow and vacuum variability, the ease of reading the dials, and the ergonomic design of the handpiece.

If you know an aesthetician who has been using a certain type of machine, ask for his or her opinion. Usually you will get a realistic assessment of a particular machine's nuances in its real-world application. Brochures and salespeople are trying to sell their product, but a recommendation based on experience can prove invaluable in the search.

Next, consider which features produce certain types of results. Have these features been examined and documented in peer review studies that validate their advertised results? If so, who sponsored the study? If the manufacturer sponsored the study, the results may be skewed.

Finally, while researching structural elements, consider the filtration system, crystal supply, and crystal disposal. Does the machine accommodate an all-in-one system with crystal supply and disposal reservoir combined? This is preferable to separate components, because it makes the crystal change easier and cleaner.

By evaluating the features, you will begin to hone in on the price you will need to pay to achieve your **goals**. The next step in our development plan is to evaluate costs and set the retail price for the treatment. If you are going to buy a more expensive machine, make sure you can translate that into a higher retail price and subsequently a better treatment.

Now that you know the **fixed price** of the various machines, you will need to examine the variable costs needed to perform the service. For example, how many clients will you be able to treat with each crystal pack? What about disposable tips? Are there any other variable expenses?

A thorough understanding of microdermabrasion-related costs will help prepare you to calculate the retail price point for the procedure per area and per client.

goals
General statements of anticipated business outcomes resulting from well-stated objectives.

fixed price
Price that remains the same, usually for a set time period.

Buying microdermabrasion equipment is a little like buying a car. Be sure you get all the extras you can (a bonus case of crystals or extension on the warranty, for example). However, do not get duped into buying something you do not want or need.

Machine Warranties

When buying your machine, keep warranties in mind (for repairs and maintenance). Your warranty should be for no less than one year with options for renewal. Be sure you get, in writing, the company's procedure for "down machines"—those that are broken or otherwise inoperable. Will the manufacturer or reseller provide a comparable loaner? Will the loan be free, or will it be a rental? A broken machine without prompt service or replacement can be a revenue disaster. If a machine breaks and you have to wait for service or send the machine back to the manufacturer without a replacement, you will be forced to cancel clients or scramble to offer other treatment choices. This will have catastrophic consequences on revenue, client retention, and employee moral. If the manufacturer does not have a replacement machine, offer to bridge the repair gap; you will most certainly need to have a contingency plan to avert the aforementioned consequences.

Hiring and Training

Knowing whom to train can be straightforward in small spas that have few available or qualified staff members. However, in larger spas where several qualified aestheticians are employed, part business savvy and part intuition will be needed when selecting how many or which staff members to train. You might think that having many staff members trained will allow more procedures to be performed; however, unless the volume of microdermabrasion business allows all qualified aestheticians to remain busy, you will have many people performing few procedures. As you now know, microdermabrasion is highly technique-sensitive, meaning the more you do, the better you become at it.[3] Until client volume warrants training additional staff, limit the training to a few individuals who are your microdermabrasion "experts." This limitation will also make your clients feel that they are getting this treatment from the most qualified staff. Remember that because microdermabrasion is technique-sensitive, those with superior eye-hand coordination and knowledge of the client selection process will excel.

Although creating an expert will be cost-effective during the delicate introductory period, it is not without potential disadvantages. Concentrating microdermabrasion training to a limited few risks the possibility of client defection should those staff members leave. This might be particularly true if the client's major reason for coming to your medical spa is for microdermabrasion. The antidote to this would be the various other services that the client receives. Although noncompete clauses, penalties, and threat of legal action can discourage departing staff from pilfering the client list, the fact of the matter is that clients have a right to transfer care. They will be less likely to do so, however, if they receive various other services from other staff members, thus spreading around the loyalty.

You may never know that a staff member is going to leave; sometimes, it just happens unexpectedly. You can plan ahead to recover your training costs if the employee leaves, for example, by inserting a training fee into the contract. Regardless, training is a cost of doing business, and spa owners should hone their ability to make good employee choices. As a potential business owner or spa manager, you will strive to create customer loyalty to the spa or company rather than just to the aesthetician. Simultaneously, of course, you will hope that the working environment and benefits of employment create employee loyalty.

Cost Analysis

A part of owning or operating a spa business involves doing some "number crunching." In the case of adding a new microdermabrasion

> Wear and tear, changes in technology, and flexibility are all considerations when evaluating the financing options for your microdermabrasion machine. Once you have all the information in place for the purchase, talk with your accountant to be sure you are making the best deal for your company. A professional opinion on subjects like these can keep you out of financial trouble.

service to your spa, this number crunching will come in the form of performing a cost analysis. A cost analysis weighs the expense of offering a procedure as a basis for pricing the service fairly. To make money you have to understand how much it will cost to provide the procedure to your clients. A cost analysis has two separate components: (1) **direct costs** and (2) **indirect costs**. Direct cost is a breakdown of all the costs that directly relate to implementing a microdermabrasion procedure; in other words, all costs that are incurred exclusively by the microdermabrasion treatment. These costs are offset only by payments from clients who receive this treatment. We will mostly be discussing direct costs related to microdermabrasion in this text. Because it can be confusing, a few examples may be helpful.

Direct Costs

As we have stated, *direct costs* are those costs associated directly with offering a microdermabrasion procedure. These direct costs will be the cost of the regular purchase of crystals, disposable tips, filters, and reservoirs; maintenance expenses; specific marketing for the microdermabrasion procedure; and costs associated with training, insuring, and compensation of applicable employees. In other words, direct costs are those that you incur solely as the result of microdermabrasion (Table 11–2).

Costs are always changing and usually increasing. You need to evaluate your costs at least every six months to make sure they have not gone up. For example, crystals may be more expensive now than the last time you purchased them. You uncovered some of the cost information when you were shopping for your machine and putting together your contract. If not, now is the time to figure out the profitability.

Indirect Costs

With your direct costs analyzed, add your standardized indirect cost formula (total **overhead costs** divided by the number of procedures performed). You now have an idea of how much you will need to make for microdermabrasion treatment to be profitable to your business. Herein lies the trickiest part: How do you price your product to make it enticing enough to achieve your goals of profitability (and sustainability)?

Pricing Strategies

As you have come to realize, pricing a microdermabrasion service is not as cut-and-dry as some might think. Once you have conducted your cost analysis, you have a baseline. Factoring in the direct and indirect

direct costs
Costs that are directly and exclusively attributable to a specific product or service.

indirect costs
Cost necessary for the functioning of the organization as a whole but that cannot be directly assigned to one service or product.

overhead costs
Indirect costs.

Common indirect costs are rent, telephone, business telephone book advertising, and other generalized marketing.

Indirect costs are sometimes referred to as *overhead costs* and are applied to all procedures based on treatment time. Most spas have a standardized overhead cost per hour.

Table 11–2 Direct Cost–Single Microdermabrasion Treatment	
Revenue per Procedure	$125.00
Time per Procedure	60 minutes
Direct Cost of Sales	
Crystals	$1.00
Disposable tip	2.00
Reservoir	3.00
Equipment lease	4.12
Maintenance contract	2.00
Peel supplies	0.75
Mask supplies	0.75
Clinical supplies (gauze, cleanser)	2.00
*Marketing campaign	2.08
Clinical employee wage	22.50
Clinical employee benefits	4.50
Total Direct Costs	**$44.70**

*Marketing campaign is based on $5,000 annually and 2,400 microdermabrasion visits per annum. To find the annualized cost of any item, multiply by the visits per annum.

costs, you will have a figure that is the cost to the spa for performing each treatment. Given that the spa is in business to make money, the price should be set higher than this figure. But how much higher? To determine this you will want to determine which pricing strategy you want to employ.

Pricing strategies may seem like they are part of the marketing plan; however, pricing is quite different and should be evaluated independent of marketing. The theories and implementation of pricing strategies can be very sophisticated. For our purposes we will focus on four distinct pricing strategies: (1) price and costs, (2) price and competitors, (3) price and customers, and (4) price and business objectives. These pricing strategies will drive your business objectives, compared with promotional pricing, which is an occasional price break that may be used to move overstock inventory, for example.

Pricing and Costs

A business that offers microdermabrasion has to ensure the revenue it generates will cover the costs or, in other words, yield a profit. Several different pricing tactics can be used to cover costs and should be evaluated based on different business models. In the medical spa and day spa sector, one usually thinks first of **premium pricing**. This pricing strategy uses high prices to communicate the uniqueness of the product or service. With premium pricing you will need to back up your premium claim with a premium service. Your machine, ancillary offerings, and technique must warrant this pricing strategy. Also, the aesthetician and others in the spa must be able to articulate with confidence knowledge that will assist the client in his or her purchase. Clients must feel that they receive value for the price they paid. Otherwise, you will just outprice yourself from the market. Therefore, this pricing strategy is not recommended for those just entering the market.

The next type of price strategy that might be used in the spa area is **penetration pricing**. In penetration pricing, the price is set low to allow access into the market by gaining market share. This strategy creates break-even costs or even a loss for the business. As the name might indicate, this is the ideal pricing strategy for those just entering the market.

Next is **economy pricing**. Economy pricing keeps all costs low to provide the lowest cost to the customer. This is a very popular strategy, made famous by Wal-Mart. This strategy is one that offers the lowest profit margin for small independent spas. A viable option in some instances, it is not recommended for the faint of heart.

Product-bundling pricing is a tactic that is commonly used in the day spa and is finding its way into the medical spa. This is similar to the concept of *packages,* but product bundling is more sophisticated than packages. This type of pricing combines multiple services, such as microdermabrasions and facials bundled together. For product bundling you look at the costs and determine how much discount can be taken in exchange for collecting the fee in advance. Product bundling can also help the spa to be efficient in scheduling and increase spa use by knowing the number of clients who have packages and predicting the number of clients who should be scheduling appointments. Although many other different types of pricing strategies exist, these four are the most familiar and most commonly used in our industry. When considering product-bundling pricing, look at the operating costs per treatment as a benchmark. The direct costs of the treatment will not be affected by bundling, but overhead figures can be manipulated.

Before choosing a pricing strategy, evaluate your business objectives for the year. Your objectives might include maximizing profits, attracting

premium pricing
Pricing strategy in which the price is set high to compensate for a high-quality product, usually with a high production cost as well.

penetration pricing
Pricing strategy in which the price is set low to allow for introduction into an existing market.

economy pricing
Low pricing of a product or service as a means to entice customers to buy.

product-bundling pricing
Pricing strategy in which one or more products or services are offered at a discount.

new clients, achieving a revenue goal, preventing further competition, or maintaining or increasing market share. A business could use each of these pricing models at different times during the year to execute its plan.

Pricing and Competitors

Entrepreneurship and *competitiveness* are often synonymous. For competition to translate into success, a microdermabrasion business owner needs to negotiate a fine line between "active interest" and "nosy neighbor." By collecting small amounts of information, you can catch a glimpse of what the competition is doing with pricing, menu offerings, and compensation. The ability to collect and accurately translate this information into useful operational information for practical use is a valuable skill for sizing up your own spa business. The processes by which you choose to gather information obviously need not be extreme or invasive. However, being watchful of advertising, word of mouth, or public presentations should give a fairly complete picture from which to draw your conclusions. Furthermore having microdermabrasion at neighborhood spas can be the most valuable experience of all.

Pricing and Customers

In retail business, it is said that the price of an item is the price the customer will pay,[4] meaning that the price of a product is consumer-driven. It is no less true in the spa and medical spa businesses. An important first step in setting your microdermabrasion prices is understanding your customers. Because microdermabrasion can be competitive, your customers may already be having the treatment at another spa. This is one of the few areas in which a customer survey is recommended. However, elaborate data collection is not necessary. Pricing surveys should be focused on price sensitivities about procedures, product, and value. In our environment, perceived value tracks closely with the price the client will pay.

Surveys can be tricky to put together. Preparing the questions in a manner that does not influence the answer can sometimes be difficult. Therefore, a professional should prepare surveys that influence significant decisions, such as pricing. Otherwise, the information you get will be exactly what you thought it would be, because you asked the question to get the predicted answer.

Pricing and Business Objectives

Pricing microdermabrasion to facilitate your business's growth and profitability is a smart business tactic. However, when companies drastically cut prices in an effort to attract customers, the end result can be disastrous. To avoid using desperate, last-option pricing decisions,

Some simple survey questions might include:

- Have you ever had microdermabrasion?
- If not, would you consider having the treatment?
- How much do you think is reasonable to pay for microdermabrasion?

consider implementing a standard pricing policy. A standard pricing policy is a document that is controlled by the spa manager or spa director and is a list of all the prices. The initial prices are calculated through a mathematical formula based on cost and a specific markup percentage. When prices are increased, a standard price increase formula is used. This is far more effective than saying, "We should charge 50 cents less, because that is what ABC spa is charging." Furthermore, running a special or packaging services can make the spa more competitive and interesting than other spas.

Standard pricing policies help the company meet its yearly business objectives. The yearly objectives are part of the annual business plan, which is a complex document that includes a budget, a marketing plan, and a growth plan (which includes isolated development plans for specific services). It gives focus and depth to the business growth.

When a spa adds a service such as microdermabrasion, creating an isolated development plan for the growth of the procedure within the spa ensures success. When you use a model such as the one depicted here, you will want to make the information detailed and appropriate to your individual situation.

KEEPING THE MICRODERMABRASION BUSINESS MOVING TOWARD PROFITABILITY

For your new microdermabrasion service to thrive, you will need to keep up with the trends, regulations, and competition associated with your new service (or even the spa industry at large). These are collectively referred to as your *business landscape*. The business landscape will be the deciding factor in many areas, most notably marketing your microdermabrasion program accurately and effectively.

Three deeply intertwined aspects of evaluating your business landscape are the (1) marketplace, (2) clients, and (3) competition. Independently and consequentially, these three components are in a state of constant change. By identifying the present conditions of each, you have defined the current landscape. The marketplace is different in every city; sometimes it is even more localized than your *city* and maybe your *local community*. Therefore, to have a firm grasp on the marketplace, you must understand your city and local community.

With a comprehensive understanding of local dynamics, narrowing the general population down to your business's client base is the second and most misunderstood component of the business landscape.

standard pricing policy
Business document that outlines the specific price range of a given product or service, preferred pricing strategy, and circumstances under which each might change.

yearly business objectives
Part of the annual business plan that identifies the goals a business would like to attain during a given fiscal year.

annual business plan
Growth plan that outlines business objectives, marketing plans, and budgets for the period of one fiscal year.

marketplace
Any environment in which two or more people buy or sell a product or service.

Making a profit is the main reason for being in business. Understanding pricing strategies, how the competition prices, and what the market will bear in your client demographic requires insight, skill, and intuition, but it will ensure you stay in business.

understanding your client
Component of the business landscape during which a business evaluates and acquaints itself with its target demographics.

understanding your competition
Component of the business landscape during which a business evaluates the competition in terms of pricing, procedures, demographics, and promotions.

indicators
Key value used to measure performance over time as it relates to an organization's progress achieving its goals.

database
Electronic compilation of extensive categorical information relevant to business processes such as marketing or inventory.

Understanding your client will have a domino effect on marketing, pricing, and many other components that are critical to the success of your business.

Finally, although knowing your marketplace and your clients will have significant role in your daily operations, **understanding your competition** does not. Therefore, it should not have an equal share of consideration. Worrying about your competition could become a distraction (or an obsession) that will only harm your practice. You should limit your understanding of the competition to the few bits of information you really need to compile your prices, menu, and promotions.

In addition to keeping current with your business landscape, moving forward includes accurate and regular monitoring and daily tracking of operations and business risks. Establishing **indicators** and goals, and understanding your financial statements, plays a pivotal role. Most important are indicators and goals; you should review them weekly to evaluate the performance of the spa and individual aestheticians. This review will pave the road to spa success. In the following sections, we discuss the issues of your business landscape in more detail.

Understanding the Client

Understanding your client is helpful when designing your marketing and development plans. We have discussed how this affects your development plan; after all, if the demand does not exist, then no need for marketing. With regards to marketing, most marketing principles are general and are considered *the norm,* because they have proven to change or modify consumer behavior. However, with a well-thought-out interpretation of your potential clients, you will be able to tailor your campaign to your client base, as opposed to broader populations. Enhanced collection and analysis will help you refine your campaign from conception to implementation.

An analysis of the existing client base will give you a composite sketch of your target demographic. The information you should seek includes service preferences, price sensitivity, age, household income, knowledge of the industry, referral source, and preconceived notions of the facility and services.

Take note of the existing clients in the current **database** who might be interested in microdermabrasion (based on your composite sketch criteria). This can be done in two ways: (1) through a survey or (2) by a mathematic analysis based on growth. If you use a survey, the process is very simple. Create a survey that clients can fill out while waiting for their treatment. Filling out the questionnaire can include a microdermabrasion treatment offer at an introductory promotional price.

Sample Three-Month Development Plan

JANUARY

Objectives	1. Begin training programs. 2. Evaluate spa database.
Tactics	1. Schedule training with spa educator. Discuss with the manufacturer times for spa meetings and educational presentations. 2. Create a criteria selection form for spa database evaluation.
Goals	1. Complete training by February 25th. 2. Have a list of potential clients from the database that is ready for a marketing campaign by the end of January.
Costs	1. Training wages for all participating employees. Projected extra wage cost is 84 hours @ 22.00/hr = 1,848 + taxes. 2. Front desk training wages for the analysis. Projected extra wage cost is 25 hours @ 15.00/hr = 375 + taxes.

FEBRUARY

Objectives	1. Develop multipronged marketing campaign. 2. Evaluate the progress of the training to ensure we are on target. 3. Develop spa goals.
Tactics	1. Develop e-mail, in-house, and radio strategies. Develop and print literature for microdermabrasion, including informational literature, *what to expect* literature, and pricing information. 2. Evaluate testing that has taken place in the training. Observe classroom and clinical training. 3. Analyze the potential number of available clients.
Goals	1. All literature will be ready by February 20th. All marketing campaigns will be ready to launch February 20th. 2. Ensure no glitches exist in the training process. Evaluate the model "reviews" of the procedure. 3. Create client goals and revenue goals.
Cost	1. Budget $2,500 for printing literature. Budget $5,000 for first 3-month wave of microdermabrasion marketing.

Continued

Sample Three-Month Development Plan—cont'd

MARCH

Objectives	1. Discuss the goals with the staff.
	2. Evaluate progress and schedule.
	3. Understand the immediate success and opportunities of the spa performance.
Tactics	1. Meet with the staff and introduce the goals and bonus program for the microdermabrasion launch.
	2. Create a daily *hot sheet*.
	3. Review feedback questionnaires from clients about the new treatment.
Goals	1. Get the staff excited and willing to participate in the growth of the new treatment.
	2. Use the daily hot sheet to ensure the goals are being met.
	3. Evaluate questionnaires for opportunities.
Cost	1. Budget $2,000 for staff bonuses.

Those who are not in the spa during the time you are doing the survey can be called or e-mailed with the survey.

Using the mathematic approach is useful and effective. Knowing the number of clients you currently have in your database, you can realistically project the potential number of clients who will cross over to micro-dermabrasion. Keep the number low, for example, 2 to 5 percent of the database. Of course, this figure will depend greatly on the services you already provide and the general client type who frequents your spa.

With this information in hand, create an in-house campaign to capture these clients to treatment. Current clients will be the first to experience the treatment and enjoy your microdermabrasion treatment. To further improve the number of microdermabrasion clients, create a referral offer for those who experience the treatment and refer a friend.

Understanding the Competition

Your competition is everywhere, even outside your business sector. Like it or not, the *ideal* is the marker against which the commonplace is compared. Your waiting area will be compared with the most exquisite furnishings fit for royalty. Your customer service will be held up to virtually unattainable standards, and your treatment programs will be expected to surpass the abilities of the leading plastic surgeons. This is just the way the customer or client thinks. This does not suggest that your microdermabrasion business must settle for mediocrity; rather, it should ground you against putting undeserving emphasis on "keeping up with the Joneses" or overreaching your own business goals. Your microdermabrasion business success will be served best by an internal motivation to satisfy your own client. Other microdermabrasion spas across town and the Fortune 500 conglomerates across the globe are all your competition, but you must shrink your description of the competition down to a bulleted list of information which can facilitate your individual business goals.

The competition across town or across the hallway can be distracting. You may want to know what they are doing, who their clients are, and what treatments they offer. It is important to know what your competition is doing, but do not be obsessed with them. The few key points that you should know about your competition are their pricing, common procedures, demographic target, and promotions. Once you know these things or have an idea of the direction of their business, stay informed but leave it alone. Use your time efficiently by growing your own business, not by paying attention to someone else's.

Competition across the country is important because it gives you an idea of the direction of the industry at large. Look for a couple of very progressive businesses on each coast and in the middle of the country. Stay on top of what they are doing, including their pricing, procedures, promotions, written materials, and Web site promotions. Also, read the trade magazines and stay involved with professional organizations. This will help you to keep up with the trends and fads that are developing in the industry and adjust your business if you wish.

Marketing

Creating marketing strategies and watching them *bring in the clients* can be very rewarding at times; at other times, it can be disconcerting. Business growth followed by success is dependent on innovative and effective marketing. The marketing plan you create should use as many tactics as possible, because each of them will have a different reach, appeal, and anticipated affect on the practice. These tactics should include direct mail (including e-mail), Web site, newspaper, radio, and in-house strategies, such as literature (Table 11–3).

Direct Mail

Direct mail is a commonly used tactic to introduce new services. The spa or spa usually sends out a card or letter with an offer attached.

Table 11–3 Marketing Strategies

Marketing Strategy	Breadth of Market Reach	Cost	Cost to Acquire Risk
Direct mail	Low	High	High
E-mail	Low	Low	Low
Web site	High	Moderate	Low
Newspaper	Moderate	High	High
Billboard	Moderate	Moderate	Moderate
Radio commercial	Moderate	Low	Low
Regional magazine	High	High	Moderate
Local-affiliate television commercials	High	High	Moderate

Direct mail has a success rate of 1.5 percent or less. The average spa may believe this to be a terrific way to introduce a service or product, but it can be expensive, as you will see in the following example.

If you send out 1,000 cards you will get, at best, 15 clients through the door. If the direct mail piece cost $2.00 per card plus postage, the total per card is $2.37. The total cost for the mailer will be $2,420. That means each of the 15 clients who come through the door must spend $161.33 to cover just the cost of the mailer. That is before you begin to cover the overhead or make any money. An unexpectedly low yield could end up being very costly. Although direct mail can be successful, with this and all strategies, do the math to make sure the ends justify the means.

Another very common means to direct mail your clients is by e-mail. It is to your advantage to make it easy and rewarding for your existing clients to volunteer their e-mail addresses for in-house marketing and promotional use. By far, e-mail is the most cost-effective means of communicating with your clients. You can develop regular e-mail–only specials and introduce new offerings with little effort and surprising results. When you put promotional signs in your office that say, "Ask about our e-mail–only specials," you will be surprised how many people will give you their e-mail addresses, because no one wants to be left out when a special is available. Furthermore, this is an inexpensive and easy way to contact your clients immediately. Some e-mail–only specials can bring in clients and help you reach your weekly goals. For instance, on a slow week, send an e-mail offering a discount on, for example, microdermabrasion, only if the client schedules an appointment in the next 24 hours. Just watch your phone lines light up!

This is not to say that all direct mailings are successful. On the contrary, some are a gamble. Consider taking proactive steps to decrease the risk by trimming the fat from your mailing pool. Send direct mail, including e-mail pieces, only to those clients who have responded positively to an in-house survey or who have been into the spa in the last six months. A well-thought-out database should be able to do as much with little time. In addition, consider a *cross-selling direct mail campaign* that combines one treatment (for example, Restylane or Botox) with a promotional microdermabrasion treatment. Because of the unpredictable nature of direct mailings, mail the offer to a selected number of more qualified clients rather than your entire database.

Web sites

Any 21st-century business owner knows the value of maintaining a Web site. In doing so you make your business, its services, and its contributions to the greater industry available to a worldwide audience. In fact, the World Wide Web lends itself to a unique spin on marketing: voluntary marketing. Rather than soliciting potential clients, or upselling existing ones, voluntary marketing is when the potential client actively seeks you out and researches your products and services. Once they contact you, they have already made the decision to buy. Therefore, the design, content, and resources offered on your Web site should be readily available and easy to use.

Getting a Web site up and running can be complicated, often wrought with bugs. Designing and building a Web site ought to be left to a professional. They can monitor, repair, or add or delete content quickly, often on demand. Once it is up and running it can be just as useful to existing customers as it is to drawing in new ones. Appointments can be set or changed, accounts paid, and products ordered. Also, any document printed and distributed onsite can also be made available for download. This includes informational literature, homecare instructions, and pricelists.

Like other marketing devices, it is recommended that your Web site be consistent in its design and overall message. This assists in creating your brand identity, and helping your clients recognize you. Colors, fonts, monikers, and images ought to be the same on your letterhead, your marketing devices, and your Web site!

Newspaper

While antiquated, newspaper advertising is tried and true. In most cities, every day, literally hundreds of ads for plastic surgery, spas, and medical skin care can be found. If you intend to use this medium, you will need to stand out. Is your ad special, or is it just one in the maze of many? Are you participating in *advertorials* (ads that are formatted and read like an editorial)? What is the competition offering in the ad closest to yours? Newspapers can be an expensive tactic to acquire new clients. As with all marketing tactics, the question that must be answered when it comes to newspaper advertising is, "What is the **cost to acquire**?" In other words, how much money must be spent to get one new client to walk through the door? Taken one step further, how many appointments did it take for the client to spend enough money to cover the cost of the newspaper ad and begin to produce a profit for your spa? Add into the financial mix the variable costs of ad design and any additional marketing, and you may find that newspaper ads are pretty expensive unless you can really attract a number of clients.

Radio

Radio advertising is a viable option for smaller markets. In larger metropolitan areas like Los Angeles or New York, the reach of the radio station may be too great to merit radio advertising. In other words, a large percentage of potential clients are simply too far away to consider driving to your spa. Even under this condition, radio will provide great name recognition and tremendous branding, but the important question to ask is, "What is the objective of radio advertising?" If the objective is to attract clients, the larger your city is, the greater the risk of unsatisfactory new client yield. Having said that, radio may work well in smaller communities, especially if a morning drive time slot is available and the host is willing to do a live advertisement or, better yet, a testimonial.

There are other ways to use radio which don't necessarily involve direct advertising, yet still can involve use of your name and brand. You can sponsor events, or even sponsor a program on your local affiliate of National Public Radio.

In-House Strategies

In-house strategies are among the most effective and low-cost means of attracting new clients and increasing revenue. By implementing cross selling, **powering the client database**, and **referral programs**, you can create a sophisticated, layered initiative to generate additional revenue, as well as flex your knowledge of your business.

First, learn and implement **cross selling**. This is a tactic that will begin to build your practice by moving an active client in one category

---

cost to acquire
Average cost per new customer of any one marketing strategy.

powering the client database
In-house marketing strategy that involves innovative and detailed use of information already contained in a business database to increase traffic.

referral programs
In-house marketing strategy that rewards an existing client for referring a new one.

cross selling
Term that describes the process of selling related peripheral items to a customer.

to an additional category or categories. For example, an injection client, one who is only in the spa for Botox or dermal fillers, may be open to the opportunity of experiencing microdermabrasion. In fact, he or she may be getting microdermabrasion at another spa or spa. Cross sales can be made in a couple of ways: You can offer a gift certificate, followed by a discount on a package sale, or cross selling can happen subtly when you combine procedures in a package. For example, when a client buys a facial package, include a couple of microdermabrasion treatments. Almost everyone can benefit from microdermabrasion, so it really is a win-win proposition.

Powering the database uses your existing database to uncover potential candidates for microdermabrasion. This requires investigative work on the part of the staff, but it is worth it. It can cost 10 times more to gain a new client than keep an old client,[5] so get to work on those clients you already have in your database. Look through the database and find out which clients have not visited the spa for a while. Evaluate the number of "lost clients," and create a cross-selling campaign to draw them back into the spa.

A referral program will help you to discover new clients. Most spas experience at least a 30-percent referral rate. In other words, each month, 30 percent of your new clients are referred by happy clients. Do you reward those clients who send you business? If not, why not? Referrals are the easiest new clients you will get; they are presold because their friends have told them that your spa was the best. Create a referral program for your established clients. Use gift certificates or cash rewards, and everybody wins!

Literature

Having literature available for the procedures you offer is an essential part of the in-house marketing campaign. Original literature specific to your practice can be informational, educational, and identifiable. If you do not print original literature, then be sure to have literature that is supplied by the manufacturer. If the manufacturer does not supply literature or brochures, several vendors create "boilerplate" literature that will work just fine. The important thing is that the literature is accurate and available. Included in the literature category should be *post-treatment* instructions. Even if these are printed on your copy machine, you can still customize and dress up the presentation. However, the content is what is important, and function should take obvious precedence over form. Written post-treatment instructions are important to ensure the client follows your instructions and that no misunderstandings occur.

> The best form of advertising is word of mouth or experience-based. They are reliable, affordable, achievable, and manageable. Try to make each client satisfied enough to want to tell at least one other person to use your spa.

Selling Microdermabrasion Treatments

With all of these marketing and advertising ideas in mind, how does one actually sell microdermabrasion treatments? It is more than the individual advantages of your machine or your personal style as that type of industry jargon would be foreign, if not boring, to the potential client. As with any procedure or product, *knowledge* is the key to success. Before you ask yourself, "How do I sell this treatment?" you must ask, "How much do I really know about this service?" Assuming you are well-versed in microdermabrasion, what you need is an organized plan to communicate the features and the benefits to the client. The *features* are how the program works, and the *benefits* are what it will do for the client. Organize your information by discussing the features first, and conclude with the benefits (Table 11–4). The features for microdermabrasion include a good home-care program, use of inert aluminum oxide crystals (or salt or diamonds) to polish and exfoliate the skin, stimulation of dermal collagen remodeling, and peeling dry skin associated with the treatments. The benefits are improved tone, texture, pigment, and appearance of fine lines. Additionally, and this cannot be stressed enough, talk to your clients. Do not just hand them a written program, collect their money, and give them the bum's rush. When you talk, your knowledge comes through and the client will begin to trust you and develop a much-needed rapport.

Business Risks

Just as the aesthetician needs insurance, so does the spa. A conversation with your insurance agent will direct you to the best approach and company.

In our litigious society, merely owning a business (let alone having a staff and equipment) makes a business susceptible to risk. Each year, a business should evaluate the potential business risks that could be damaging to the earning power of the company. Among the potentially harmful business risks are government regulations, technology changes, the borrowing power of the company, and possible litigation. Make sure alternative plans are in place, should the company face a problem.

Table 11–4 Organizing Your Knowledge to Sell Your Treatment
What is microdermabrasion?
What makes your treatment unique?
What are the features of your machine?
Why do you prefer these features?
What home-care programs are associated with treatment?
What are the benefits of your microdermabrasion program?

State Government Regulations

State government regulations are a very real risk for the medical spa and luxury spa sector. For example, restrictions are being put on who can perform microdermabrasion and under what circumstances. The spa director, as well as any practicing aesthetician, should be aware of the changes in government regulations. They should also know their state regulations concerning combination peels, and acids that are used with microdermabrasion. Furthermore, aestheticians should know how to look up state guidelines on the government Web sites, and find out what laws are changing and if they will be affected. If the state in which you live is considering new laws about microdermabrasion that will affect your career or business, you have the right to make comments to the regulatory boards or legislators to promote and protect your profession.

Technology Changes

Technology advancements are happening every day. Improvements in handpieces, crystal management, and filters make a new machine more attractive to the aesthetician. Clients are far more sophisticated than ever before, and their demands for the newest technology may also drive the decision-making process of the spa.

Liability Issues for the Spa

Another important issue to investigate is malpractice insurance. Is this procedure going to be covered by the physician's policy, or does the medical spa have a separate policy that will be covering the aestheticians performing microdermabrasion? Ask questions about training requirements. Sometimes, insurance carriers require additional training for employees providing microdermabrasion. If the insurance is not going to be covered by the physician or the spa (but by the aesthetician individually), it is absolutely critical that a copy of the policy be available to the physician and the medical spa.

Indicators and Goals

Company history speaks to the traditional history, such as, "This is where we came from, and this is what we look like now." More importantly, company history is about the comparatives of indicators and goals. Although these categories may initially feel financial in nature, the reality is that indicators and goals really speak to history and the ability to exceed against the historical goals.

Setting goals for the spa and aesthetician is appropriate. The goals should reflect the number of client calls, the number of clients scheduled, the number of clients treated, the referral patterns, and other important indicators for the spa. These goals should translate directly into the revenue goal for the spa.

The goals you set up should be attainable; otherwise, everyone gets discouraged. Failure is a bad feeling and one that you do not want in your spa. If the microdermabrasion procedure is being brought into an already-established practice, the goals can be a little more aggressive because you have an already-established client base. If on the other hand, your spa is a start-up, then conservative numbers are in order. The goals should be set for six months and evaluated monthly. This way, you can determine how successful the process is and if you need to add additional advertising or marketing.

Set your goals and let the front desk and aesthetician know the goals. Some managers like goal setting to be a collaborative process. This only works if you, as the manager, stretch your employees to accept goals that seem a bit out of reach. Employees are a bit more conservative than managers, so do not be surprised if you find that your goals are a little higher than your employees'. Your goals might initially be broken down by (1) how many clients are scheduled, and (2) how many clients are treated. Once you get these numbers you can extrapolate the revenue. For example, if the goal is 50 clients and the price for the microdermabrasion is $125, then your revenue goal is $6,250 per month. This is just a treatment goal; the product goal also exists. For example, does every ticket need a product sale of at least $25? We know this will not happen, but the average product sales on microdermabrasion tickets may come out to $25, and that is what you are looking to accomplish—a focus on additional sales.

Indicators track the progress of business goals. Daily or—at the longest interval—weekly reviews of each aesthetician's hot sheets will provide you with daily (or weekly) goal progress reports.

Without a weekly or daily hot sheet you do not have the opportunity for improvement. A hot sheet for microdermabrasion might include the number of new clients scheduled, number of clients seen, number of clients rebooked, average ticket revenue, and the breakdown between product and service revenue. You also might be interested in the referral pattern. The indicator hot sheet should be the tool to evaluate, redirect, and grow the business. Over time, it will be the comparative you use to measure your progress. Indicator sheets are simple in form. They need only the information you are looking for and should not be cumbersome. Refer to the following Indicator Sheet.

Business Recordkeeping

Recordkeeping is a broad category and includes business recordkeeping and recordkeeping for client treatments. We will be discussing business

---

indicator hot sheet
Daily or weekly progress report that measures and provides daily insight into a business's or employee's performance.

Initially, you may find that daily review of indicators is not necessary. In that event, a weekly sheet will do. However, do not extend this past a week. It is too easy to forget about the growth process. At the end of the month you will get the numbers, and they could be disappointing; however, by that point, nothing can be done to improve the numbers for the month.

Indicator Hot Sheet

	Week One	Week Two	Week Three	Week Four	Actual	Goal
Number of new clients booked						
Number of clients seen						
Number of clients rebooked (after treatment)						
Number of packages sold						
Revenue per ticket						
Service revenue per ticket						
Product revenue per ticket						

recordkeeping in this section. The records that should be kept for a business can be extensive, but with the computers and programs available today it is much easier. An organized business should include many different *sets* of information; each of these categories of information should be filed and organized monthly. Included in the financial information should be tickets (cash and credit card), inventory, purchases, **accounts payable (AP)**, and **accounts receivable (AR)**. Other records that should be organized and available include insurance records (health and liability), lease contracts, rent contracts, human resources records, marketing files, and client database.

It is important to keep financial information organized and up-to-date. It is the history of the company's performance and a road map to the future. Each year, a notebook should be dedicated to your financial reports; it should be divided into the 12 months and include a 13th tab for a *year-end* report.

All tickets should be kept with a notation whether the payment was by cash or credit card. Refunds should also be documented on a ticket and processed accordingly. It is helpful to have a computer program that does all of this for you. If you do, a detailed printout should be made at the end of the month and placed in the notebook.

Inventory should be done monthly. The worksheets to do the inventory and the computer printout should be filed in your notebook. **Purchasing** is the acquisition of products, supplies, and other purchases

accounts payable (AP)
All accounting responsibilities associated with the recording and payment of all vendor-related business expenditures.

accounts receivable (AR)
All accounting responsibilities associated with the recording and allocation of all payments received by the business.

purchasing
Structured process a business undergoes to acquire materials needed for operation.

you made in the month. A record of this (usually through a purchase order system) should be placed in your monthly notebook.

AP and AR reports should be placed into the notebook every month. It is unusual to have an account receivable, because clients usually pay when the service is provided; however, if you do have house accounts, the amount owed by your clients should be very small. Other records are really files that should be kept at your fingertips and updated as required. Additional information that is accumulated should be placed into these files. These files do not change each year. They should stay with the timeless files, that is, files do not need to be updated each year (e.g., lease files, insurance files), and they should always be kept at hand.

Reading Income Statements

income statement
Financial statement that summarizes the revenues generated and the expenses incurred by an entity during a period of time.

balance sheet
Document that states a business's assets and liabilities on a given date.

deferred revenue
Money that the organization has received but not yet earned as of the closing date on the balance sheet; the amount is carried as a liability until the organization provides the goods or services for which the money was received.

cost of goods sold (COGS)
Direct costs of materials used in the products a business makes or sells.

The **income statement** is an important document. It is one of the documents a bank will ask to see when you are getting a loan or signing a lease. It is also a document that you should review monthly. Review the *indicator hot sheet* in tandem with income statements, and then file them in the monthly notebook.

Learning to read an income statement is easy. Start at the top, and look at the *revenue* or *income* line. This will tell you how much money you have collected. It includes all the packaged treatments redeemed but should not include the revenue from packages sold—that revenue goes on to the **balance sheet** in a category called **deferred revenue**. The revenue line can and should be broken into different types of revenue (such as facials, peels, and microdermabrasion) so that you know how much money you collected in each category. The next line is **cost of goods sold (COGS)**; these are the direct costs and, like the revenue, should be broken into categories that respond to the revenue. The next line should be gross margin. *Gross margin* is the amount of money you made before overhead costs. General costs should include personnel, marketing, rent, telephone, and a general category. Finally, you come to a line called *income before taxes*. This is the amount of money you really made before paying Uncle Sam. A good computer system will allow you to look at the aforementioned categories with a percentage attached. This is important because it helps you to understand the ratios at which the company is performing.

Understanding the Balance Sheet

The balance sheet is the partner document to the income statement. Banks really like this document because it tells them about your value: your assets and your liabilities. When you look at the balance sheet, the first category is usually the *assets;* this includes equipment you own, cash in the bank, and other assets. The next page is the *liabilities,* which lists the company debt. The balance sheet is a detailed snapshot of the company and helps anyone valuing the business to be clear about its status.

Whether you are a single aesthetician renting a booth or a director of a multisite business, it may always seem that money slips through your fingers. Reviewing the income statement monthly and the indicator hot sheet daily will help you to avoid some of this frustration. When you review these documents, be sure to evaluate them against your budget. Budgeting is the discipline you create to ensure that the money goes to the categories you want and does not ooze out into other places. However, sometimes it seems that, despite your best efforts, you cannot seem to direct the flow of cash. This usually means that you have a flawed budget or that costs are out of control. If this is happening, you may need to have a professional accountant look at the books and help you to locate the problem. Keeping money where it belongs requires discipline and daily evaluation.

> The revenue on the income statement does not match the cash to the bank. Revenue on the income statement will reflect all treatments, including redeemed package visits, which do not have cash attached because the package is generally prepaid.

■ CONCLUSION

Starting a new business or adding to your existing business can be exhilarating and full of challenges, but it is never as easy as it seems. Those who are successful follow the intricate steps of business development, analysis, and the daily monitoring of progress. Microdermabrasion is a worthwhile procedure—one that will bring improvement to the client's skin and an expansion of the menu offerings. A well-thought-out and carefully implemented microdermabrasion plan will make a business more competitive and certainly more successful.

▶ ▷ ▷ Top 10 Tips to Take to the Spa

1. Look for a manufacturer with a well-established reputation.
2. Consider a short-term lease or purchase agreement, so the machine can be traded in when newer models come onto the market.
3. The more frequently the procedure is performed, the more expert the aesthetician becomes; use microdermabrasion often to become an authority.
4. Become an expert at understanding your client.
5. Develop a feature and benefit communication style to increase sales.

6. Recognize the potential business risks for microdermabrasion.
7. Use goals to achieve success.
8. Use indicators to measure success.
9. Keep organized business records.
10. Learn to read financial statements.

Chapter Review Questions

1. Operating a microdermabrasion business includes what key components?
2. What is the purpose of starting a microdermabrasion business? Which of the above components are necessary to accomplish this?
3. Where should a business owner or operator begin when considering adding microdermabrasion to their spa menu? Be specific about what is involved in the onset.
4. What role does the competition play with regards to beginning a microdermabrasion service? What about clients? The marketplace?
5. Which resources should you consider when purchasing a microdermabrasion machine? Who ought to be consulted? How will this affect training?
6. What fixed costs are associated with offering a microdermabrasion service? Direct costs?
7. What are indicators? Goals? How do they relate to one another?
8. True or False: All microdermabrasion machines are the same.
9. True or False: A warranty should include a replacement provision while your machine is being repaired.
10. True or False: Not all aestheticians need to be trained on the new microdermabrasion service.
11. What is a cost analysis? How does one determine if a microdermabrasion service is appropriate for their particular spa?
12. How do you learn about the demographics for microdermabrasion?
13. Identify the different pricing strategies? When is each appropriate?
14. Why is marketing an indirect cost of microdermabrasion?

15. What are income statements?

16. How do you keep money from slipping through your fingers?

17. Discuss writing a business plan to implement microdermabrasion.

18. What is the optimum price for your microdermabrasion service? Who determines this price?

19. What are the benefits of a standard pricing policy? How often should it be reviewed?

20. Identify the parts of the annual business plan. How does each contribute to the success of your enterprise?

21. How can your database assist you in reaching your business goals?

22. What options are available to a business owner/operator to market their microdermabrasion service? When is each appropriate?

23. What business liabilities exist for a spa offering a microdermabrasion service? How can these risks be circumvented?

24. How can a spa owner/operator use goals to motivate staff to sell? Clients to buy?

25. Why is an income statement important for a spa? How does it apply to the microdermabrasion service?

Chapter References

1. How to buy a microdermabrasion system without getting skinned. (2001, August) [Online]. *Cosmetic Surgery Times.* Available: http://www.cosmeticsurgerytimes.com.

2. How to buy a microdermabrasion system without getting skinned. (2001, August) [Online]. *Cosmetic Surgery Times.* Available: http://www.cosmeticsurgerytimes.com.

3. Brown, L. (2003, March). *The cosmetic spa: The role of microdermabrasion in skin care* [Online]. Available: http://www. skinandaging.com.

4. Canada Business Service Centre. (2004, February 15). *Setting the right price* [Online]. Available: http://www.cbsc.org.

5. Keller, K. L., Sternthal, B., & Tybout, A. (2002). Three questions you need to ask about your brand. *Harvard Business Review, 80*(9).

Glossary

A

Ablation removal of epidermal or dermal skin from the body; usually associated with the presence of a wound.

Absorbents products that pass through the skin.

Accounts Payable (AP) all accounting responsibilities associated with the recording and payment of all vendor-related business expenditures.

Accounts Receivable (AR) all accounting responsibilities associated with the recording and allocation of all payments received by the business.

Acetic Acid mild organic acid derived from vinegar.

Acid Mantle thin coating on the stratum corneum that is intended to protect the skin from infection and has a pH of 4 to 6.5.

Acidic anything that has a pH less than 7.0.

Acne an inflammation of the sebaceous glands and hair follicles.

Acquired Immunodeficiency Syndrome (AIDS) opportunistic infections that occur as a result of the final stages of HIV and the associated compromise of the immune system.

Actinic Keratoses potentially precancerous lesions of the skin, generally from sun exposure.

Acute having a rapid onset with a short but severe course.

Adipose Cells cells that contain stored fat in connective tissue.

Aging Analysis examines how aging physically presents itself in the skin, particularly, to what sorts of damaging conditions the skin has been exposed in the past and the results of that damage; considers both intrinsic and extrinsic aging modalities.

Alkaline anything that has a pH greater than 7.0.

Alpha Hydroxy Acids (AHAs) mild organic acids used in cosmeceutical products; AHAs "unglue" cells in the epidermis, allowing keratinocytes to be shed at the stratum granulosum and providing skin with a healthier texture.

Aluminum Oxide Crystals common type of abrasive crystals used for microdermabrasion.

Amino Acids organic compound that contains an amino group and a carboxylic group.

Ampoules a container for liquid solutions.

Anagen Phase hair growth phase in which growth is actually occurring.

Anatomy study of the body structures.

Annual Business Plan growth plan that outlines business objectives, marketing plans, and budgets for the period of one fiscal year.

Anthranilates weak UVB filters that mainly absorb in the near-UVA portion of the spectrum.

Antimicrobials agent that halts or prevents the development of microorganisms.

311

APIE Problem-oriented charting aid that emphasizes assessment, planning, implementation, and evaluation.

Apocrine Sweat Glands larger of the sweat glands that are housed in axillary (underarm), pubic, and perianal areas.

Appendages anatomic structures associated with a larger structure; for the skin, appendages include hair follicles and sweat glands.

Ascorbic Acid see *Vitamin C.*

Ascorbyl Palmitate fat-soluble form of ascorbic acid.

Astringents drying agents that shrink and contract the skin.

Atrophic Scars flat, small, round, and generally inverted scars; usually seen in acne or chicken-pox scarring.

Avascular lacking in blood vessels; thus having a poor blood supply.

Ayurveda Indian theory dating back to 2500 B.C., known as the science of living. Ayureda defines the essentials that were perceived as being necessary to health.

Azelaic Acid antibacterial agent that is usually used for acne treatment and has shown promise in minimizing dyschromia; kills the bacteria that infect pores.

B

Balance Sheet document that states a business's assets and liabilities on a given date.

Basal Cell Carcinoma slow-growing tumor that generally does not metastasize; the most common form of skin cancer that usually occurs in regions of repeated sunburn.

Basal Layer see *Stratum Basale.*

Benzophenones chemical absorbers that respond to UV light by generating a free radical capable of rapid polymerization.

Bloodborne Pathogens infectious substances present in the blood that can cause infection or disease.

Body Dysmorphic Disorder (BDD) psychosocial disease that causes individuals to be inappropriately concerned with their appearance.

Botox® (*Clostridium Botulinum*) trade name for small doses of the botulism toxin that are injected into the wrinkle-causing muscles; toxin blocks the release of the chemicals that would otherwise signal the muscle to contract, thus paralyzing the injected muscle.

Burns skin injury that occurs as a result of intense thermal, electrical, or acidic agents.

C

Camphors used topically as an anti-itch agent; derived as a gum from evergreens native to China and Japan.

Carbohydrates one of a group of chemical substances (including sugars) that contain only carbon, hydrogen, and oxygen. Common in fruits, grains, and nuts;

Carbolic Acid see *Phenol.*

Career Plan action taken by a professional to set goals and to ensure their realization.

Catagen Phase intermediate stage in the hair growth phase.

Cavitation the formation of gas bubbles in a liquid.

Cellulitis potentially serious infection of the skin that presents as a small red area surrounding a skin injury; those at risk include the elderly and those with compromised immune systems.

Ceramides class of lipids that do not contain glycerol.

Charting Formats any method meant to document or record the events, consequences, or abnormalities associated with a procedure.

Chi concept originally theorized by the Yellow Emperor of China's Han Dynasty; according to Chi, nature has a delicate balance, and it describes illness as an imbalance.

Chronic disease or occurrence showing little or no improvement over a long period of time.

Cinnamates derivative of cinnaminic acid that is useful for protection against low levels of UVB rays; makes sunscreens waterproof.

Citric Acid alpha hydroxy acid derived from citrus fruit, such as oranges and grapefruit.

Cleansing Agents products that remove foreign matter and excretions from the skin's surface. Common ingredients in cleansers include detergents, surfactants, and antimicrobials.

Client Information Sheet document used to gather social, personal, and demographic information.

Clinical Indications conditions suited for a particular treatment or procedure based on specific indicators.

CO_2 Laser aggressive type of laser used for skin resurfacing that vaporizes skin and causes thermal injury, allowing for improved collagen production.

Cocamidopropyl Betaine foaming agent used in shampoos and cleansers.

Collagen water-soluble protein found in connective tissues. Particularly, type I collagen forms a network in the epidermis and is credited with providing skin with its tensile strength and firmness.

Collagen® bovine-based dermal filler that acts as a synthetic collagen.

Collagenase any enzyme that catalyzes the hydrolysis of collagen.

Comedones typical small lesions associated with acne breakouts; usually raised and red in color.

Consultation initial visit with a professional during which the client and the professional both investigate whether a specific treatment or service is warranted and if the desired outcome is achievable.

Contaminated act of making an item or compound nonsterile or impure.

Continuing Education Units (CEUs) any certified training or event that is intended to build or add skills.

Contraindications any sign or symptom that a particular treatment that would otherwise be advisable would be inappropriate.

Corneocytes act as cellular glue in the epidermis, holding cells together.

Cornified hardening or thickening of the skin.

Corundum naturally occurring aluminum oxide.

Cosmeceutical a product that does more than decorate or camouflage but does less than prescription drugs; term originally coined by Dr. Albert Kligman.

Cost of Goods Sold (COGS) direct costs of materials used in the products a business makes or sells.

Cost to Acquire average cost per new customer of any one marketing strategy.

Cross Selling term that describes the process of selling related peripheral items to a customer.

Crow's-Feet dynamic rhytids next to the eyes, caused by repeated muscle movement from expression over time.

D

D-Alpha Tocopherol see *Vitamin E.*

Database electronic compilation of extensive categorical information relevant to business processes such as marketing or inventory.

Deep-Epidermal Wounding injury that reaches deep into the epidermis, as with peeling solutions.

Deferred Revenue money that the organization has received but not yet earned as of the closing date on the balance sheet; the amount is carried as a liability until the organization provides the goods or services for which the money was received.

Dermabrasion predecessor to microdermabrasion that used a wire brush or a diamond-coated wheel to resurface the skin to the papillary dermal level.

Dermal-Epidermal Junction superficial side of the dermis that is connected to the epidermis.

Dermis second layer of skin that is responsible for attaching the skin to the subcutaneous structures of the body.

Desmosomes small hair-like structures in the spiny layer of the epidermis.

Desquamation shedding of cells, such as at the stratum corneum.

Detergents synthetic cleansing agent that acts as a wetting agent and emulsifier.

Diamond Crystals type of microdermabrasion crystals that are comprised of diamond particles, the strongest material on Earth.

Diamond-Encrusted Tips reusable microdermabrasion system that has varying wands for specific regions and coarseness.

Dibenzoylmethanes UVA ray absorber.

Differentiate to make something stand out or be unique compared with something that would otherwise be similar.

Dimethicone silicone oil consisting of dimethylsiloxane viscous polymers.

Direct Costs costs that are directly and exclusively attributable to a specific product or service.

Downtime industry jargon for recovery time.

Dynamic Rhytids wrinkling that occurs because of facial movement.

Dyschromia discoloration of the skin.

E

Eccrine Sweat Glands smaller of the sweat glands that reside all over the body.

Economy Pricing low pricing of a product or service as a means to entice customers to buy.

Elastin protein responsible for giving tissue its elastic qualities.

Eldopaque® four-percent concentration of hydroquinone; bleaching agent used to treat hyperpigmentation.

Emollients products that have a softening or soothing effect on the skin.

Environmental Protection Agency (EPA) governmental agency set up to protect human health and the environment.

Epidermal Cells cells found in the outermost layer of skin.

Epidermis top layer of the skin.

Epithelialization growth of new skin over a wound.

Epithelium membranous tissue covering internal organs and lining skin appendages.

Erbium Laser less aggressive type of laser that causes less thermal injury while still causing epidermal and papillary dermal injuries.

Ergonomically Correct being consistent with body contouring so as not to inflict long-term damage (as with repeated use of poorly designed office equipment or devices).

Erythema spot on the skin showing diffused redness caused by capillary congestion.

Ester water- and fat-soluble.

Exfoliate to remove dead skin cells and other debris from the skin's surface to give it a healthier sheen.

Extrinsic Aging changes that are brought on by the effects of the environment and our choices relating to them, specifically sun exposure.

F

Fibroblasts cells that produce connective tissue.

Filaggrin synthesizes lipids (fats) that are thought to serve as "intercellular cement"; important component of NMF.

Fitzpatrick Skin Typing method of skin typing that considers skin's complexion, hair color, eye color, ethnicity, and the individual's reaction to unprotected sun exposure.

Fixed Price price that remains the same, usually for a set time period.

Folliculitis infection of the hair follicle, such as ingrown hairs.

Four Humors early medical concept originally postulated by Hippocrates, which stated that the character of a person is determined by the specific balance of the four fluids (black bile, yellow bile, blood, and phlegm) that he perceived as running through the body.

Free Radicals atoms with an unpaired electron.

Full-Thickness Wound wound that penetrates to such a depth in the upper reticular dermis or subcutaneous tissue and is associated with slower healing; scarring will develop.

Fungal Infections any infection caused by the kingdom of organisms that includes yeasts and molds.

G

Gel Solution semisolid material that is easily absorbed in the skin without the irritation associated with other cream-based solutions.

Glabella area between the eyebrows with underlying muscle groups that cause creasing (frown lines) as a result of repeated squinting or frowning over time.

Glogau Classification of Aging Analysis system of aging analysis that calculates the degree of aging-related damage and assigns numeric typing; considers both intrinsic and extrinsic aging.

Glycerin humectant that is a natural by-product of the soap-making process.

Glycolic Acid alpha hydroxy acid derived from sugar cane; has a small molecular size that allows for easier penetration into the skin.

Glycosaminoglycans (GAGs) polysaccharide chains, most prominent in the dermis, that bind with water, smoothing and softening the surface from below; most abundant GAG is hyaluronic acid.

Goals general statements of anticipated business outcomes resulting from well-stated objectives.

Granulocytes white blood cells involved in immune response; include neutrophils, eosinophils, and basophils.

Ground Substance consists mainly of GAGs (hyaluronic acid, chondroitin sulfate, and dermatan sulfate); involved in maintenance and repair of dermis.

H

Health History Sheet document used by medical professionals to gather information on past and present health conditions, as well as likelihood for future conditions; includes allergies, medical conditions, and prescription information.

Health Insurance Portability and Accountability Act of 1996 (HIPAA) federal regulation that dictates procedural protocols to protect client privacy.

Hepatitis caused by multiple viruses defined as hepatitis A, B, or C; it is a contagious inflammation of the liver with possible chronic consequences, particularly with hepatitis C.

Herpes Simplex (HSV) infectious disease caused by HSV-1, characterized by thin-walled vesicles that tend to occur repeatedly in the same place on the skin's surface.

Herpes Zoster virus responsible for both shingles and chickenpox.

Hippocrates Greek physician and "father of medicine," who created the Hippocratic oath and theorized the four humors.

Hippocratic Oath oath taken by all doctors relating to the practice of medicine; created by Hippocrates.

Histamine amino acid histidine, found in the body and released from mast cells as part of an allergic reaction.

Human Immunodeficiency Virus (HIV) virus that causes acquired immunodeficiency syndrome (AIDS); see *acquired immunodeficiency syndrome (AIDS).*

Humectants moisturizing agent.

Hyaluronic Acid acid that occurs in intercellular ground substance of connecting tissue; plays an important role in controlling tissue permeation, bacterial invasiveness, and intracellular transport.

Hydroquinone safe, topical bleaching agent that inhibits the production of tyrosine within melanocytes; topical agent used to decrease the hyperpigmentation on the skin.

Hyperkeratinization thickening of the horny layers of skin, particularly the palmar and plantar areas.

Hyperpigmentation overproduction and over-deposits of melanin.

Hypertrophic Scars overly developed scar tissue that rises above the skin level, often overfed by an abundance of capillaries; will usually regress over time.

Hypodermis layer of subcutaneous fat and connective tissue lying beneath the epidermis.

Hypopigmentation lack of production of melanin from melanocytes.

I

Image Businesses type of business in which the way the public views the company is based largely upon how things look, or how they are perceived, more than actual performance.

Impetigo skin infection from staphylococcal or streptococcal bacteria.

Impressions initial and potentially lasting opinions or judgments of a person, place, or thing.

Income Statement financial statement that summarizes the revenues generated and the expenses incurred by an entity during a period of time.

Indications any sign or circumstance that a particular treatment is appropriate or warranted.

Indicator key value used to measure performance over time as it relates to an organization's progress achieving its goals.

Indicator Hot Sheet daily or weekly progress report which measures and provides daily insight into a business's or employee's performance.

Indirect Costs cost necessary for the functioning of the organization as a whole but that cannot be directly assigned to one service or product.

Inflammatory Phase early wound healing phase during which blood and fluid collect and substances begin to fight infection and promote healing.

Insult injury or a trauma to tissue.

Integumentary System skin and its appendages (nails, hair and sweat and oil glands).

Intense Pulsed Light (IPL) machine that uses a variety of filters to diminish areas of color, both red and brown, on skin.

Intrinsic Aging changes that would occur over time without the effects of any environmental factors.

Inventory itemized list of merchandise or supplies on hand.

Ischemia localized restriction of blood flow usually caused by an obstruction of normal circulation.

J

Jessner's Solution peel solution for the skin that is 14 percent resorcinol, 14 percent salicylic acid, 14 percent lactic acid in ethanol.

Juvéderm® trade name for hyaluronic acid dermal filler.

K

Keloid Scars scar formation in which tissue response is excessive in relation to normal tissue repair.

Keratin protein cell found in the skin, hair, and nails; insoluble in water, weak acids, or alkalis.

Keratinization progressive maturation of the cell in the movement through the stratum corneum.

Keratinocytes any cells in the skin, hair, or nails that produce keratin.

Keratolysis separation of the skin cells in the epidermal layer.

Keratolytics products or agents that loosen horny skin layers.

Keratoses any condition of the skin characterized by excessive horny growth.

Kojic Acid bleaching agent derived from bacteria on a Japanese mushroom; usually used in conjunction with hydroquinone.

L

Lactic Acid alpha hydroxy acid derived from milk.

Lamellar Granules control lipids that produce NMF.

Langerhans' Cells cells possessing processes (dendrites) that detect pathogens; involved in immune response. Type of macrophage common to the epidermis.

L-Ascorbic Acid water-soluble vitamin C.

LED Light Emitting Diode. Used in lasers and electronic devices.

Lentigines flat brown spots appearing on aged or sun-exposed skin; commonly called liver spots, they are not related to any liver disease.

Lesions an area of injured tissue.

Leukocytes white blood cells without granules involved in immune response; include lymphocytes and monocytes.

Lipids fat or fat-like substances, insoluble in water.

Lymphatic Drainage drainage of lymphatic fluids.

Lymphocytes white blood cells involved in the body's immune system; their numbers increase in the presence of infection.

M

Machine Features in relation to microdermabrasion, the specific components of a machine that separate it from its competition; some features include type of filtration system, type of crystal supply system, ergonomic handpieces, and portability.

Macrophage part of the immune system in the skin; scavengers that clear debris in tissue injury.

Magnesium Ascorbyl Phosphate water-soluble and fat-soluble form of vitamin C; it is a vitamin C ester.

Malic Acid alpha hydroxy acid derived from apples.

Malignant cancerous, or harmful to one's health.

Malnutrition any condition that causes a lack of nutritional substances for the body to use and distribute.

Marketing Strategies planned use of marketing elements and media pathways to create a strategy to introduce new clients or reactivate former clients.

Marketplace any environment in which two or more people buy or sell a product or service.

Mast Cells large tissue cell present in the skin that produces histamine and other acute symptoms of allergic reactions.

Medical Waste waste resulting from medical activity that includes human blood and blood products, and used or unused sharps (syringes, needles, and blades).

Melanin pigment that protects skin from ultraviolet damage.

Melanocytes cells in the epidermis that produce pigment.

Melanoma malignant, darkly pigmented mole or tumor of the skin.

Melasma Gravidarum "Mask of pregnancy" from an overproduction of melanin.

Melquin® three-percent concentration of hydroquinone; bleaching agent used to treat hyperpigmentation.

Merkel Cells cells that are usually close to nerve endings and may be involved in sensory perception.

Microdermabrasion nonsurgical aesthetic skin procedure that uses tiny crystals to strike and exfoliate the skin.

Mission Statement written statement of a business's individual philosophy.

Modulate to regulate or adjust to an adequate proportion.

Moisturizers agent that replenishes moisture to the skin.

Muscle Memory ability of muscles to behave the same way after a repeated action.

N

Natural Moisturizing Factor (NMF) compound found only in the top layer of skin that gives cells their ability to bind with water.

Necrosis death of cells when tissue is deprived of blood supply.

Neutral having a pH that is exactly 7.0; neither acidic nor alkaline.

Neutrophils most common type of white blood cells that kill bacteria and discourage infection.

Nicotinamide member of the vitamin-B complex that has been shown to decrease TEWL.

Nonsurgical Aesthetic Skin Care any noninvasive procedure that is intended to improve overall skin health and appearance.

O

Occupational Safety and Health Administration (OSHA) federal agency responsible for defining and regulating safety in the workplace.

Octyl Methoxycinnamathe chemical agent found in sunscreens.

Open Systems in microdermabrasion, the first machines allowed for the escape of crystals and crystalline dust particles. Originally these particles were thought to be a risk factor for Alzheimer's disease, but this has since been disproved. Most modern machines are closed systems that do not allow particulate emission.

Organelles microorganisms responsible for functions within the cell.

Overhead Costs indirect costs.

Oxidized prolonged and damaging exposure to oxygen; oxidized materials are usually brown in color.

P

Papain protein-cleaving enzyme derived from papaya and certain other plants.

Papillae projections from the dermis into the epidermis that hold them together.

Papillary Dermal Wounding any injury to the skin that reaches deep enough to cause bleeding.

Para-Aminobenzoic Acid (PABA) cousin of the B complex that is found in animals; most common use is as an effective sunscreen.

Parsol 1789® preferred sunscreen ingredient that protects against photodamage and premature aging of the skin from exposure to UVA light.

Partial-Thickness Wound wound that penetrates only the epidermis or the upper layer of the papillary dermis; tend to heal quickly and without scarring.

Pathogens agents that cause disease, namely bacteria and viruses.

Penetration Pricing pricing strategy in which the price is set low to allow for introduction into an existing market.

Perception process by which individuals use their senses to make decisions or gather information.

Petrolatum semisolid mixture of hydrocarbons obtained from petroleum; used in medicinal ointments and for lubrication.

Phenylbenzimidazole Sulfonic Acid chemical agent found in sunscreens.

Pheromone chemical substances that, when released, may affect the behavior or physiology of a recipient.

Photodamage damage caused by repeated and unprotected sun exposure over time; also called solar damage.

Photographs necessary component of skin-care treatment program that accurately documents the original skin condition to prove or disclaim treatment results.

Photomodulation to use controlled light therapies to regulate irregularities of the skin.

Physiology study of body function.

PIE problem-oriented charting aid that emphasizes planning, implementation, and evaluation.

Pilosebaceous Unit hair follicle and accompanying sebaceous glands and arrector pili muscle.

Pinpoint Bleeding small entry to the papillary dermis.

Positive Pressure specific vacuum pressure applied while administering a microdermabrasion treatment.

Post-Inflammatory Hyperpigmentation (PIH) dyschromia associated with injury to the skin.

Postmitotic Cells cells that have completed mitotic division.

Potential of Hydrogen (pH) scale by which a material is characterized as being acidic (pH less than 7.0), alkaline (greater than 7.0), or neutral (7.0).

Powering the Client Database in-house marketing strategy that involves innovative and detailed use of information already contained in a business database to increase traffic.

Preauricular in front of the ear.

Premium Pricing pricing strategy in which the price is set high to compensate for a high-quality product, usually with a high production cost as well.

Preservative agent used to prevent spoilage.

Pretreatment any process that will aid or facilitate a future procedure.

Pricing Strategies process by which a business determines the best way to price products or services to entice customers while allowing for profit

Product-Bundling Pricing pricing strategy in which one or more products or services are offered at a discount.

Professional Ethics set of guidelines that should set a framework for professional behavior and responsibilities.

Progressive Improvement Plan (PIP) administrative document that is intended to record a problem and the actions that will be taken to improve the problem and prevent its reoccurrence.

Proliferative Phase phase of wound healing during which replacement of protective epithelial tissue occurs over the old wound site.

Protein class of complex compounds that are synthesized by all living creatures; proteins are broken down into amino acids for use, including the rebuilding of tissue.

Pseudofolliculitis Barbae form of folliculitis commonly seen as a result of shaving or waxing.

Psoriasis chronic skin disease characterized by inflammation and white scaly patches.

Purchasing structured process a business undergoes to acquire materials needed for operation.

R

Radiesse® trade name for dermal filler used to improve laugh lines around the mouth.

Rashes general term for a topical eruption of the skin.

Realistic Expectations belief that a certain outcome is within the realm of possibility or is likely based on unbiased examination of evidence presented.

Red Bagging slang term that means placement of a medical waste material into an appropriately marked and sealed biohazard receptacle.

Reepithelialization replacement of protective epithelial tissue.

Referral Programs in-house marketing strategy that rewards an existing client for referring a new one.

Reflexology system of massage in which certain body parts are massaged in specific areas to favorably influence other body functions.

Remodeling Phase phase of wound healing during which collagen is assembled to replace skin.

Renova® tretinoin that is meant specifically for aging; recommended for clients with drier skin.

Restylane® trade name for hyaluronic acid dermal filler.

Rete Pegs anatomic feature that holds the dermis and epidermis together.

Reticular Dermis sublayer of the dermis that connects the dermis to the epidermis and is home to the skin's appendages (nails, hair, glands).

Reticulin water-soluble protein in the connective tissue framework of reticular tissue.

Retin A Microsphere® a gentler Retin A, based on an advanced delivery system.

Retin A® (Tretinoin) keratolytic agent used to treat acne and reverse photodamage.

Retinols vitamin A derivatives that must first convert to retinoic acid before being useful to the skin.

Retinyl Palmitate vitamin A derivative that must first convert to retinoic acid before it can be useful to the skin; also thought to be useful for collagen synthesis.

Rhytids wrinkles.

Ringworm popular term for dermatomycosis caused by species of fungi from the Microsporum family.

Rosacea adult form of acne that produces redness, swelling, and obvious telangiectasias.

Rubin Classification of Aging Analysis system of aging analysis that calculates the degree of photodamage and assigns a numeric level; considers only extrinsic aging.

S

Safety Bill of Rights original name of OSHA.

Safety Coordinator specially designated person in a business who is responsible for updating the OSHA safety manual as warranted.

Safety Manual OSHA document that outlines the hazardous materials and equipment specific to each location, as well as the safety protocols for each.

Salicylates salt derivative of salicylic acid that is used as a chemical agent in sunscreens.

Salt Crystals type of microdermabrasion crystals that are made from sodium; thought to be more irritating than conventional aluminum oxide crystals.

Scars marks left in the skin or on an internal organ as a result of deep tissue trauma; scars result from injury, disease, or medical procedures.

Sebaceous Glands small glands usually located next to the hair follicle in the dermis that release fatty liquids onto the hair follicle to soften hair and skin.

Seborrheic Keratosis benign skin tumor common in the elderly; thought to develop from prolific epidermal cells.

Selenium chemical agent resembling sulfur; helps protect the skin from solar-induced skin cancers.

Shingles sudden, acute inflammation and blisters, linked to herpes zoster.

Skin Condition fundamental skin classification in which an individual's skin is grouped according to the degree of moisture retention, its reaction to products or environment, or both.

Skin History Sheet document used to gather information on a client's past and present skin health; includes past treatment, sunburns, and conditions that are necessary for treatment.

Skin Turgor flexibility of the skin.

Skin Typing more detailed skin classification that gives indications as to how a certain skin type will react to various treatment conditions.

Slough to cast off skin, feathers, hair, or horn.

SOAP problem-oriented charting aid that emphasizes subjective data, objective data, assessment, and planning.

SOAPIER problem-oriented charting aid that emphasizes subjective data, objective data, assessment, planning, implementation, evaluation, and revision.

Sodium Lauryl Isethionate similar to sodium lauryl sulfate but not as irritating; less effective as an emulsifier.

Sodium Lauryl Sulfate common ingredient in household detergents and soaps; most commonly used as an emulsifier.

Soiled any item that is contaminated or formerly in contact with medical waste.

Spa Protocols any set of rules or guidelines established by a spa for safe practice; guidelines will vary by location but are expected to be observed by aestheticians working within the individual spa.

Squamous Cell Carcinomas (SCCs) malignant cancer of the epithelial cells.

Standard Pricing Policy business document that outlines the specific price range of a given product or service, preferred pricing strategy, and circumstances under which each might change.

Static Rhytids wrinkling that occurs without reference to facial movement.

Stem Cells a stalk-like cell that is unspecialized; gives rise to specialized cells.

Stratum Basale lowest layer of the epidermis (or basal layer); houses germinal cells and regenerating cells for all layers of the epidermis.

Stratum Corneum superficial sublayer of the epidermis; varies in thickness over the body.

Stratum Granulosum thin, clear sublayer of the epidermis.

Stratum Lucidum sublayer of the epidermis characterized by the appearance of granules and the disappearance of the nucleus within the skin cells.

Stratum Spinosum sublayer of the epidermis intertwined with desmosomes.

Subcutaneous beneath the skin.

Sun Protection Factor (SPF) determines the amount of time an individual can be in the sun with protection from a sunscreen before burning. SPF is difficult to understand and varies from one individual to the next, depending on skin type.

Sunscreens any agent that protects the skin from harmful UVA and UVB light, helping to protect skin from photodamage including skin cancers and dyschromia; blocks rays either by physical or chemical means.

Suppurate to form or discharge pus.

Surfactants surface-active agent that lowers surface tension.

T

Tartaric Acid alpha hydroxy acid derived from grapes.

Technique-Sensitive exact protocols and processes must be observed to obtain an optimal outcome; however, because of individual variations in pressure or style, different aestheticians may get different results, even if protocol is observed.

Telangiectasias small visible capillaries;

Telogen Phase stage of hair growth during which the hair is at rest.

Therapeutic Program program for home use complete with the necessary prescriptions, topical vitamins, and sunscreens.

Tinea Corporis body ringworm.

Titanium Dioxide physical sunscreen that scatters light rather than absorbing or filtering it.

Transepidermal Water Loss (TEWL) process by which our bodies constantly lose water via evaporation.

Tretinoin see *Retin A*.

Trichloroacetic Acid (TCA) chemical used in peel solutions that dissolve aging cells to make room for newer, healthier ones.

Tyrosine enzyme that produces melanin in melanocytes; overproduction of melanin is associated with hyperpigmentation.

U

Ubiquinone (Co-Q₁₀) lipid-soluble cellular antioxidant present in virtually all cells.

Ultrasound use of high-frequency sound waves to increase the intercellular spaces of the epidermis and dermis, allowing penetration of a topical product during treatment.

Understanding Your Competition component of the business landscape during which a business evaluates the competition in terms of pricing, procedures, demographics, and promotions.

Universal Precautions actions taken to prevent the transmission of infectious diseases; involves the use of protective procedures and equipment, such as gloves and masks.

Unrealistic Expectations belief that a certain outcome is possible, regardless of merit or circumstance.

Urticaria Pigmentosa allergic reactions such as hives with a large number of mast cells.

V

Vacuum Settings adjustable setting on microdermabrasion machine that is responsible for the rate at which crystals strike the skin, as well as the subsequent elimination of used crystals and biowaste particles.

Vesicles fluid-filled containers on the skin's surface.

Vitamin B see *Nicotinamide*.

Vitamin C antioxidant that is a necessary factor for the formation of collagen in connective tissue and maintenance of integrity of intercellular cement.

Vitamin E antioxidant that has been shown to inactivate free radicals; the exact mechanism that controls this function is unknown.

Vitiligo skin disorder characterized by white patches surrounded by otherwise normally pigmented skin; most common on dark-skinned individuals from tropical regions.

W

Warts flat, cutaneous, and flesh-colored lesions caused by papillomavirus.

Wood's Lamp ultraviolet (UV) rays used to detect fluorescent material in the skin that is indicative of certain diseases or conditions.

Wound disruption of normal tissue that results from pathologic processes beginning internally or externally to the involved organ.

Wound Healing restoration of tissue continuity after injury or trauma.

Y

Yearly Business Objectives part of the annual business plan that identifies the goals a business would like to attain during a given fiscal year.

Yeast Infections viral infection caused by several unicellular organisms that reproduce by budding; oral yeast infections are common in those with compromised immune systems.

Yin and Yang concept originally devised by Fu Xi that describes the harmony between nature and its daily phenomenon.

Z

Zinc Oxide physical sunscreen that scatters and reflects light rather than absorbing or filtering it.

Index